Nurses' Work:
Issues Across Time and Place

Patricia D'Antonio, RN, PhD, FAAN, is an Adjunct Associate Professor of Nursing and the Associate Director of the Barbara Bates Center for the Study of the History of Nursing at the University of Pennsylvania. She is also the editor of the *Nursing History Review,* the official journal of the American Association for the History of Nursing. Dr. D'Antonio's research and writing in nursing history have been recognized by awards including the "Best of the *Journal of Nursing Scholarship*—Profession and Society," the Barbara Brodie Nursing History Fellowship from the University of Virginia, and the Lavinia L. Dock Award from the American Association for the History of Nursing.

Ellen D. Baer, RN, PhD, FAAN, is Professor Emeritus of Nursing, Associate Director Emeritus, and Chair of the Advisory Board of the Barbara Bates Center for the Study of the History of Nursing at the University of Pennsylvania. Dr. Baer has been a Fulbright Senior Scholar at the University of Athens in Greece, a Visiting Professor at New York University, and held the Hillman Term Professorship in Nursing at the University of Pennsylvania and the Wallace Gilroy Professorship of Nursing at the University of Miami. Her research and writing in nursing history have been recognized by the Centennial Nursing Heritage Award from the American Nurses Association, the Lavinia L. Dock Award from the American Association for the History of Nursing, the Distinguished Nurse Researcher Award from the Foundation of the New York State Nurses' Association, the Agnes Randolph Dillon Award from the University of Virginia, the Media Award from the American Academy of Nursing, and distinguished alumni awards from New York University and Columbia University.

Sylvia D. Rinker, RN, PhD, is a Professor of Nursing in the School of Health Sciences and Human Performance at Lynchburg College in Lynchburg, Virginia. She is a member of the Board of Directors of the American Association for the History of Nursing, where she serves as a member of the Strategic Planning Committee and as Chair of the Lavinia L. Dock Award Committee. Dr. Rinker is also the archivist for the Xi Upsilon Chapter of Sigma Theta Tau International at Lynchburg College and on the Advisory Board for the Women's Studies/Gender Studies minor at Lynchburg College. She was the Associate Director of the Center for Nursing Historical Inquiry at the University of Virginia from its founding in 1991 until 1998. Her highly regarded historical scholarship was recognized with the Teresa Christy Award from the American Association for the History of Nursing.

Joan E. Lynaugh, RN, PhD, FAAN, is Professor Emeritus of Nursing at the University of Pennsylvania and Director Emeritus of the Barbara Bates Center for the Study of the History of Nursing. She currently serves as Vice Chair of the Visiting Nurse Society of Greater Philadelphia. A prolific researcher, writer, and editor, Dr. Lynaugh's distinguished career in nursing has been recognized by the Centennial Nursing Heritage Award from the American Nurses' Association, the Lavinia L. Dock Award from the American Association for the History of Nursing, the Agnes Dillon Randolph Award from the University of Virginia, the Distinguished Alumni Award from the University of Rochester, and the President's Award from the American Association for the History of Nursing in 2000. She was designated a Living Legend by the American Academy of Nursing in 2005.

Nurses' Work: Issues Across Time and Place

Patricia D'Antonio, RN, PhD, FAAN
Ellen D. Baer, RN, PhD, FAAN
Sylvia D. Rinker, RN, PhD
Joan E. Lynaugh, RN, PhD, FAAN
Editors

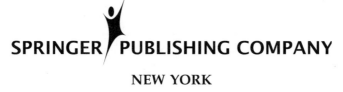

SPRINGER PUBLISHING COMPANY

NEW YORK

Springer Publishing Company, LLC.
11 West 42nd Street
New York, NY 10036

Acquisitions Editor: Sally J. Barhydt
Production Editor: Phil Bugeau
Cover design: Joanne E. Honigman
Composition: Graphic World Inc.

07 08 09 10 / 5 4 3 2 1

Cover Photos: Left—M. Adelaide Nutting. From Lavinia Dock and M. Adelaide Nutting's *A History of Nursing From the Earliest Times to the Present Day With Special Reference to the Work of the Past Thirty Years*, volume 3 (1912). Center—A nurse at St. Mary's Hospital in Rochester, New York, circa 1950. Reprinted with the permission of the Barbara Bates Center for the Study of the History of Nursing. Right—Tom Buckley, RNC, MSN, in the neonatal intensive care unit at the University of Virginia Medical Center. Reprinted with permission of Mr. Buckley.

Library of Congress Cataloging-in-Publication Data

Nurses' work: issues across time and place/Patricia D'Antonio . . . [et al.], editors.
   p. cm.
  Includes bibliographical references and index.
  ISBN 0-8261-0211-5 (alk. paper)
    1. Nursing—History. I. D'Antonio, Patricia, 1955-

RT31.N86 2006
610.73—dc22
                            2006045037

Printed in the United States of America by Edwards Brothers.

Contents

Contributors

Emily K. Abel, PhD, Professor of Public Health and Women's Studies at the University of California, Los Angeles

Patricia E. Benner, RN, PhD, FAAN, Professor and Chair of the Department of Social and Behavioral Sciences at the University of San Francisco School of Nursing, where she also holds the Thelma Shobe Endowed Chair in Ethics and Spirituality

Agnes S. Brennan, RN, late Superintendent of the New York Training School at Bellevue Hospital

Barbara L. Brush, RN, PhD, FAAN, Associate Professor and Director, Division of Health Promotion and Risk Reduction Programs at the University of Michigan School of Nursing

Elizabeth Capezuti, RN, PhD, FAAN, Associate Professor and Co-Director, The John A. Hartford Foundation Institute for Geriatric Nursing at New York University College of Nursing

Cynthia A. Connolly, RN, PhD, Assistant Professor in the School of Nursing and in the History of Medicine and Science at Yale University

Lynne M. Dunphy, RN, PhD, Assistant Dean and Associate Professor at the Christine E. Lynn College of Nursing at Florida Atlantic University

Diane Hamilton, RN, PhD, Professor at the Western Michigan University School of Nursing

Virginia A. Henderson, AM, RN, FRCN, late Senior Research Associate Emerita at Yale University School of Nursing

Arlene W. Keeling, RN, PhD, Centennial Distinguished Professor of Nursing and the Director of the Center for Nursing Historical Inquiry at the University of Virginia

Marie O. Pitts Mosley, RN, EdD, Consultant and retired Associate Professor at Hunter-Bellevue School of Nursing and Howard University School of Nursing

Mary Adelaide Nutting, RN, late Director of the first graduate education program for nurses at Teachers College, Columbia University, where she remained until 1925

Frances Reiter, RN, MA, late Professor of Nursing and Dean of the Graduate School of Nursing at the New York Medical College

Linda E. Sabin, RN, PhD, Professor of Nursing in the School of Nursing at the University of Louisiana at Monroe

Margaret D. Sovie, RN, PhD, FAAN, late Director of Nursing at the Hospital of the University of Pennsylvania and Associate Dean for Practice at the University of Pennsylvania School of Nursing

Cynthia Toman, RN, PhD, Assistant Professor in the School of Nursing and Associate Director of the AMS Nursing History Research Unit at the University of Ottawa

Jean C. Whelan, RN, PhD, Adjunct Assistant Professor of Nursing at the University of Pennsylvania

Foreword

Nurses' Work: Issues Across Time and Place is an unusually perceptive collection of classic and historical scholarly nursing articles on the work of nursing—whether that work be done by informal caregivers or professional nurses. Taken together, historical scholarship tells nurses how the practice of nursing has changed over time and how these changes have shaped the self-understanding of nurses and those for whom they have cared. These collected works demonstrate the primacy of practice and the relationships between work and the knowledge embedded in that work. The authors claim a seat for nurses at the policy tables because of the significant societal contributions of nursing work: ". . . a practice at the unique intersection of individual need and community resources, of family wishes and social customs, of local acts and global initiatives. . . ." (D'Antonio, p. xvi).

Emily Abel's work on family caregiving in the 19th century, provided primarily by women, demonstrates the intensive nature of caring for the sick, particularly the bedridden patient. Through careful scholarly attention to women's diaries, Abel weaves the concrete embodied story of caregiving provided by women in the neighborhood and by family caregivers. In the past, no women could be assured an uninterrupted career outside the home due to the traditional expectations that women would do the work of nursing within the family. Public nursing work, as the remarkable cultural invention it is, becomes clearer in the progression of these historical accounts of nursing work. Women would extend their established work of caregiving within the family to strangers outside the home, first to neighbors and then to those who were displaced from their families and placed in institutions established for nursing care. It is not accidental that the nursing profession's domestic past influences today's nurse when nurses seek to bridge the gap between the separation of the social and the medical so integral to Cartesian scientific medicine.

Just as the work of the nurse took place first in the home, nurses' work today involves assisting patients and/or families in restoring the connections and identities that get disrupted during illness, injury, and institutional care. Identities are social before they are personal. Individual identities are disrupted by ruptures in social functioning and belonging caused by illness, injury, and are often further disrupted by the separation and stigma unfairly associated with illness and disabilities. Care and caregiving work includes the aim of restoring one's sense of social identity and belonging. Patricia D'Antonio points out the early bid for dominance, building on hierarchical class structures that separated the working class "professed nurse" and middle- and upper-class "ladies." Nightingale, drawing on her Christian tradition, reestablished the vision of the work of caring for strangers outside the home as a "calling."

This vision of nursing work as a "calling" influenced its ambivalent relationship between money and power. Tracing the economic changes in nursing work, articles in Section 2 reveal the ambivalence and necessity of making public nursing work viable economically. Diane Hamilton's recovery of the humanizing public health work of the Metropolitan Life Insurance Company's Visiting Nurse Service left a legacy that can still be seen today in community-based home nursing care. Likewise, the professional nurse registries have evolved over time, and it is enlightening to read of the ingenuity of early nurses as chronicled and interpreted by Jean Whelan.

Technology is never neutral, and the historical articles present in Section 3 draw out some of the significant sources of new technologies' influences on nursing work, and thus, nurses' knowledge. From the preventoriums designed to prevent full-blown tuberculosis in children exposed to the disease, to the radical responsibility of nursing patients "cocooned" in iron lungs during the epidemics of polio from 1929 to 1955, it is clear that new, significant knowledge was developed along the way. Reading historical articles helps us understand the influence of the social environment on disease and should redouble our efforts at including social sciences and humanities in the education of nurses today. Reading Section 3 should stimulate and enrich historical studies of the role of nursing care in other technologies such as transplantation surgeries in which treating mouth ulcers and suppressed immune systems relies heavily on the work of nurses.

Section 4 gives an intellectual history of nurse scholars' understanding and public articulation of the nature of nursing work. One is reminded that what is so close at hand may be the most difficult to see and articulate. Nurses have struggled to show the craft, knowledge, science, and wisdom of nursing practice in a societal context where highly technical medicine is valorized and described—at the expense of a clear vision of the work of nursing required to provide the safe passages of patients through today's complex health care institutions and the lack of adequate attention to the care of multiple chronic illnesses. The authors succeed in bringing the knowledge embedded in the practice of nursing in from the margins. It is their hope to have nurses feel renewed and empowered by a deeper understanding of the past. We owe them a debt for their success and a promise to continue this scholarly exploration of the past wisdom of the practice of nursing in order to better understand the centrality of nursing work to a good society. Every nursing student and practicing nurse will be enlightened by reading this work.

Patricia E. Benner, RN, PhD, FAAN

Preface

This collection of chapters explores the historical context of enduring issues in the essence of nurses' work: clinical nursing practice. It builds on the success and warm reception of our first award-winning anthology, *Enduring Issues in American Nursing*. But where that volume looked inward at the issues of identity, authority, and knowledge that shaped the development of the nursing profession, this anthology looks outward toward those who shaped its actual work. Nursing is what nurses do when they are with patients, families, groups, or communities. But what of the ease with which different groups with different backgrounds and different relationships to patients also claim the title *nurse?* What of the constant tension between private interest and professional self-determination that confounds the nurse's relationship with money? What about the clinical implications of the amazing responsiveness of nurses to social, scientific, and technological change? And what of the ways in which different nurses in different times and places thought about the meaning of clinical practice?

Nurses' Work: Issues Across Time and Place brings together a rich body of historical scholarship that encourages readers to think about these questions, and raise new ones. Our collective experience has been that nurses have become strikingly more sophisticated in their concept of a "usable past." Where once we may have turned to histories of valiant struggles and sure lines of development, we now seek studies that help clarify the possibilities and problems, the challenges, and the contradictions we confront in our own clinical practice. We hope our readers find insight into their own practices in these readings. We also hope that they take from these readings a sense of clinical practice as a wonderfully complicated, messy, sometimes idiosyncratic, but always critically important world of people, places, politics, and processes. And, finally, we hope our readers come to understand history as a methodology that more fully develops the complexities, ambiguities, and keenly felt sense of responsibility that characterizes clinical moments—those spaces defined by time and place where practitioner and patient meet to consider how to create change.

Certainly, the belief in the primacy of clinical practice—the work of nursing—has always defined the mission of the profession. The strength of such a belief unites the diversity of nursing's educational programs, practice initiatives, research agendas, and knowledge paradigms. Clinical practice is why, for example, students sit in classrooms, practitioners try out different staffing arrangements, investigators probe data for sound evidence, and questions abound about the nature of nursing knowledge. We may disagree about where the classrooms should be located, the conditions necessary for clinical innovation, the parameters for evidence-based practice, and if there is, indeed, such a thing as a distinct body of nursing knowledge. But we know that our assessments (and, yes, our diagnoses), decisions, interventions, advocacy, research, and scholarship make a profound difference in the experiences of patients in our care.

As importantly, the belief in the primacy of clinical practice influences how we, as a profession, think about many significant and enduring issues. It influences who we identify as our patients and how we think about our constantly negotiated and renegotiated relationships with other professionals and with family caregivers who also have vested interests in our patients' welfare. The belief in the primacy of practice also influences how we put our learning, interventions, research, and scholarship into action. It affects how we organize our care, how we decide to be paid for our care, how we engage with the policies and politics of care, and how we decide what works in diverse health care settings and why. And our commitment to the primacy of our particular practice—a practice at the unique intersection of individual needs and community resources, of family wishes and social customs, of local acts and global initiatives—is the reason we demand an influential seat at the proverbial table, wherever it might be.

Historically, nursing has tended to think about clinical practice in fairly structural ways. We think about practice as differentiated by expertise and discuss the differences between generalist and advanced nursing practice. We also think about practice as differentiated by clinical foci and emphasize the different knowledge and skill sets necessary for psychiatric nursing practice, surgical nursing practice, or community health nursing practice. Finally, we think about practice in relation to the site within which it is delivered and speak to its place in hospitals, homes, and hospices. We now know much from this approach to clinical practice. We know how nurses negotiated access to patients who needed their work both within and outside of institutional walls, and we know of their battles to claim the right to determine the parameters of "good nursing care."

Many of the documents and essays in *Nurses' Work: Issues Across Time and Place* do acknowledge the usefulness of this way of thinking about clinical nursing practice. Indeed, historians have long been interested in the work that nurses did. But scholars now analyze more than just the work itself: They look at not only what nurses did but why their care took the form it did. They raise questions about the reciprocity between the assigned tasks and the shared worksite values that influenced decisions about how those tasks would be performed. They tease out the threads of common interests around which nurses joined to build a sustaining work culture. And, most importantly, they cast patients as equally important actors in shaping the work of nurses.

The chapters in *Nurses' Work* draw on this rich body of historical scholarship. For conceptual clarity, the editors approach questions about clinical nursing practice by focusing on four themes that we believe best capture issues related to nurses' work across historical time and geographic place. In the four sections of the book, these themes address (1) who does the work of nursing, (2) who pays for the work of nursing, (3) what the real work of nursing is, and (4) how our nursing predecessors have struggled with the relationship between work and knowledge. We approach these themes in two ways: first, through an introductory essay to each section that focuses on the question raised and places it within a broader context; and second, through chapters that represent the interpretations of historical leaders and contemporary scholars. We do not claim the final word on the history of clinical practice or on the work of nurses. Perhaps we might claim the first—with a wish that our readers will take the opportunity to immerse themselves in the historical literature, develop their own perspectives, and reemerge invigorated and ready to tackle the issues of nurses' work today and in the future.

Patricia D'Antonio, RN, PhD, FAAN
for the editors

SECTION 1

Those Who Do Nurses' Work

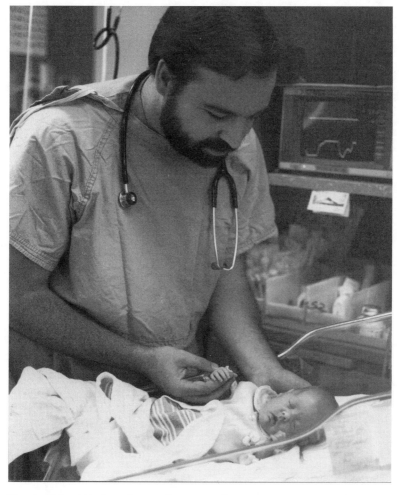

Tom Buckley, RNC, MSN, in the neonatal intensive care unit at the
University of Virginia Medical Center. Reprinted with the permission of
Mr. Buckley.

Introduction

Patricia D'Antonio

Who does the work of nursing? On the one hand, the answer seems relatively straightforward. Historically, the actual work of nursing has rested primarily with women: with mothers, daughters, sisters, and neighbors caring for sick children, spouses, parents, and friends in their homes. Indeed, the seemingly irreducible connection between one's gender and one's innate capabilities, loving responsibilities, and ordained duty framed the late nineteenth-century drive to professionalize the work of nursing. At a time when debates over higher education and independent careers for women provoked controversy and dissent, nursing leaders capitalized upon the image of nursing as traditional women's work and successfully forged a new profession, new life paths, and new opportunities around the idea of nursing as, yes, women's work, but now scientifically informed women's work performed by a cadre of hospital-trained, not family-denoted, nurses.

But professionally trained nurses, as we know, never have and still do not do all the work of nursing. Who does the work of nursing? Now, any simple answer seems elusive and even controversial. Many different men and women with different backgrounds and different relationships to patients also claim the title *nurse* and do some of the work of nursing. Hence, even if the image of nursing has been framed by notions about women's traditional responsibilities, how that duty finds its form in actual clinical practice changes across time and place. The articles in this section consider these changes.

Emily Abel, for example, looks at the intergenerational family nursing work of Emily Hawley Gillespie, a nineteenth-century Iowa farm woman, and her daughter Sarah Gillespie, a teacher torn between her commitment to her own work and her responsibilities to her sick mother. Over the time we come to know them, both Emily and Sarah assumed that they would render nursing care wherever and whenever it was needed. And they both did. But as their individual stories unfold, we enter into a world where the work of nursing is extraordinarily complicated and complex. This work is as much about emotional experiences and intensely personal relationships as it is about tasks and activities. It gives both Emily and Sarah a sense of competence and mastery, as well as a sense of burden and sacrifice. It provides a space where they could repair frayed social bonds, and it sets the stage for the reopening of old emotional wounds. Emily and Sarah often feel alone and isolated—but would they welcome the introduction of a professional nurse?

As I suggest in my chapter on the relationships between and among more urban nineteenth-century women, nurses, and physicians, the answer may well be yes, but only under certain circumstances. Here we see how long before professional nursing leaders brought their vision of scientific nursing work to the hospital bedside, an earlier generation of physicians and women reworked fundamental assumptions about that work at the bedsides of patients in their homes. This reworking drew on increasingly meaningful gender and class relationships that resonated with those emerging in nineteenth-century America: Physicians would supervise middle-class nursing women, who would in turn supervise the hired nurse. Thus, Emily and Sarah might indeed welcome a professional nurse into their home, but they might also have insisted on maintaining a meaningful managerial role in that care: one based on their own status, education, and, more importantly, personal knowledge of their sick kin. Indeed, the giving and taking of the prerogatives of nurses' work on the basis of class and personal connection can still be heard in debates about contemporary nursing practice. What kinds of nurses should do what kinds of work? How might one reconcile the tension between the head work and the hand work of nursing? And how does the professional nurse's expertise compete with or complement a family's sense of personal knowledge?

Still, as Linda Sabin reminds us, we must be careful not to always conflate nursing with women's work. Sabin calls our attention to the tradition of male caregivers in the nineteenth-century American South. The nursing work that occurred in communities such as those in Mississippi and Florida has received relatively little attention in nursing's historical literature. But what a rich picture they present. Now we see how white men interpreted their socially ascribed roles as "protectors" and "leaders" of dependent women, children, and African American slaves to include the work of nursing, particularly during times of epidemics, panics, and quarantine. These white men were quite a diverse group, who nursed for many different reasons: some to live up to a Southern code of honor, others to protect property and business interests during epidemics, and still others to earn relatively substantial salaries. Theirs was usually not a life calling, but their legacy remains important.

African Americans, of course, had their own strong traditions of care and nursing work. Marie Pitts Mosley's chapter on the nursing work of Jessie Sleet, Elizabeth Tyler, and Edith Carter vividly captures the care of these three professional public health nurses. Mosley's work, of course, adds race to our consideration of the work of nurses: These pioneering African American nurses reached out to their own communities of color in New York City and worked with them to transcend the educational, occupational, economic, and racial barriers that compromised their health and social well-being. Her work, though, has broader implications. The work of Sleet, Tyler, and Carter superbly illustrates what all nurses know about their practice. Nurses' work exists at the intersection of family needs, social norms, changing expectations, and scientific knowledge. Thus, when we look historically at who does nurses' work, we do not find a simple answer. As the chapters in this section suggest, the answer lies in the idea of nurses' work as a wonderfully rich process that is entrepreneurial, contingent, and a constantly contested activity defined by the people in need of care, the place of care, the social setting, and the needs, desires, and ambitions of the patients, families, practitioners, and communities that claim ownership (or are assigned ownership) of that work.

CHAPTER 1

Family Caregiving in the Nineteenth Century: Emily Hawley Gillespie and Sarah Gillespie Huftalen, 1858–1888

Emily K. Abel

On October 14, 1871, Emily Hawley Gillespie, an Iowa farm woman, wrote in her diary: "Mrs. Houghton & I sat up all last night with old Mrs. Stephens, 74 yrs, she died 10 minutes past 9 this morning, we lay her out in black dress—I came home this afternoon."[1] Although studies of nineteenth-century health care providers have proliferated during the past twenty years,[2] few investigate the care delivered by family and friends. Most historians pass quickly over informal care, noting only those domestic healing practices that were later absorbed into the formal system of health delivery.[3] Studies of women healers still concentrate on the few

Funded by the UCLA Center for the Study of Women. The diaries of Emily Hawley Gillespie and Sarah Gillespie Huftalen are quoted with permission of the State Historical Society of Iowa. The author also wishes to thank Karen Anderson, Suzanne L. Bunkers, Carole H. Browner, Judy Nolte Lensink, Mary Rothschild, Regina Morantz-Sanchez, and Margaret K. Nelson. An earlier version of this chapter was presented at the 65th annual meeting of the American Association for the History of Medicine, Seattle, Washington, May 2, 1992.
This chapter was originally published in the *Bulletin of the History of Medicine*, 1994; 68:573–599. Copyright Johns Hopkins University Press. Reprinted with permission.

exceptional women who can be considered forerunners of contemporary female health professionals.[4] Although it is commonplace to note that most care was delivered by women at home, we know little about women's work as caregivers.

A Midwife's Tale by Laurel Thatcher Ulrich greatly enlarges our understanding of "social medicine" in the late eighteenth and early nineteenth centuries. Ulrich demonstrates that caring was a "universal female role" and that midwives worked closely with a broad network of neighborhood women. Nevertheless, Ulrich focuses on a woman who had earned recognition as a healer.[5] In this chapter, I try to illuminate the nineteenth-century world of caregiving by examining the lives of Emily Hawley Gillespie and her daughter Sarah between 1858, when Emily's diary began, and 1888, the year she died. Although neither Emily nor Sarah had exceptional experiences or skills, both routinely incorporated care for birthing women, the sick, and the dying into their daily lives.

Various friends and relatives rendered care to Emily whenever she was in need. When Emily's health began to fail in the mid-1880s, Sarah assumed primary responsibility for nursing her mother. Because each woman kept an extensive diary, we can explore that caregiving experience from the point of view of the recipient as well as the caregiver.

Like other primary sources, these diaries have limitations as well as advantages. Many entries consist solely of short, matter-of-fact statements, noting daily events rather than revealing intimate thoughts. Although Emily wrote virtually every evening, Sarah was not nearly as conscientious. During periods when she was most intensively involved in rendering care, she often failed to write at all. Moreover, although each diary provides an important check on the account of the other, it cannot be considered an independent production. Emily bought Sarah a diary in 1877. The two often wrote together at night and presumably discussed some of what they were writing. On at least two occasions, Emily opened Sarah's diary, read the last entry, and appended encouraging remarks. When Emily was very ill, she dictated her comments to Sarah. Nevertheless, these diaries do enable us to examine many events from the perspectives of both mother and daughter.

Emily and Sarah Gillespie were hardly alone in devoting much of their time to nursing the sick. Other diaries, letters, and memoirs reveal that despite the stereotype of the delicate Victorian woman, nineteenth-century women were intimately acquainted with pain, illness, and death. They dressed wounds, changed bandages, held basins for vomiting patients, and emptied chamber pots.[6] Nursing care dominated women's lives for many reasons. One was the high incidence of disease and disability.[7] Moreover, although some men participated in nursing care, the reigning ideology assigned the work of caring exclusively to women.[8] Few medical services relieved women's burdens. When the first government survey was conducted in 1873, the nation boasted only 120 hospitals, most of which were custodial institutions that served the deserving poor.[9] Skepticism about medical interventions deterred some patients from relying on physicians. Without telephones or automobiles, summoning physicians involved considerable time and effort.[10] When nursing schools were established during the last decades of the nineteenth century, their graduates provided care to patients in private households. But hiring nurses was an option only for the very affluent.[11] As Emily's and Sarah's accounts reveal, women's responsibilities for care not only disrupted their lives but also enabled them to acquire extensive medical knowledge and skills, brought them into sustained contact with fundamental aspects of human existence, and bound them to a broad network of friends and kin.

EMILY HAWLEY GILLESPIE

Emily Gillespie was born in 1838, the oldest of four children of Hial Newton Hawley and Sarah Baker Hawley, Michigan farmers. From an early age, she participated in household and farm labor. Because her parents' farm was less prosperous than the average, she also was compelled to take advantage of the few opportunities for young women to make money. In addition to teaching school, sewing for neighbors, and peddling books, she nursed invalids.

When she was in her early 20s, she wrote frequently of her fear of death. At least one of her nursing experiences may well have sharpened her sense of vulnerability. In May 1860, she spent the night with a neighbor suffering from consumption. "Am at Mrs. Wiley's this evening," she wrote. "Poor woman, I do pity her, she took my hand & said 'your hand will be like mine sometime; mine was once like yours'" (EHG, May 20). The absence of other people in the house appears to have added to Emily's terror. "I alone with one almost dying," she complained (ibid.). At other times, Emily could draw comfort from the presence of the women around her. Two months later, in July, she wrote, "Called at Mrs. Wileys, she is no better. I with Mrs. Converse, Mrs. Evans and Mrs. Culver sit up with her to night, how sick she is" (EHG, July 1). A few days later, she wrote, "Edna & I, Harriet Sutherland, Adison and Augusta Stone & Maria Dawes sit up to night with the corpse. Mrs. Wiley died this morning about 4" (EHG, July 5). Then, Emily noted, "The Dr's. came this morning to dissect Mrs. Wiley, her heart & lungs were grown fast. Right lung all gone & left one except a part about the size of a hickory nut" (EHG, July 6). It is unclear whether Emily actually witnessed the autopsy. If she did, her presence would have enormous historical significance. Ulrich notes that during the late eighteenth and early nineteenth centuries, doctors sometimes called midwives to watch dissections. "As guardians of women and children," Ulrich writes, "midwives presumably ensured proper reverence for the bodies. From the doctors' point of view, inviting midwives to observe was perhaps a professional courtesy, a way of including them in an important educational event. At the same time, it helped to validate the activity and perhaps to reassure anxious relatives."[12] Perhaps Emily seemed like an appropriate family representative because she had cared for Mrs. Wiley before her death. It also is possible that Emily's graphic description of physical deterioration helped her cope with her anxieties. As Elizabeth Hampsten notes, working-class women in the nineteenth century frequently wrote about death and decay with a frankness that startles readers of the twenty-first century.[13]

Emily left home in June 1861 at the age of 23 to work as a housekeeper for her uncle, an innkeeper in a small town in Iowa. Fourteen months later, she married James Gillespie, a 25-year-old farmer. The marriage was not happy. James was subject to deep depression and uncontrollable rage and occasionally threatened suicide. By the early 1880s, Emily feared for her own safety. After James had one of his "bad spells" in October 1883, she wrote, "It makes my blood run cold & I shake like a leaf" (EHG, October 4). Driving with him in a carriage the following April, she felt "perfectly terror struck" (EHG, April 19). In December she wrote that the children "dare not leave me alone with him" (EHG, December 19). Emily also worried that James would expel her from the farm, depriving her of a livelihood as well as a home.

In addition, marriage confined Emily to a life she had hoped to avoid. From an early age, she had aspired to become a lady.[14] As a farm woman, she engaged in a constant round of grueling labor. James plowed and planted the fields, chopped wood, churned the butter, cared for the horses, and repaired the farm equipment. But Emily kept a vegetable garden and did all the housework. Although James built their house, she cleaned it, painted the walls, laid flooring and carpeting, and constructed closets. During the last decades of her life, a variety of store-bought goods and household appliances lightened her burdens. She no longer spun and wove cloth or made soap and candles. In addition, she benefited from technological advances. She bought a wringer for washing in 1878, a new coal stove in 1882, and a sewing machine in 1883.

But her housework continued to be far more arduous than that of many middle-class urban women.[15] Long after they could buy ready-made clothes, she continued to sew overalls and shirts for her husband and son. Instead of sending out her laundry, she devoted one day to washing and another to ironing. She canned the vegetables and fruit and baked the bread that more affluent urban housewives bought in stores. Moreover, in order to pay for the manufactured goods that were available, she had to increase her workload. To obtain cash, she sold butter, eggs, honey, vegetables, and poultry. In July 1883, she noted that she had 118 turkeys, 78 chickens, and 20 birds (EHG, July 26). In addition to feeding them regularly, she built and cleaned their cages, chased them when they escaped onto neighbors' land, and protected them from skunks, gophers, and cats. In 1877 Emily wrote that the "only happiness" of farm women "lies in their children. with fond hopes that *they* may rise higher, that *they* perhaps may be an ornament to society" (EHG, August 29).

Emily's son Henry was born in 1863 and her daughter Sarah in 1865. Although both worked on the farm from an early age, Emily encouraged them to seek upward mobility through education. She paid their tuition at a private academy where they could associate with "young Ladies & gentlemen," carefully supervised their school work, and urged them to enter such "noble" professions as teaching and medicine (EHG, November 10, 1879). In 1886, she declared that Henry and Sarah were her "reward" for "all the sorrows" of her marriage; "pure & noble minds with high aims, no more could be asked" (EHG, August 28).

Despite the enormous burdens Emily shouldered as both a farm woman and a mother, she assumed as a matter of course that she would render care whenever it was needed. In addition to nursing her husband and children through assorted illnesses, she cared for a variety of extended kin and neighbors. The following represent examples of her activities. "Oh! Oh!! Oh!!! what awful news again," Emily wrote in August 1868. "Uncle got hurt in the reaper—we went to see him, he is in dreadful pain" (EHG, August 21). Once again, she described bodily affliction in lavish detail, writing that "about 3 inches flesh, bones, arteries, cords & all" had to be removed from her uncle's arm (ibid.). She continued to visit her uncle regularly during the succeeding 3 weeks.

In 1869, Emily commented that "they sent for me" to attend the birth of Nell Thomas, a neighbor (EHG, July 22). Because both infant and maternal mortality rates were high during this period, death frequently followed closely upon birth. In September Emily wrote, "[S]tay at Mr. Thomas' most all day, their Baby is *sick*" (EHG, September 7). She returned to the Thomas house the following day to attend the baby's burial (EHG, September 8). Two months later, Emily again had responsibility for nursing a critically ill patient. In 1869, she noted that James's brother "come & tell us Ma is worse, we go & stay most all day, come home & do chores, then go back. I stay all night, James went home" (EHG, November 5). The following day she wrote, "Ma died just 23 minutes of 2 o'clock this morning—died without a struggle" (EHG, November 6). In 1871, she "sat up" all night with Mrs. Stephens, an elderly woman, and then helped to lay her out (EHG, October 14).[16] In September 1872

Emily assisted Mrs. McMillen when she gave birth to a boy (EHG, September 22), and in March 1873 she spent the night watching Mr. Stephens, who had been sick for several months: "He died this morning half past three" (EHG, March 21).

Some observers note that the work of nineteenth-century farm women gave them the satisfaction of honing skills and demonstrating competence.[17] Caregiving offered similar opportunities. When Emily was still living at her parents' house, she described her prowess in dispensing medicine: "Aunt Mary came here," she wrote in 1858, "she has not spoken loud in fourteen weeks. I gave her a teaspoon of 'Chamberlains Relief' & in about half an hour she talked aloud;—she was so pleased that she cried" (EHG, November 25). Emily exhibited similar self-confidence whenever James became ill. On one such occasion in 1863, she pronounced, "I have made up my mind tis a 'nervous fever'" (EHG, August 18). Two days later she noted, "I wash him & make him some catnip tea, rub his stomach with liniment he said he felt better" (EHG, August 18). In January 1868 she again made her own diagnosis and decided what treatment to administer: "I think he has symptoms of infection of the bowels," she wrote. "have kept hot cloths wet with vinegar across him all day" (EHG, January 6).

Emily also felt competent to act on her own when Henry hit his thumb with an axe and "cut it nearly off" in May 1884. "Deara-me it is too bad," she wrote. "He held it on while I done it up. I hope it will grow on again without leaving too bad a scar" (EHG, May 13). This entry reminds us that women's domestic healing practices could involve far more than administering garden herbs. In this case, Emily performed the equivalent of a surgical procedure.

To be sure, some medical emergencies were beyond her abilities. A physician amputated Emily's uncle's arm. Judith Walzer Leavitt notes that nineteenth-century women increasingly summoned doctors to officiate at births,[18] and it therefore is not surprising that Emily frequently noted the presence of doctors at many of the deliveries she attended. Because women continued to give birth at home, however, Emily worked alongside doctors and retained some power to make medical decisions.[19]

In providing Emily with a sense of mastery, caregiving resembled much of her other work. But in one important respect, Emily's responsibilities for care were unique. Most household and farm labor isolated her from the community around her. She often complained that the constant demands of work left little time for socializing. Moreover, although she received some help with her chores, first from her sister Harriet and then from her daughter Sarah, she never shared tasks with neighborhood women. Emily's success as a farm woman also separated her from the broader community. Partly as a result of her efforts, she and James became increasingly prosperous. Although they lived with James's parents at the time of their marriage, they were able to move to their own land in 1864 and to build a new house in 1872. Their farm thrived during the agricultural depression of the 1870s, when many others failed.

As Emily's fortunes rose, she spurned those she left behind. She attributed the plight of others to their personal failings. Jealously guarding her possessions, she responded with rage when neighbors sought to borrow farm implements. One of her sharpest grievances against James was that he was too generous toward his extended family and neighbors, helping anyone in need. Believing that "charity begins at home first," Emily wanted him to focus on bettering his immediate family (EHG, September 23, 1879).

Nor did Emily view the farm as a joint enterprise with her husband. The two fought bitterly about the amount of work each did. Emily complained that James imposed an excessive workload on her and deprecated her economic contributions to the family. Moreover, instead of sharing the money she earned with James, she spent it herself.[20] Although James had no interest in acquiring the trappings of the genteel life, she improved her home with $50.40 of new carpets in 1880 (EHG, December 16). James, she scornfully noted, considered them "too nice" (EHG, June 22). She adorned herself and her children as well, buying silk, cashmere, and velvet to make clothes. In February 1886, the cost of Sarah's new dresses was $43.84 (EHG, February 17). Emily's most prized possession was a carriage, which she had wanted for years and finally bought for $65 in 1885 (EHG, September 16). "It is splendid," she wrote after riding in it for the first time, "but James is *too harsh* for anything so *fine*" (EHG, September 27).

If farmwork ruptured social bonds, caregiving helped to restore them. The sufferings of others elicited Emily's tenderness and sympathy. Whenever James fell ill, she expressed a warmth and solicitude that was absent from her diary at other times. In August 1863 she wrote, "'Tis sad when he is sick. . . . I read him the letter I wrote to my folks. I had said in it a few words about his being sick; the tears came trickling from his eyes" (EHG, August 16). And she expressed admiration for his courage: "O, how good he is; he said he did not know but he was as ready to go now, as ever, if his time had come, and if he found out he must die, he would settle up his business & die in peace with all. O, with what composure of mind he talks, O, God I pray that when I die I may be as well prepared to go as James is" (EHG, January 20, 1863). James's second major illness, in 1868, prompted equally loving comments: "O my prayer is that he may get well, for O, Lord . . . wilt Thou spare him to me a while longer for I feel I have no other friend on Earth. . . . Ah me all seems bad when dear ones are sick. James groans so mournfully" (EHG, January 6).

Caregiving also enabled Emily to exhibit concern for her sister Harriet, who came to Iowa in September 1869 and stayed with Emily for 2 years. Although Harriet taught school, she also helped with the housework. Emily's two children were young, and she was grateful for her sister's assistance. After Harriet married John McGee in November 1871 and moved to his farm, the two women continued to exchange goods and services. Emily attended Harriet in October 1872 when she had a stillbirth and again in August 1873, when Harriet's first daughter was born (EHG, October 1; August 24).

The relationship cooled considerably when Harriet's fortunes declined. When Harriet and John owed "debts to the amount of twenty-six hundred dollars" in October 1876, Emily noted that they had been "advised to do different" (EHG, October 1). But Emily continued to assist at Harriet's confinements. In May 1878 she wrote, "Harriet has another Boy it was born to day tween four & five o'clock. I have been there all day." The agony Emily witnessed moved her: "Ah what suffering one can endure," she wrote (EHG, May 16). The relationship between the sisters continued to deteriorate after Harriet and her husband lost their farm. When Harriet failed to return a garden tool promptly, Emily wrote,

> I wanted to dig some roots in the garden this afternoon. our potatoe-fork was down to Harriets. I was provoked that I had to go after it when I was so tired. . . . [W]hen I work & get things to use I do not like to have them gone when I want them. . . . I hope . . . it may learn them a lesson that they can not always expect some one of their relatives to help them. They must work to a better advantage for them-selves. (EHG, May 9, 1881)

When Emily helped Harriet after an abortion in 1882, she again expressed a sense of commonality with her sister.[21] "She looks very bad indeed. I am really sorry for her." Emily wrote, "Ah me! such is the life of most women" (EHG, March 19). Although conflicts continued to erupt between the sisters, Emily did not doubt that she would offer assistance to Harriet in any crisis. In August 1883 Emily vowed never to visit Harriet again "except that she sends for me or any of them are sick" (EHG, August 26).

Caring activities also bound Emily to a large female network. We have seen that despite the contempt Emily displayed for many of her neighbors, she routinely attended their childbirths, sat up with their dying, and nursed their sick. When she went to neighbors' homes to dispense such services, other women occasionally did the housework she left behind. When Emily provided assistance to Harriet during a delivery in October 1872, for example, Harriet's sister-in-law Lilly went to Emily's house to bake her bread and prepare James's dinner (EHG, October 1).

Moreover, births, illnesses, and deaths frequently were communal events. Although Emily performed most farm chores by herself, she typically shared caregiving tasks with others. In October 1873 she wrote, "go with Harriet to see Isabelle, she is sick, her baby 1 week old" (EHG, October 11). When Emma Brook's husband died in January 1886, Emily spent the day at her house with three other women. One was Mrs. Chapman, with whom Emily had previously enjoyed a close bond, but from whom she had recently become estranged. In May 1884, Emily had complained that Mrs. Chapman appeared "unfriendly toward me" (EHG, May 23). When she had invited Mrs. Chapman to visit her the following September, the latter had declined, pleading an excess of work (EHG, September 13). As Emily cleaned the Brook house and cooked the dinner, however, she healed the breach in the relationship: "Mrs. Chapman and I had a good visit," Emily reported later in the day. "I asked her to come & see me she invited me to come & see her. I mean to go too" (EHG, January 14, 1886). Emily's experiences as a recipient as well as a giver of care tied her to a female community. Her diary entry for September 4, 1863, read:

> ah, me, what I have to write for this day; was real sick all night (last night), did not sleep a minute . . . about daylight James sent for some help to take care of me. Pa went, got Mrs. Lewis, Mrs. Coats, Mrs. Parliman & Margaret, Ma *was* here. Mrs. Lewis was the Dr. (paid her $2.00) she is a real good woman Baby was born about half past ten A.M. . . . about three o'clock I felt that all was well; was lying comfortably in bed; the boy beside me, the Ladies, all but Margaret went home. Mrs. Lewis kissed me, O, she seemed like one kind deliverer, & they were all kind.

It is likely that, despite Emily's use of the term *Dr.*, Mrs. Lewis was the midwife.[22] Although male physicians officiated at some of the deliveries Emily attended, she marshalled the help of women alone. The presence of James's mother, "Ma," also is noteworthy. By this time, Emily and James had been living at the home of his parents for almost a year, and the relationship between Emily and her in-laws had grown increasingly conflictual. Emily accused them of compelling James to work too hard and paying him too little. Nevertheless, to Emily's surprise, Ma attended the birth. It was customary for one woman to remain at the home of the birthing woman for several days to provide practical assistance; in this case, the helper was James's married sister, Margaret Doolittle.[23]

The women who attended Emily's second confinement confronted death as well as birth. "Ah. ah," Emily wrote on July 7, 1865. "Can it be possible that we have a little daughter born this morning—that weighs 5 lbs. 7 oz—her twin brother did not live to even breathe." Once again,

Mrs. Lewis delivered the baby, and James's mother provided assistance, despite growing tensions between her and Emily.

When Emily became seriously ill in 1886, an even broader array of neighbors and kin offered their services. Sarah reported that during the first 2 weeks, six women sat with Emily through the night, one as many as four times. Many others came during the day to provide both nursing and practical assistance.

It would, of course, be impossible to determine what combination of altruism and self-interest underlay the network of support between Emily and other women. To some extent, the mutual assistance of nineteenth-century women operated like an insurance system, spreading the risks of trouble. When Emily rushed to her neighbors' homes in times of crisis, she knew she was making an investment in her own future. When her neighbors watched her at night and did her housework, they were repaying her for services previously rendered.

Nevertheless, some evidence suggests that Emily did not view other women solely as instrumental resources for discrete tasks. Although she focused narrowly on her own well-being when she worked on the farm, her activities as a caregiver appear to have sprung at least partly from a sense of attachment to others. We have seen that she expressed rare warmth and sympathy toward those she tended. When others ministered to her needs, she assumed that they too were acting out of affection and concern. After listing various women who visited her in the late spring and summer of 1886, she wrote, "All the neighbors all round every where they all seem every one like real true friends far different than ever before" (EHG, June 3). The visits of Mrs. Chapman were especially precious. The two women had reestablished their friendship while working together at the home of a bereaved neighbor the previous January. Mrs. Chapman's care in June 1886 cemented their bond: "She was here yesterday," Emily wrote. "She was talking about how Her & I used to visit together & she cried about it . . . and as soon as I can ride am going up there" (EHG, June 3).

Nevertheless, it is important not to romanticize women's ties of interdependence. We have seen that conflicts continued to erupt between Emily and Harriet after Emily provided assistance during childbirth. Harriet visited Emily daily and "sat up" with her on at least two occasions in May and June 1886, but Emily did not welcome her sister's ministrations. On June 3, she wrote, "That Harriet comes up every day but most everytime she comes has something to say about the past that makes it unpleasant Im fraid all the time when [she] comes here that when I get well that there will be something." After seeing Harriet the following October Emily exclaimed, "No! I did *not* have a *good* Visit with her" (EHG, October 20). Nor did the help provided by James's sister Margaret Doolittle overcome the rift between her and Emily. Margaret had stayed with Emily and helped with the housework after Henry's birth in 1863, but whatever closeness may have developed between the women at that time vanished when Margaret sided with James in his battles with Emily. Like many other relatives and friends, Margaret visited Emily when her health failed in the spring of 1886. But that summer James left home, and when Margaret appeared at the Gillespie door in October, Emily threatened to have her arrested.

SARAH'S RESPONSIBILITIES

Sarah's activities as a caregiver resembled those of Emily. Until Sarah left home in 1883, the two women shared the rhythms of daily life. Sarah helped her mother can tomatoes, plant strawberries, sell eggs, honey, and butter in town, prepare supper, cut carpet rags, and sew clothes. Sarah also shared her first major nursing experience with her mother. On October 3, 1884, Sarah's brother Henry was helping to rebuild a church in a nearby town when he suffered an accident: "O dear I can hardly write in my journal," Emily wrote. "Last Friday noon Mr. Morse came for me to go to Manchester that Henry was hurt. O, O, he had fallen from the church spire—I could not be thankful enough that he was not killed . . . the first place he hit anything was 9 ft. then 20 ft. to the roof & from there it was 45 ft. *Oh, terrible*. I have been with him all the time . . . it is too bad, terrible to think of, to fall 74 feet, not a bone broken . . . he is seriously hurt it seems as if he is bruised in every place . . . it is indeed the hardest time in my life" (EHG, October 6). According to Sarah, for the first 4 days and nights, "he was fanned & rubbed every second by myself & Ma. He was taken to Mrs. Nell Smiths where he boarded. . . . He was literally covered with black & blue spots and had to be bathed in hot water—and cold clothes kept on his head. O such pain and suffering as he endured. He was light headed a couple of times at night and we had to work so hard to keep him alive" (SGH, October 19).

The two women were attentive to each other, not just to Henry. Sarah described Emily's response as well as her own: "Ma did not cry but was as white as a corpse, She is almost sick at best" (SGH, October 19). Emily noted that "it is very hard" for Sarah too (EHG, October 12). While Emily stayed with Henry during the day, Sarah returned to the farm each morning to do the household and farm chores. She described her workload and complained about the toll that caring took on her own health:

> I can't tell how many washings & ironings I have done. But a doz. pillow slips had to be changed each day besides sheets & clothes & I [remember] washing & ironing 23 slips one day when I came home & then baking a doz. pumpkin pies & making cake & washing all the dishes

making the beds & to see to every thing else. . . . I wrenched my back lifting & turning Henry & now my left wrist is 'gun' out. He can not turn
over or get on or off the bed without lifting. (SGH, October 19).

But there were compensations. After recounting all the housework
she did, Sarah commented, "Why I am stronger than I thot I was" (SGH,
October 19). She also believed that she was uniquely equipped to minis-
ter to Henry's needs. Although many friends offered to "sit up" with
Henry, she noted that she "couldn't trust such a care to anyone" (ibid.).
And it is likely that Sarah knew that Emily considered her indispensable:
"O what would I do without her," Emily wrote shortly after the accident
(EHG, October 6). Henry was able to return to the farm on October 11
and to walk with the aid of crutches by October 19, although, as noted
in the entries above, he continued to need substantial care from both his
mother and Sarah for several more weeks.

Sarah's sense of responsibility for Emily began even before Henry's
accident. Although Emily prided herself on offering protection to her
children, she appeared much weaker in Sarah's diary than in her own.
Sarah was well aware that Emily suffered intensely from James's out-
bursts and threats of violence. "Poor Ma," she wrote often; or, "I feel so
sorry for her." After one of James's "fits" in 1882, Sarah described her
mother as "nervous & trembling as an autumn leaf" (SGH, March 10).
Although we lack Henry's account, both Emily's and Sarah's diaries suggest that he too viewed his mother as an object of pity. Emily frequently
expressed her determination to appear strong and in control before her
children. Whenever they witnessed an attack of "nerves," she vowed to
act "pleasant" in the future. But she also was grateful whenever Sarah
and Henry responded to her problems, and appears to have been aware
that her neediness tied them to her.

During the spring and summer of 1884, when Emily was 46, Sarah
first began to notice her mother's physical ailments. She wrote that Emily
appeared "sickly" and that her hands were "numb." Emily wrote, "My
fingers & hands have had a queer feeling for some time. I will be glad if
they get their natural feeling & thankful, too, they feel as if the cuticle
was about worn out" (EHG, September 9). Two weeks later she noted
that a local doctor had corroborated her self-diagnosis: "Dr. Sherman
said I must bathe my hands in alcohol, that the cuticle was so thin just as
I thought" (EHG, September 23). Emily attributed her physical problems
to the burdens she shouldered and especially to the stresses engendered
by James's violent and erratic behavior: "Ah! James. Had you have
treated me as half human I do believe I should have been in better health
now, but instead of being a protector, you have hundreds of times almost
broke my heart" (EHG, May 11, 1886).

Because Sarah's caregiving responsibilities were intertwined with her teaching career, they must be described together. Although teaching was one of the few respectable occupations open to nineteenth-century women, it had numerous disadvantages. It paid poorly, conferred little security, and was physically and emotionally demanding. Teachers often had large and unruly classes with students of vastly disparate ages. Many teachers viewed their work solely as a way of making money before marriage and happily abandoned it on their wedding days.[24]

But Sarah invested great hopes in her career. She enjoyed making an independent income and had a strong sense of mission about the work. After her first day at a new school, she wrote that her students "had been used to do about as they pleased, whispering, chewing gum, & a general shuffling noise." She vowed to "work diligently to overcome these formed habits" (SGH, November 16). She took equal pride in the attention she devoted to teaching the fundamentals of spelling and arithmetic. Sarah also found happiness in her life away from the farm. Most of the homes in which she boarded had a son or daughter her age. One taught her to play the organ, another to sew a lace pattern. Together they went sleigh riding, visited friends, and held impromptu parties. She was always pleased to see her mother again, but she occasionally found days at home dreary and was glad to return to her hosts.

Emily watched closely over Sarah's teaching career, preparing arithmetic problems Sarah could use in the classroom, consoling her during periods of discouragement, giving her hints about enforcing discipline, and offering her rest at the farm on weekends. But even with Emily's help, Sarah did not enjoy undiluted success. Especially in the beginning, she confronted several major setbacks. She failed her first teaching certification examination and had to remain home as her friends departed for jobs. Although she received a certificate the following year, she did not immediately find a post. During her first term as a teacher, she found it difficult to exercise discipline and was not rehired for the following term.

Sarah first felt secure as a teacher during her second term, from November 1884 to March 1885. Her growing professional confidence, however, coincided with increased anxiety about her mother. When Sarah left for school, she confessed that she did not "like to leave Ma so miserable" (SGH, November 30). And, indeed, as soon as Sarah departed, Emily's health grew worse: "My hands feel real bad & in fact I have a singular feeling all over; when I rub my flesh it gives a peculiar sensation—a shudder—almost hurts, my nerves must be in a bad condition. I hope I may be better sometime" (EHG, December 3). During the next few months she complained that the problems had spread to her feet and head.

Soon after Sarah returned to the farm for a vacation in the spring of 1885, Emily described her condition this way: "I have a nervous chill &

fever every day when I move around it seems as if my head would almost burst & every time my heart beats I can hear and feel the flow of blood on the top of my head so much that the sound is some of the time unendurable" (EHG, April 6). Sarah reported that she "kept cold water" on Emily's head (SGH, April 8). Emily also found relief in a remedy she prescribed for herself: "I feel better when I eat dandelion greens," she commented (EHG, April 30). Before leaving, Sarah recruited a "hired girl" to do some of the housework she left behind.[25] Sarah's worries intensified during her third term. Although she was "glad" to see the family with whom she boarded, she wondered how her mother was faring in her absence. "Ma was sick abed and had a burning fever when we came away—I do hope & pray she may get better soon" (SGH, May 3). Returning home for a visit a few weeks later, she commented, "I tell you I've cried more than once since Fri. evening when I first saw her this time. Something must be done for her" (SGH, May 24). She found that her mother had increased difficulty walking and could feed the turkeys only by lying down (EHG, May 21). Back at school, Sarah recorded her concerns about leaving Emily with only the hired girl to help: "Ma has the dropsy to her body—Im so afraid it will get all over her—& wish I knew what could be done to help her. She did not sleep she said her feet & legs pain her so badly—Now if I was there Id rub them for her—But there is nothing done for her at all" (SGH, June 4).[26] Emily also compared the hired girl invidiously with Sarah. When Sarah returned from school in July, Emily wrote, "Sarah wash, mop & do up the work before eleven A.M. O so much nicer than it has been done for three months" (EHG, July 27).

During Sarah's fourth term as a teacher (November 1885 to March 1886) Emily's condition continued to deteriorate. Early in 1886 she wrote that when she tried to move a chair, she "fell flat upon the floor. I could have cried for its very discouraging to be so weak" (February 5). Returning to the farm for a weekend, Sarah reported that she found Emily "ever so much weaker" (SGH, February 6). Sarah also had to contend with the intense hostility between her parents. Emily complained that James purposely aggravated her condition. He drove the carriage too fast when they were together, refused to supply her with the proper food, and made her faint by cleaning a kerosene lantern too close to her room. During her vacation in the spring of 1886, Sarah chastised her father for his behavior, watched over her mother, rubbed her swollen legs, and brought the food she desired. The day before Sarah left, Emily again stressed her dependence on Sarah: "She *is* such a *blessed good* girl. if it were not for her it seems as if I would almost starve, and no one else to do the slightest errand" (EHG, April 17).

When Sarah began a new term in April 1886, she increasingly was torn between her responsibilities as a daughter and as a teacher. On her last day at home, she wondered whether she "ought to go & leave" her mother (SGH, April 18). When she arrived at her boarding place, she described herself as "very homesick" because she had left her mother "failing so badly" (ibid.). Her spirits rose when she entered the classroom: "Seems like home again. Think we will have a good school" (SGH, April 19). But the following day she noted that her students thought she was "crosser" than she had been the previous term: "I guess I am worrying about Ma," she explained. "Wish I might see her" (SGH, April 20). By month's end, Emily wrote that she could "hardly walk" and that she felt "entirely broken down, both nerve & muscle and courage" (April 30). The same day, Sarah commented in her diary, "Ma is just dying for want of care I'm almost a mind to give up my school." When Sarah returned for a short visit, Emily noted that Sarah "dreads to leave me feeling so bad" (EHG, May 2). Sarah wrote, "Don't believe I'll try to teach any more for I have to worry so much. I'm thinking of Ma every minute" (SGH, May 3). Two days later, however, she again dwelt on the joys of her job: "We had a splendid school today. Seems as though I could take them in my arms & kiss them all" (SGH, May 5).

Sarah returned to the farm for the weekend 10 days later. She slept with her mother on the night of Saturday, May 15. When she awoke the following morning, she discovered that her mother "did not realize anything" (SGH, May 18). Although Emily soon regained consciousness, she continued to require around-the-clock care for several weeks. Sarah resigned her job and stayed home to nurse her mother. Emily reported that Sarah "comes every minute to see how I feel" (EHG, May 21). Sarah also described the services she rendered. She wrote that Emily "had been to weak to sit up much for 2 or 3 days. But has to be rubbed & hot flannels Kept on & hot teas & a great deal of care" (SGH, May 20). Whenever death seemed imminent, Sarah "sat up" in order to forestall "sinking spells." Although neighbors and a "hired girl" provided some assistance, Sarah frequently was alone at night. She often noted that she slept just 1 or 2 hours. On June 2, 1886, she slept from 11:30 P.M. to 12:30 A.M. and from 2:15 to 3:45 A.M. (SGH, June 3). At month's end, she wrote that she undressed and went to bed for the first time in 6 weeks (SGH, June 28). The following week, however, she cared for her mother between two and six times each night (SGH, July 8). She reported that her eyes ached and that she was sick herself as a result of "irregular sleep" (SGH, 22 June 1886).

Sarah accepted without question that her primary duty as a daughter and a woman was to provide this nursing care. Because she felt strongly attached to her mother, caregiving was a labor of love. Nevertheless, she also longed to be back at school. Four days after this crisis began she wrote, "It makes me cry to think of them (My pupils)"

(SGH, May 20). Two weeks later, a rumor that she would be rehired the following term "much pleased" her (SGH, June 6). She also was glad to learn that the students preferred her to the replacement and the director thought that the school was not functioning well in her absence.

Henry had been working in Kansas City, Missouri, when the crisis began and returned on May 19, finding another job in the vicinity. Although he lived at the farm and cared for his mother when he could, he was away most days. Sarah complained that her father intensified rather than alleviated her burdens. According to her account, James was indifferent to her difficulties: "Pa does not seem to think but that I can work all night & all day," she commented bitterly (SGH, May 26). She was "provoked" when he would not relieve her even "1 hr. of the night" (SGH, June 10). When James asked Sarah not to bother him and allow him to sleep, she remarked indignantly, "I thot I needed rest if any one" (SGH, June 17). James left home a few weeks later, and he and Emily never again lived together.

Sarah also received relatively little assistance from formal health providers. Hospitals were scarce in Iowa in the 1880s; those that existed served people without family to care for them. During May and June 1886 physicians from town occasionally stopped by the house, left medicine, discussed Emily's prognosis, and offered advice. On June 28, Sarah noted: "Dr. Fuller said for me to get asparagus root & steep it & put in a drop or two of alcohol to keep it & let Ma smell of it." It seems likely that Sarah took this recommendation seriously and attempted to follow it. Most of the time, however, she administered remedies without a doctor's direction.

Emily loathed the enforced dependency of an invalid. In August 1886 she wrote, "I pray I may walk again and be so that I can get around & wait upon myself. . . . To be helpless is *so bad* I can not tell *how* bad" (EHG, August 7). The following month she explained why she had neglected her diary: "each time when I felt like writing no one was near to ask for pen & ink and Book, or were busy. It seems to me a *deep, sorrowful & bad afflication* that I *can not* wait upon myself" (EHG, September 5). In October she complained, "I could sew some but can not get any of my things to get any thing to do & to ask for every thing I want *is surely* the hardest work I ever done" (EHG, October 2).

But her children's attentiveness also gave her enormous pleasure. Shortly after becoming seriously ill, she wrote, "I have lived for them & now they have sacrificed time & money, and they can not do too much for me" (EHG, May 21). She expressed her gratitude again: "The Children have been so kind & faithful to care for me. doing & watching. . . . *I thank Henry & Sarah* for their watchful care" (EHG, August 4).

Nevertheless, Emily also worried that the work was a strain on Henry and Sarah: "Sarah sits up most nights & does a good deal of cooking & it is too much for her" (EHG, June 3). It is likely that she also had concerns about Sarah's teaching career. Emily had wanted Sarah to achieve the upward mobility that had been denied to her. But Sarah was now marooned on the farm and engulfed in domestic obligations. Rather than pursuing professional success, she was repeating the narrow pattern of her mother's life.

Emily slowly regained her health throughout the summer and early fall of 1886, and Sarah was able to return to school in November. She wrote only sporadically in her journal during the next few months. Emily's diary, however, indicates that she continued to experience new health problems. As a result of lying down so much, her hip joints became sore, and at the end of December she burned her foot. Although Henry and a hired girl tended to her regularly, she was convinced that Sarah alone could meet her needs. When Sarah returned for a vacation early in 1887, she reported that she "put on a poultice of potato, changing it often during the day." At night, she applied "bread & milk & sugar" (SGH, March 11). The following day, Emily noted that her sore foot had greatly improved: "I verily believe my foot might not have ever healed and got well had not Sarah have come home to take care of it" (EHG, March 12).

It was not unusual for family members to rely on unorthodox practitioners as well as members of the regular medical profession,[27] and during this 1887 vacation, Sarah sent for a "magnetic doctor"[28]: "I believe he can cure Ma" (SGH, March 19). She was not immediately disappointed. Two days after his arrival, she wrote, "Ma is constantly better. It is wonderful what the simplicity of rubbing will do. And it is not so simple either, for there is the will & the magnetism which develops and enshrouds the healer & is passed from him to the patient" (SGH, April 10). Emily expressed even greater faith in his powers, writing that her hair was not as white as before and that she felt he could almost bring "the dead back to earthly life" (EHG, April 12). He stayed at the house for 5 weeks, administering a total of 33 treatments (SGH, April 25). His presence added to Sarah's burdens. She had to cook his meals; when he expressed distaste for her food, she had to help him find other places to eat. Because James refused to pay his fee, the responsibility fell on Henry and Sarah. Most seriously, because Sarah often lacked the protection of her father and brother, she was vulnerable to sexual harassment: "Dr. Munson is a free-lover," she complained. "I do not believe in his doctrine. . . . The idea of an old man wanting to kiss & hug me—Its surely unreasonable & below my dignity" (SGH, April 20).

Sarah accepted another job for the term beginning in April 1887 but deferred opening the school to stay home an extra week. Instead of boarding in the community, she traveled the 9 miles between the farm and school each morning and evening in order to tend her mother. While she was away, Henry and the hired girl shared responsibility for Emily's care. When the hired girl left abruptly, Sarah had to find a replacement. This, too, was an onerous job. She wrote, "Saturday morning at 9 o'clock I drove to town for the mail as I heard nothing from Mrs. McFarland, the woman who wished to work for us. I concluded to drive to Dorsetville for her. . . . A Scotchman led [the horse] past a brush fire. . . . The place where they said Mrs. Mc was, she was not, for she had gone 7 mi. farther to Lamont. I engineered the way & drove there. . . . I saw Jas. Grey and he found out for me where Mrs. Mc was" (SGH, April 25). They did not reach the Gillespie farm until 8 P.M. As Emily commented, it was "a real hard jaunt for Sarah" (EHG, April 25).

When the school term ended, Sarah returned home and devoted herself to her mother's care. She later wrote, "School closed the 25th of June. . . . I was very tired that Saturday night & thankful too, for I felt as though my school days were ended, not thankful for my own sake as much as Ma's & Henry's. Ma was so glad to have me with her again" (SGH, November 6). Emily was aware of Sarah's mixed emotions, noting that Sarah would "so much rather teach than to stay" (EHG, June 29). Sarah did not return to the classroom until several years after her mother's death in March 1888.

Although Sarah's departure from school freed her from the burden of reconciling the competing demands of work and home, it also deprived her of her primary way of limiting her caregiving responsibilities. As Emily worsened, Sarah spent her days bathing her mother, lifting her from bed, turning her over, dressing her, and helping her use the bed pan. In addition, Sarah gave Emily catnip tea, bathed her hip in smart weed water, and cleaned her bed sores. Two weeks before Emily died, Sarah wrote, "Her bed-sores are very painful—one which is a trifle better now is 3 in. deep & 21/2 in. in diameter. I have to cut out the 'puss' & cleanse them often & it fairly makes my veins refuse to carry the blood some-times" (SGH, March 15). Even when Sarah did not provide direct care, she could not escape the sight of her mother's deteriorating body. In February, she suddenly lost her appetite when she saw her mother lying in an unusually convoluted position: "She was in a terrible shape. . . . Well—it spoiled my meal. I was choked & had to leave the table. I was so hungry & had some nice mashed potatoes on my plate; but somehow I was not the least hungry in less than a minute" (SGH, February 3). It is possible that Emily's infirmities affected Sarah so intensely because she identified closely with her mother. Unlike formal health providers, Sarah could not rely on a prescribed role to limit the emotional impact of her mother's suffering. Watching Emily, Sarah may have foreseen her own future.

Although various friends and relatives called and offered their services, the bulk of the work fell on Sarah. Once again she complained about her exhaustion. Because she had little time to eat, she lost weight. She also wrote about painful back problems, which she attributed to the stress of lifting her mother. Emily continued to express both concern about the burdens imposed on Henry and Sarah and gratitude for their help. In February she wrote, "Sarah is lying down to rest. She is tired it grieves my heart that she has had to get up to care for me every night" (EHG, February 19). Because Henry and Sarah frequently wrote Emily's diary for her during the months before her death, her comments served as a way of conveying sentiments to them. An entry in Sarah's handwriting at the close of 1887 read: "Sarah takes the best care of me she can" (EHG, December 28). A few weeks later Emily was able to write herself. In an entry clearly intended for Sarah to read, she stated, "Sarah is here and cares for me. . . . Dear Daughter it is to Ma more than words or pen can tell" (EHG, February 12).

We can see that the care Sarah rendered had a variety of different components. One was to offer sympathy and reassurance. Nineteenth-century attitudes about the importance of personal ties elevated this aspect of caring.[29] Because people believed that tensions and conflicts could produce disease, they thought that loving solicitude could restore health. Just as Emily attributed her illness to James's violence and indifference, she insisted that Sarah's attentive care alleviated emotional stress and thus facilitated healing. As Emily frequently stated, Sarah's kindness and attentiveness were the "best medicine."

Sarah's concern for her mother's emotional well-being also meant that Sarah had to conceal the toll caregiving inflicted. Because Emily hated being a burden, she wanted to believe that her children rendered care with "willing hearts." Six weeks before Emily's death, Sarah complained: "My side & back are very lame and, though I very much dislike to own it I feel very tired; a kind of tired sick. And if I make visible complaint, such as to lie down or go without a meal why, Ma will look so much worse & worry so" (SGH, February 2). Just as Emily took pride in being "pleasant" despite her troubles, so Sarah had to mask her own feelings.

Other aspects of Sarah's care required physical stamina and medical knowledge, not just warmth and sensitivity. When she fed her mother special teas, cleaned her bed sores, and watched for signs of death, Sarah performed skilled nursing care. Sarah also did "dirty work."[30] According to Emily, a doctor brought a "rubber attachment—for urinal purposes" to the house in November 1887; because Emily was extremely frail at this time, Sarah must have helped her mother use it (EHG, November 7). Her own diary indicates that she also had to clean up vomit, excreta, and blood. Emily had believed that Sarah was too "fine" to participate in such "unpleasant" farm chores as milking cows and feeding hogs. Female delicacy, however, could have no place in the sick room.

Emily's illness also left Sarah with a staggering amount of household and farm labor. Even when caring for her mother "night and day," she rose at 5:30 A.M. to prepare Henry's breakfast, fed more than 200 turkeys, baked bread and pies, mopped the kitchen, washed the family's clothes, and took berries to the market. "Dear me," she wrote in March 1887, "the clockstrikes 8 & now I've my dishes to wash & Ma's foot to dress. Beds to make. etc, etc" (SGH, March 26). Finally, Sarah helped her mother financially. Although she had to forfeit her own income, she and Henry paid the fees of at least one doctor.

Caregiving clearly imposed serious costs on Sarah's life. She twice withdrew from the workforce and once postponed the opening of school. Preoccupation with her mother's well-being also prevented her from adhering to the high standards she set for herself. When her students found her "crosser" than usual, she feared she was violating her own code of professional behavior. Even when Emily lay dying in March 1888, the offer of a new teaching job sorely tempted Sarah, much as she tried to convince herself otherwise: "No—I can not teach no use to think of it now," she wrote 9 days before her mother's death (SGH, March 15). But it is possible that Sarah's involvement in caregiving also enhanced her self-esteem. We saw that she found new reserves of strength when nursing her brother after his accident. As the primary caregiver for her dying mother, Sarah had to manage difficult situations, make decisions on her own, and exercise skill. And Sarah received not just appreciation from her mother but also recognition from experienced practitioners. After Emily's death, Sarah proudly noted that a local doctor "requested me to assist him in an operation" and then offered to recommend her as a "skilled nurse" (SGH, October 22).

CONCLUSION

It is important to exercise caution in generalizing from this case study. Emily and Sarah were native-born white women living in the rural Midwest, and their experiences undoubtedly were very different from those of women in other social groups. Moreover, many aspects of their experiences expressed the particularities of their personalities and relationship. The deterioration of Emily's marriage, coupled with the tensions in her female friendships, made her especially dependent on her daughter. Although Emily encouraged Sarah to pursue individual achievement and furthered her career in many ways, Emily also expected Sarah to respond to her own neediness. Because Sarah had long been solicitous of her mother's well-being, caregiving represented an extension of previously established patterns in the mother–daughter relationship, not an abrupt change.

But in several ways, Emily and Sarah were typical of other women of their era. Throughout the nineteenth century, caregiving commonly dominated women's lives. Because the average life span was short, the need for parent care often arose when daughters were relatively young.[31] Many nineteenth-century women who left home to seek paid employment relinquished their jobs when family members became ill; even entry into a career rarely excused single daughters from the duty to care.[32]

Despite the rise of a vast system of health care in the United States since the 1880s, care for sick and disabled people is still predominantly a private responsibility. Researchers consistently find, for example, that families and friends deliver 70% to 80% of long-term care to the frail elderly.[33] Moreover, recent government policies have sought to reimpose care for sick and disabled people on private households. Between the mid-1950s and the mid-1970s, state mental hospitals discharged the majority of their patients; a 1978 study reported that two thirds of them returned to receive care from their families.[34] The establishment of a prospective payment system for acute hospital care has resulted in a drop in the average length of stay, shifting care back to the home.[35] And various measures attempt to reduce the size of the nursing home population and thus increase family responsibilities for frail elderly people.[36]

But such policies are not simply returning to nineteenth-century methods of caregiving. A complex series of historical changes have profoundly altered the content and meaning of informal care. As a result of the advent of mass-produced labor-saving devices, few contemporary caregivers have such difficult and unrelenting household chores as Sarah. The emergence of a formal system of health care delivery also has transformed family caregiving. Sarah never considered the possibility of taking her mother to a hospital or employing a trained nurse. Although physicians occasionally stopped by the house, they left major responsibilities in her hands. If the development of the health care system has lightened some aspects of caring work, it also has undermined women's traditional skills. Women who deliver care to family members today frequently do so under the direction of skilled medical providers.

As a result of the loosening of the bonds of kinship and community, women are less likely to feel responsible for ensuring the well-being of such an extensive network of relatives and neighbors. One reason caregiving consumed Emily's energies is that she nursed a large number of people in addition to her immediate family. Despite her strained relationships with many members of her community, she responded immediately to their calls for help. In turn, the services she rendered helped to strengthen her bonds to her neighbors. Moreover, caregiving was a social endeavor, and both Emily and Sarah shared many tasks with other women. Because women today are less likely to be able to rely on community structures of support, caregiving has become a lonelier activity.[37]

Nevertheless, some aspects of this story have a contemporary ring. The defaults of men helped to determine the amount of care Emily and Sarah delivered. According to their accounts, James felt no responsibility for his wife's care. Although Henry's attention to Emily helped to ease Sarah's burdens, the siblings did not share caregiving equitably. Henry filled in when Sarah was unavailable and provided relief when her obligations became too great. The primary responsibility, however, rested with Sarah. Caregiving was women's work in the broader community as well. When sickness visited households, men often fetched doctors and escorted female neighbors and relatives to and from their homes. But women alone provided the great bulk of direct nursing services. Today, as in the nineteenth century, gender determines the allocation of caregiving obligations; more than three fourths of adult children caring for parents, for example, are women.[38]

This story also reminds us that caregiving is embedded in relationships and cannot be considered apart from them. Women who care for each other or share caring responsibilities often become closer. But closeness can breed tensions and conflicts, as well as warmth and solicitude. By assisting Harriet during childbirth and after an abortion, Emily mended some of the rifts in their relationship, but by the spring of 1886, the difficulties between the sisters had become too great to enable Harriet to be an adequate caregiver. Although Harriet twice sat up with Emily at night and visited regularly during the day, Emily derived no comfort from her sister's presence. Sarah's strong sense of attachment to her mother created a different set of problems. Sarah experienced Emily's pain as if it were her own and responded with enormous sensitivity to Emily's conflicting needs. As a result, caregiving was often an overwhelming experience. Because many contemporary policymakers idealize family care, it is important to recognize that the intensity of intimate relationships can impede as well as foster the delivery of care.

NOTES

1. The diaries of both Emily Hawley Gillespie (EHG) and Sarah Gillespie Huftalen (SGH) are located at the State Historical Society of Iowa in Iowa City. This essay builds on the analysis of Emily Hawley Gillespie's diary by Judy Nolte Lensink in *"A Secret to Be Burned": The Diary and Life of Emily Hawley Gillespie, 1858–1888* (Iowa City: University of Iowa Press, 1989), and of Sarah Gillespie Huftalen's diary by Suzanne L. Bunkers in *"All Will Yet Be Well": The Diary of Sarah Gillespie Huftalen* (Iowa City: University of Iowa Press, 1993).

2. For reviews of some of this literature, see Ronald L. Numbers, "The History of American Medicine: A Field in Ferment," *Rev. Amer. Hist.*, 1982, 10: 245–63; John Harley Warner, "Science in Medicine," in *Historical Writing on American Science: Perspectives and Prospects,* ed. Sally Gregory Kohlstedt and Margaret W. Rossiter (Baltimore: Johns Hopkins University Press, 1985), pp. 37–58.

3. These include Charles E. Rosenberg, *The Care of Strangers: The Rise of America's Hospital System* (New York: Basic Books, 1987); Paul Starr, *The Social Transformation of American Medicine: The Rise of a Sovereign Profession and the Making of a Vast Industry* (New York: Basic Books, 1982).

4. See, for example, Judy Barrett Litoff *American Midwives: 1860 to the Present* (Westport, Conn.: Greenwood Press, 1978); Barbara Melosh, "The Physician's Hand," *Work Culture and Conflict in American Nursing* (Philadelphia: Temple University Press, 1982); Regina Markell Morantz-Sanchez, *Sympathy and Science: Women Physicians in American Medicine* (New York: Oxford University Press, 1985); Susan M. Reverby, *Ordered to Care: The Dilemma of American Nursing; 1850–1945* (New York: Cambridge University Press, 1987).

5. Laurel Thatcher Ulrich, *A Midwife's Tale: The Life of Martha Ballard, Based on Her Diary, 1785–1812* (New York: Alfred A. Knopf, 1990).

6. Among the many letters, diaries, and memoirs that discuss nineteenth-century women's caregiving experiences are Nannie T. Alderson and Helena Huntington Smith, *A Bride Goes West* (New York: Farrar & Rinehart, 1942); Eleanor Allen, *Canvas Caravans, Based on the Journal of Esther Belle McMillan Hanna* (Portland, Ore.: Binfords & Mort, 1946); Susan S. Arpad, ed., *Sam Curd's Diary: The Diary of a True Woman* (Athens: Ohio University Press, 1984); Sarah Connell Ayer, *Diary of Sarah Connell Ayer* (Portland, Maine: Lefavor-Tower, 1910); M. S. Bailey, "A Journal of Mary Stuart Bailey, Wife of Dr. Fred Bailey from Ohio to California, April–October 1852," in *Ho for California! Women's Overland Diaries from the Huntington Library,* ed. S. L. Myres (San Marino, Calif.: Huntington Library, 1980); Nannie Stillwell Jackson, *Vinegar Pie and Chicken Bread: A Woman's Diary of Life in the Rural South, 1890–1891,* ed. Margaret Jones Bolsteri (Fayetteville: University of Arkansas Press, 1982); Harriet Connor Brown, *Grandmother Brown's Hundred Years, 1827–1927* (New York: Blue Ribbon Books, 1929); H. Carpenter, "A Trip Across the Plains in an Oxen Wagon, 1857," in Myres, *Ho for California!;* Amelia Akehurst Lines, *To Raise Myself a Little: The Diaries and Letters of Jennie, A Georgia Teacher, 1841–1886,* ed. Thomas G. Dyer (Athens: University of Georgia Press, 1982); F. M. Eddy, "An American Spinster," in *Victorian Women: A Documentary Account of Women's Lives in Nineteenth-Century England, France, and the United States,* ed. Erna Olafson Hellerstein, Leslie Parker Hume, and Karen M. Offer (Stanford, Calif.: Stanford University Press, 1981), pp. 155–57; M. Edwards, "Letters to Sabrina Bennett," in *Farm to Factory: Women's Letters, 1830–1860,* ed. Thomas Dublin (New York: Columbia University Press, 1981), pp. 82–87; Anne Ellis, *The Life of an Ordinary Woman* (Boston: Houghton Mifflin, 1929); Annie Fields, *Life and Letters of Harriet Beecher Stowe* (Detroit Gale Research, 1979); Margaret A. Frink, *Journal of the Adventures of a Party of California Gold-seekers (Indiana to California, 1850)* (privately printed, 1897); C. Haun, "A Woman's Trip Across the Plains in 1849," in *Women's Diaries of the Westward Journey,* ed. Lillian Schlissel (New York: Schocken, 1982), pp. 165–86; Virginia Wilcox Ivins, *Pen Pictures of Early Western Days* (privately printed, 1905); Joel Myerson and Daniel Shealy, eds., *The Selected Letters of Louisa May Alcott* (Boston: Little, Brown, 1987); Hallie F. Nelson, *South of the Cottonwood Tree* (Broken Bow, Nebr.: Purcella, 1977); Agnes Just Reid, *Letters of Long Ago* (Caldwell, Idaho: Caxton Printers, 1936); L. A. Rudd, "A Woman's Trip Across the Plains in 1848," in Schlissel, *Women's Diaries of the Westward Journey,*

pp.187–98; Lillian Schlissel, "The Malick Family in Oregon Territory, 1848–1867," in *Far From Home: Families of the Westward Journey,* ed. Lillian Schlissel, Byrd Gibbens, and Elizabeth Hampsten (New York: Schocken Books, 1989), pp. 3–106; Martha Farnsworth, *Plains Woman: The Diary of Martha Farnsworth, 1882–1922,* ed. Marlene Springer and Haskell Springer (Bloomington: Indiana University Press, 1986); *Caleb and Mary Wilder Foote: Reminiscences and Letters,* ed. Mary Wilder Tileston (Boston: Houghton Mifflin, 1918).

7. Judith Walzer Leavitt and Ronald L. Numbers, "Sickness and Health in America: An Overview," in *Sickness and Health in America: Readings in the History of Medicine and Public Health,* ed. Judith Walzer Leavitt and Ronald L. Numbers (Madison: University of Wisconsin Press, 1985), pp. 3–10.

8. See Mary P. Ryan, *Cradle of the Middle Class: The Family in Oneida County, New York, 1790–1865* (Cambridge: Cambridge University Press, 1981); see also Robert L. Griswold, "Anglo Women and Domestic Ideology in the American West in the Nineteenth and Early Twentieth Centuries," in *Western Women: Their Land, Their Values,* ed. Lillian Schlissel, Vicki L. Ruiz, and Janice Monk (Albuquerque: University of New Mexico Press, 1988), pp. 15–33; for an analysis of the relevance of the domestic code to nineteenth-century farm women, see Nancy Grey Osterud, *Bonds of Community: The Lives of Farm Women in Nineteenth-Century New York* (Ithaca, NY: Cornell University Press, 1991).

9. Morris J. Vogel, *The Invention of the Modern Hospital: Boston, 1870–1930* (Chicago: University of Chicago Press, 1980), p. 1.

10. John B. Blake, "From Buchanan to Fishbein: The Literature of Domestic Medicine," in *Medicine without Doctors,* ed. Guenter B. Risse, Ronald L. Numbers, and Judith Walzer Leavitt (New York: Science History Publications, 1977), pp. 11–30; James H. Cassedy, "Why Self-Help? Americans Alone with Their Diseases, 1800–1850," in *Medicine without Doctors,* pp. 31–48.

11. Melosh, "The Physician's Hand" (n. 4), pp. 77–112; Reverby, *Ordered to Care* (n. 4), p. 98.

12. Ulrich, *A Midwife's Tale* (n. 5), p. 251.

13. Elizabeth Hampsten, *Read This Only to Yourself: The Private Writings of Midwestern Women, 1880–1910* (Bloomington: Indiana University Press, 1982); for an analysis of the way that graphic descriptions of bodily parts could assuage the fears of nurses, see Melosh, "The Physician's Hand" (n. 4), pp. 54–60.

14. For an analysis of Emily's aspirations, see Lensink, *"A Secret to Be Burned"* (n. 1).

15. See Ruth Schwartz Cowan, *More Work for Mothers: The Ironies of Household Technology from the Open Hearth to the Microwave* (New York: Basic Books, 1983); Alice Kessler-Harris, *Out to Work: A History of Wage Earning Women in the United States* (New York: Oxford University Press, 1982), pp. 110–12; Susan Strasser, *Never Done: A History of American Housework* (New York: Pantheon, 1982).

16. Because few Americans had access to professional funeral services before the end of the nineteenth century, the responsibilities of caregivers frequently continued after death (see James J. Farrell, *Inventing the American Way of Death, 1830–1920* [Philadelphia: Temple University Press, 1980]).

17. See, for example, Glenda Riley, *Frontierswomen: The Iowa Experience* (Ames: Iowa State University Press, 1981); Strasser, *Never Done* (n. 15).

18. Judith Walzer Leavitt, *Brought to Bed: Child Bearing in America, 1750–1950* (New York: Oxford University Press, 1986); see Marilyn Ferns Motz, *True Sisterhood: Michigan Women and Their Kin, 1890–1920* (Albany: State University of New York Press, 1983).

19. See Leavitt, *Brought to Bed* (n. 18).

20. Many other farm women also assumed that the money they earned was theirs to spend alone. See Sarah Elbert, "The Farmer Takes a Wife: Women in America's Farming Families," in *Women, Households, and the Economy,* ed. Lourdes Beneria and Catharine R Stimpson (New Brunswick, NJ.: Rutgers University Press, 1987), pp. 173–97; Joan M. Jensen, *With These Hands: Women Working on the Land* (Old Westbury, NY: Feminist Press, 1981), pp. 32–33.

21. As Lensink notes, it is impossible to determine whether Harriet had a miscarriage or an intentional abortion ("*A Secret to Be Burned*" [n. 1], p. 422n).

22. Ibid., p. 40.

23. See Leavitt, *Brought to Bed* (n. 18).

24. See Polly Kaufman, *Women Teachers on the Frontier* (New Haven, Conn.: Yale University Press, 1984).

25. Nineteenth-century families that could not afford domestic servants frequently recruited neighborhood women to help out in times of trouble. Unlike servants, hired girls occupied the same social status as their employers, and they typically spent their days together. See Faye E. Dudden, *Serving Women: Household Service in Nineteenth-Century America* (Middletown, Conn.: Wesleyan University Press, 1983).

26. Dropsy referred to the abnormal accumulation of fluid in any part of the body (*Dorland's Illustrated Medical Dictionary,* 26th ed. [Philadelphia: W. B. Saunders, 1981], p. 405).

27. See Susan E. Cayleff, *Wash and Be Headed: The Water-Cure Movement and Women's Health* (Philadelphia: Temple University Press, 1987); Ronald L. Numbers, "Do-It-Yourself the Sectarian Way," in Risse et al., *Medicine without Doctors* (n. 10), pp. 49–72; William G. Rothstein, *American Physicians in the Nineteenth Century: From Sects to Science* (Baltimore: Johns Hopkins University Press, 1972); Starr, *Social Transformation* (n. 3).

28. Magnetic doctors believed that the application of mild electrical charges could cure disease (Lensink, *"Secret to Be Burned"* [n. 1], p. 426n).

29. See Charles E. Rosenberg, "The Therapeutic Revolution: Medicine, Meaning, and Social Change in Nineteenth-Century America," in Leavitt and Numbers, *Sickness and Health in America* (n. 7), pp. 39–52.

30. See Mary Douglas, *Purity and Danger: An Analysis of Concepts of Pollution and Taboo* (London: Routledge and Kegan Paul, 1966).

31. Life expectancy was 49 years in 1900, compared with 75 in 1984 (Jacob S. Siegel and Cynthia M. Taeuber, "Demographic Perspectives on the Long Lived Society," *Daedalus,* 1986, 115: 77–118).

32. See M. H. Everett, "Duty Commands You," in *The Female Experience: An American Documentary,* ed. Gerda Lerner (Indianapolis: Bobbs-Merrill, 1977), pp. 172–78.

33. See, for example, Community Council of Greater New York, *Dependency in the Elderly of New York City* (New York: Author, 1978); Comptroller General of the United States, *The Well Being of Older People in Cleveland, Ohio* (Washington, D.C.: U.S. General Accounting Office, 1977); Robyn I. Stone, Gail Lee Cafferata, and Judith Sangl, "Caregivers of the Frail Elderly: A National Profile," *Gerontologist,* 1987, 27: 616–26.

34. K. Minkoff, "A Map of the Chronic Mental Patient," in *The Chronic Mental Patient: Problems, Solutions, and Recommendations for a Public Policy,* ed. J. A. Talbott (Washington, D.C.: American Psychiatric Association, 1978), pp, 11–37; see H. H. Goldman, "Mental Illness and Family Burden: A Public Health Perspective," *Hosp. Commun. Psychiatry,* 1982, 33: 557–60.

35. Katherine L. Kahn, Emmett B. Keeler, Marjorie J. Sherwood, William H. Rogers, David Draper, Stanley S. Bentow, Ellen J. Reinisch, Lisa V. Rubenstein, Jacqueline Kosecoff,

and Robert H. Brook, "Comparing Outcomes of Care Before and After Implementation of the DRG-Based Prospective Payment System," *JAMA,* 1990, 264: 1984–88.

36. Rosalie A. Kane and Robert L. Kane, *Long-Term Care: Principles, Programs, and Policies* (New York: Springer, 1987).

37. See Emily B. Abel, *Who Cares for the Elderly? Public Policy and the Experience of Adult Daughters* (Philadelphia: Temple University Press, 1991).

38. See Stone et al., "Caregivers of the Frail Elderly" (n. 33).

CHAPTER 2

The Legacy of Domesticity: Nursing in Early Nineteenth-Century America

Patricia D'Antonio

The heart of nursing is, and has been, the care of the sick. Through most of history, the responsibility for nursing has rested with women: with mothers, daughters, sisters, and neighbors who cared for their sick children, spouses, parents, and friends in the home. Here lies the domestic roots of modern nursing practice. Prior to the establishment of formal training schools, and well before the drive toward professional status through the registration movement, nursing revolved around the image and the activities of mothers caring for the sick in their own homes. In the domestic world of the early nineteenth century, the time and place where this story begins, the nursing of family and friends took place at home because most sickness, birthing, and dying centered in the home. Further, in a historical world where women's domestic duties were tied tightly to notions about women's innate capabilities and their loving responsibilities, such nursing was an almost

An early version of this chapter was presented at the Colloquium in Nursing History, University of California, San Francisco, in September 1988. The author wishes to thank Marilyn Flood and Joan E. Lynaugh for their generous comments.
This chapter was originally published in the *Nursing History Review* I (1993): 229–46.

unquestioned part of their lives. The care of a sick family member, in the words of one chronicler of the early nineteenth-century domestic world, was to be "commended" to a "woman's benevolent ministries."[1]

Yet, even as the image of nursing has been framed by the historic duty of women to care for the sick at the domestic bedside, how that duty found its form in the actual work of nursing changed in the first half of the nineteenth century. It changed as ideas about expert knowledge, correct social order, viable occupational options, and the centrality of therapeutic alliances in the caring process changed. I argue in this chapter that long before Florence Nightingale brought her vision of nursing reform to the late nineteenth-century hospital bedside, earlier nineteenth-century physicians and nursing women, at the bedsides of their patients in the home, had already reworked certain fundamental assumptions about nursing's work and nurses' relationships with physicians. I am going to argue that this reform was driven by the tension between physicians and nurses as each sought to assert the centrality of their alliance with the sick patient. The legacy of this domestic reform not only influenced the later structuring of the first nurses training schools in Philadelphia, as one particular case study, but also continues to resonate in today's debate about what kinds of nurses should do what kinds of work.

This story begins in the 1830s, a time when the best in medical as well as nursing care centered in the home. Much has already been written about the chaos of early nineteenth-century medical practice—most particularly the rise of competing medical sects; the frightening and unpredictable quality of infectious diseases, which, like most diseases, had yet to be understood as specific entities; and the growing dissatisfaction and disillusionment with the traditionally heroic measures of bleeding and purging. But it is important to remember that, through it all, physicians, nurses, and patients continued to share beliefs on certain fundamental issues. Most important, all shared what historian Charles Rosenberg has described as the central metaphor dominating early nineteenth-century assumptions about health and illness: In health the body existed in dynamic equilibrium with both itself and its environment; in illness the body lapsed into disequilibrium. And all shared, to some degree, assumptions about the efficacy of those therapeutics (stimulants, purgatives, emetics, and bleedings) that produced the visible, physiological effects (the energy, evacuations, vomiting, and relaxation) associated with the careful regulation and regaining of that delicate equilibrium.[2]

Indeed, because of such deeply shared assumptions, domestic dosing (individuals prescribing their own remedies) remained the norm. Stimulants, emetics, purgatives, and, occasionally, even opium and laudanum were within easy reach of any member of the family who wished to prepare his or her body for the upcoming seasonal change or who was plagued by minor and irritating ills.[3] Physicians of all persuasions knew, accepted, and even promoted these practices, although within limits. Philadelphia physicians compiled careful lists of therapeutics necessary for the early nine-teenth-century domestic medicine cabinet, but frequently omitted botanicals, as one physician wrote, "from a conviction that nothing is so injurious as affording the means of quackery to nurses and ignorant mothers."[4]

Such "quackery" in early nineteenth-century Philadelphia was most noticeably, but not solely, associated with the Thomsonian practitioners. The Thomsonians shared the fundamental belief in the idea of equilibrium. They believed that the cause of all disease was cold and that the only cure was the restoration of the body's natural heat. They took issue, however, with traditional therapeutics, preferring botanical preparations and steaming. The Thomsonians had lists for the domestic medicine cabinet, containing various combinations of lobelia (an emetic long used by Native Americans) and stimulating peppers. They gave considerably more responsibility to the families for the actual treatment of diseases, but they also had their limits. One practitioner, despairing over the interference of opinionated nurses, flatly declared that "Thomsonian practitioners, to have justice done to either the system of practice, or the patient, require Thomsonian nurses."[5]

One breed of nurses that traditional physicians and Thomsonian practitioners both could denounce as "quacks" were the midwives. They agreed that a long catalog of problems associated with both mother and child—ills ranging from bloody noses through childbed fever and infant convulsions—could be laid squarely at the hands of the untrained and uneducated midwife.[6] They joined to ridicule her delivery techniques, her treatment of the infant, and her language. One Thomsonian practitioner in Philadelphia, Dr. J. W. Comfort, agreed with the famous allopathic practitioner William Buchan, who protested the midwives' practice of purging the infant; Comfort chided the midwives' colloquial use of the word "economy" for the medical term "meconium." Not one to miss an opportunity, however, Comfort went on to add that while it was gratifying to see allopathic physicians "exposing the malpractice of nurses giving physic to 'purge off the meconium,'" his readers should recollect "that it was the *medical profession* that first instituted this abominable practice."[7]

Here Comfort rather casually underlined a significant connection between the midwives and the regular medical practitioners: the midwives' therapeutic traditions drew heavily from both the prescriptions of standard medical practice and their own experience. In their use of emetics and purgatives during labor, their practice of dosing of infants with castor oil and goose grease after birth, and their plan for a stimulating diet for the postpartum mother, they bound themselves both to the beliefs and to the therapeutic practices of their regular medical contemporaries. Indeed, the most strident complaint medical practitioners could lodge about midwives' actual practice was that it was outdated and hence, potentially dangerous, not that it was conceptually wrong.[8]

The ultimate efficacy of this system of belief and practice must be understood, as Rosenberg points out, in relation to its social setting and emotional context. Patients, midwives, and physicians participated in an almost ritualized patterning of relationships in the home. The shared cognitive understanding of sickness and its treatment provided a framework for a relationship in which practical therapeutics could be at once emotionally reassuring to the patient and socially legitimating to the practitioner. But using a therapeutic agent, that is, actively manipulating elements of a physiological equilibrium toward healing, depended on a "shared faith"—a "conspiracy to believe" between patient and practitioner—for its effect.[9] It depended on what we might today call the therapeutic relationship. For physicians in the early nineteenth century, the crucial problem with the midwives, as with other nurses, involved the threat they posed to the sanctity and the reciprocity of the physician–patient relationship.

Midwives were notorious for their opinionated and independent behavior at the bedside. They would refuse to assist physicians of all persuasions if they disapproved of their proposed course of treatment. One midwife, for example, told a Thomsonian accoucheur that she would leave if he persisted in his vapor bath. Another refused to administer an injection of lobelia, as "she did not approve of it." Regular physicians fared little better. They saw their orders countermanded, their medicines discarded, and their patients' sickrooms inadequately prepared for both delicate therapeutic interventions and the necessary convalescence. Worse still, midwives' descriptions of afterbirth in terms that implied a fair degree of judgment and experience—describing the flow of the lochia as "just about right," "too much that way," or "not as much as ought to be"—were perceived as entirely inadequate for proper medical assessment.[10]

The crux of the problem, however, lay within the midwife's relationship with her patient. As Joseph Warrington, a Quaker physician at the Philadelphia Dispensary, ruefully pointed out, "the opinions of the nurse are not infrequently demanded by the nervous and timid lady." Warrington initially had what he thought to be the simplest solution— refer the lady back instead to her physician for answers.[11] Few midwives paid attention. They freely answered questions from their patients and not infrequently offered their own comments on the course of therapeutics: "Dr. ——," said one midwife after watching her patient swallow a particularly noxious dose, would not have given you such a medicine." Another, observing preparations for a Thomsonian vapor bath, commented to her patient that she herself would suffer death before steaming.[12]

Warrington turned to another, more complicated solution to ensure the physician's authority: Train working-class women of good moral character as adjuncts to the physician. These nurses would still be available to care for other women in childbirth, but, unlike the midwives, they would be trained by a physician, responsible to him rather than to the parturient woman, and in important ways, they would be an extension of his more "scientific" services. In 1839 Warrington founded the Nurse Society of Philadelphia. The society trained worthy, working-class women in such areas as the management of the lying-in chamber, convalescent diet, and care of the new mother and infant. The Society sent the women into the home to assist the physician during childbirth and the mother during the postpartum period. Despite close control over the practice of these nurses, Warrington still felt obliged to carefully delineate proper spheres of authority. His training of nurses was designed, he wrote, "less with a view to create the business of nursing into an *independent* calling, than to impress those who engage in it with the importance of understanding their relations with a class of men who devote years to the acquisition of the *science* and then exercise themselves for years besides."

Relatively few working-class women agreed with Warrington's prescriptive, hierarchical ordering of roles between themselves and the physician. The physician's wish for such nurses always exceeded the number willing to work for the Nurse Society. For the nurse the promise of such a dependent role would be either a well-paid invitation into the lying-in chambers of the city's social elite, or the altruistic satisfaction of knowing that another poor, birthing woman was saved from the humiliation and the danger of Philadelphia's lying-in hospitals. One can speculate that these nursing women, knowing they could "profess" their skills on their own within their own communities, found Warrington's price too high.[13]

Physicians, though, had a clear and persistent sense of what was at stake: the challenge posed by the midwives' confidence in their own therapeutics and their own relationships with their patients undermined the fragile emotional bond between physician and patient. The physicians believed they had to have the patient's complete confidence to begin any treatment or effect any cure. For one physician, Anthony Thomson, treatment became possible only after the patient had been "impressed with the belief that [the physician] is not only duly qualified for the investigation and cure of diseases, but that he is deeply interested in the case" as well. Indeed, the proper role for family, friends, and attendants involved promoting, "in every instance, the efforts of the physician to secure the confidence of his patient."[14]

Midwives were the most obvious but by no means the only threat to this fragile confidence. Nurses in general made difficult the necessary therapeutic alliance—but here we begin broaching the thorny issue of defining just who is "the nurse." Some women, with reputations in the community as good nurses, came into families as hired help when one member took ill. These nurses, as did midwives, came to families armed with their own experience and therapeutics—cold keys for nosebleeds, sulphur for measles, and leeches for fevers.[15] More often a servant would be pressed into duty. In fact, one very erudite patient expressed her preference for the care of servants over that of her willing family: "In so far as the help is mechanical," she wrote, "the relation is sustained with the least amount of effort."[16]

More often, however, members of the family were called on to nurse. More specifically, mothers, daughters, and sisters nursed their families and, depending on these women's financial and social resources, they were aided by their friends, hired nurses, or servants.[17] It was these middle-class nurses with family ties who posed the strongest threat to the fragile relationship between the physician and his patient. Opinionated, educated, connected to the patient through emotional ties, and equal to the physician in shared middle-class background—formidable in her prescribed role as guardian of the home and preserver of its health—she presented a threatening challenge to the sanctity of the physician–patient relationship. What was the physician to do? When he would prescribe a light diet, the family would produce a rich broth. When he would allow visitors, relations would enter, survey the scene, and disconcertingly shake their heads. "I wish," said one to the patient, "you had been under dear Dr. ——; he did so much good in a case exactly the same as yours. Yes! he is the Physician I shall always recommend."[18]

The problem, of course, was hardly new. Physicians had to deal with the family from the first time they entered the home. Threats had been a useful strategy. "Nurses take care!" one late eighteenth-century English physician wrote in a book to families about nursing, reprinted in Philadelphia in 1804. "If you indulge relations at the expense of your patient's life, how will you satisfy your conscience afterwards?" Conduct within the healing relationship was fairly straightforward. "It behooves the patient," this physician continued, "to regard his [physician's] rules, the nurse to see them punctually observed, and both, to be cautious about how they deviate from them; as fatal consequences may sometimes arise."[19]

Rules described at the turn of the century had subtly changed as the Civil War approached. Obedience to the physician's orders remained the norm, confidence in his therapeutics the ideal. But the authoritarian high-handedness of the physician had yielded somewhat in acknowledgment of the growing public dissatisfaction with traditional heroic medical therapeutics and, particularly, in acknowledgment of the growing power of middle-class nursing women within the physician–patient relationship.[20]

Popular ideas about domesticity and the role of women changed in the first half of the nineteenth century as urbanization, industrialization, and immigration reshaped both the economy and the social landscape. In Philadelphia, for example, the population rose fourfold between 1830 and 1860 as a result of the devastating Irish potato famine, political upheaval in Germany, and economic depression of the countryside causing farmhand migration. Industrialization, spurred by the new technologies and the river mills in Philadelphia and other growing towns, moved much of women's traditionally domestic work out of the home and into factories. Cloth, for example, was no longer spun and woven at home; the mills along Philadelphia's Schuylkill River did a much more efficient job producing a range of fabrics for sale that no one woman could create on her own. But fabric was not the only thing being bought and sold in Philadelphia. With industrialization, work itself became a commodity to be bought and sold in the market like any other object of exchange. Economically, the early decades of the nineteenth century brought with them the emergence of a new urban middle class—those able to buy work for the factory or for the home—and its counterpoint, the urban working class, those selling work for wages.

The most compelling change in the domestic world of early nineteenth-century women, though, came as a response to industrialization's new and dramatic separation of the home and workplace. The first half of the nineteenth century redefined the purpose of the home and women's role within it. The home had lost its place in economic production—domestic tasks moved into mills, and husbands and fathers left each morning to practice their professions or trades in offices or factories—to be recast in the rhetoric of the time as a social haven from the harsh work world and as an emotional nest for the rearing of children. Women's prescribed roles changed concurrently. Time that had been spent on economic tasks was now spent on more social and emotional responsibilities. The domestic rhetoric created a "cult of true womanhood," as it has been called by historians. A "lady's" proper role, now that she could buy from factories the cloth she previously had to spin and weave, became that of guardian of her family's morals, manners, and health; she became the symbol of her family's economic prosperity. At least in the popular literature, if not always in fact, the authority and the responsibility for the ideal middle-class home had shifted from men to women by the end of the 1860s.[21]

Middle-class nursing women took this authority and responsibility to heart, turning to the resources available to them. They listened to speakers, usually other middle-class women traveling the urban lecture circuit, who outlined the then-current facts of basic anatomy and physiology, nutrition and hygiene, sexuality, and family planning. They read a growing genre of domestic medicine and nursing manuals that by 1861, when the first American edition was published, included Florence Nightingale's *Notes on Nursing*. Also, they looked to their traditional resource, the hired nurse, or what historian Susan Reverby has named the "professed nurse."[22]

Because of Reverby's research, historians know something about some of these "professed nurses." They tended to be white, native born, from rural areas, and daughters of farmers or skilled workers. They tended to enter the market at ages older than other women workers, usually pushed there by the poverty and destitution that so often accompanied the widowhood, divorce, or abandonment of working-class nineteenth-century women. And, as noted earlier, they entered the market, which, of course, was the middle-class home, armed with the practical experience gained at the bedsides of their own families and often with their own particular therapeutics.[23]

The domestic bedside of the mid–nineteenth-century patient was crowded and tense. Physicians, middle-class nursing women, midwives, and professed nurses gathered there, sharing beliefs about the causes of the illness but competing for the faith of the patient in the efficacy of their idiosyncratic therapeutics. In Philadelphia, Joseph Warrington's earlier attempt to align some working-class nurses with physicians in a hierarchical relationship had failed, but the need to assert the centrality of the relationship with the patient remained. Physicians, absorbing the domestic rhetoric of their time, saw their patients as "children"—capricious, demanding, truculent, and vulnerable in every instance particularly "to the advice of ignorant nurses and misguided friends."[24]

In this carefully worded characterization lies the thrust of the mid–nineteenth-century movement to reform the work and the role of nursing women and their relationships with physicians: professed nurses were "ignorant" and middle-class women who nursed, "misguided"; working-class women who nursed threatened the physician–patient relationship through their "prejudices" while middle-class women did so through their misleading "affection."[25] To gain middle-class allies in the fight for control of the therapeutic relationship, physicians played to increasingly meaningful class distinctions among nursing women. They sought to align the perceived chaos of relationships at the patient's bedside hierarchically—with the physician supervising the middle-class woman, who, in turn, would supervise the hired nurse.

This reform proposed a realignment that resonated with the middle-class woman's domestic experience. Popular ideas about domesticity gave the woman control of the home, but they did not ask that she actually perform the physical labor required in a home. Rather, a "lady" would hire and manage the working-class "help"—persons, both men and women, now trading their labor for money in an industrializing economy. In fact, the middle-class woman was already managing the servant, cook, washerwoman, and gardener in her home. She was now being asked to manage the nurse.

Of course, to intelligently manage and supervise one's help, a woman had to know enough about their work to recognize when tasks were or were not being performed properly. Not surprisingly, then, "education" became the operative word in the proposed reformation of alliances between physicians and middle-class nursing women. Regrettably, as one physician pointed out, "few ladies, even those who are wives and mothers, have any acquaintance with the arrangement of the sick room, and the management of an invalid; they are consequently, too often forced to be guided by, and to rely for instruction of, the nurse, instead of being able to superintend her conduct, to ascertain that she performs her duties, and to correct her feelings."[26] The plan to correct the "misguided" and the "ignorant" developed along several interrelated lines. First, mothers who nursed had to be drawn away from their alliance with other women—nurses working for pay—and into a new relationship with the physician as his eyes and ears and as his superintendent in the sickroom. Interestingly, though, she was not his hands. The physical work of caring for the patient—bathing, turning, cooking, feeding, administering treatments—remained in the hands of the hireling. That work requiring judgment and intellect—watching for changes in the course of the disease, attending to the labile disposition and temper of the patient, deciding the wisdom of pursuing one course over another if alternatives were available—would be the work of "ladies."

The alliance of ladies with nurses could hold across class lines only insofar as it was felt that hired nurses offered the ladies something of value: tried and true methods of affording relief and cure. The nurses' experience, however, next came under attack. "Experience," one physician wryly noted, "is a quality to be much and justly prized in a nurse, were the term not too frequently misapplied, and confidence placed in the nurse merely because she is advanced in years and has seen much, without any inquiry as to her capacity for observing and making proper use of what she has seen." Regrettably, he continued, "it is well known, that, in the lower ranks of society, no habit is so little cultivated as the habit of attention. Thousands pass from cradle to grave without seeing correctly a single object which passes before them, and if we reflect how essential this faculty of mind is for the improvement of intellect, the importance of not trusting the domestic management of the sick wholly to hired nurses surely requires no comment."[27] Education, on the other hand, was an attribute much prized in a nurse. Where the old and the ignorant could appeal only to experience, the educated nurse could appeal to her carefully cultivated spheres of knowledge and judgment and then apply them to the care of her patient. Working, as did the physician, within the framework of both knowledge of the laws of disease and its convalescence, and within the boundaries of her intimate knowledge of both the patient and the family, the nurse could even justify her "pausing in the plan laid down for her guidance, until the physician is sent for." Indeed, "her reasons for the deviation will be listened to by the physician; and, without lowering his dignity, a useful hint from an intelligent nurse may be adopted and acted upon, much to the advantage of the patient."[28] The problem, however, was that too few educated women knew how to "properly" care for the sick.

Where Joseph Warrington had sought to train working-class women in the 1830s, his colleague, Ann Preston, dean of the Female Medical College of Pennsylvania, and one of the founders of the Woman's Hospital of Philadelphia, set her sights on the middle-class women of the 1860s. Her idea of "proper" education involved teaching such women the scientific rules of ventilation, sanitation, and convalescent diet; she instructed through public lectures, through her book, *Nursing the Sick and the Training of Nurses,* and through a formal school, established in 1861 and the first in Philadelphia, for "the practical training of nurses" at the Woman's Hospital.[29] Her idea of "proper" education, however, like those of her medical brothers, had nothing to do with the actual diagnosis and treatment of diseases—that remained within the physician's realm. Therapeutics remained peripheral to nursing—the nurse's responsibilities would be limited to making the doses as palatable as possible. Preston, like her women physician colleagues in Boston and New York, did take special interest in the nursing education of middle-class women. However, her training of nurses emphasized a hierarchical therapeutic alliance with the women of the family in support of the primary relationship of the patient to the physician over any other possible configuration along gender lines—as did that of her medical brothers, the physicians.[30]

However hierarchically defined, Preston did advocate a new configuration of relationships based on class: all nurses should be middle class. Whether in the hospital or in the home, all nurses needed to be "high toned and well trained," as well as "enlightened and refined." Indeed, at public lectures in Philadelphia on the nursing care of the sick sponsored by the newly incorporated Woman's Hospital, women nursing at home and those nursing at the hospital sat side by side in the lecture room. Apart from sporadic ward supervision by Woman's Hospital physicians and a differing fee structure—lay women paid $2 for a course of 10 lectures, nurses in training paid 75 cents—there was little to differentiate the instruction of mothers from that of their few middle-class sisters in the hospital.[31]

While Preston had little trouble attracting middle-class women to the Woman's Hospital public lectures on nursing, she had tremendous difficulty attracting such women to the hospital training school and to hospital work. She did try; in 1855 she and Hannah Wright published a pamphlet urging single, middle-class women to consider nursing an acceptable life's work. Her book, published in 1863, was as much instructional as it was a strategy to excite those single women who read it with the value of nursing as a lady's vocation. But the numbers of women accepted for training rarely exceeded one or two during the 1860s, as "the fine combination of qualities, that union of judgment, kindliness, tact, and efficiency which makes the accomplished nurse is not always to be found in applicants."[32] There were applicants, but not the right, middle-class type. Preston had stumbled on the inherent problem in her generation's efforts at nursing reform. The reworking of relationships among physicians, middle-class nursing mothers, and working-class professed nurses at the bedside of the patient in the home was based on the assumption that the actual work of caring could be hierarchically structured on the basis of class, or its code word, education. This hierarchical ordering of middle-class nursing women with the physicians as their educated superintendents in the domestic sickroom did create a meaningful managerial role for these women. However, this ordering implicitly devalued the physical aspects of nursing care. This was now the domain of the hired help, the working-class woman. While a middle-class nursing mother had to know how to ventilate a room, how to prepare a nutritious diet, and how to keep her loved one comfortable in bed, the actual airing, cooking, turning, and bathing remained the purview of the hired help. Middle-class women would supervise such work; they would not *do* it. In 1864 Preston herself articulated the inherent contradiction in creating class-based alliances in nursing. While emphasizing publicly that "the nurse alone, who intelligently cooperates with the healing powers of nature is, in certain stages of the illness, more important and effective than the physician," she could not avoid hoping, privately and pragmatically, that an increase in the number of applicants to her training school might allow the hospital to "do away with the necessity of chamber-maids," as the necessary nursing duties included so many more menial tasks.[33]

It would be later in the nineteenth century when the reforms associated with Florence Nightingale and the trained nurse would reframe such "menial tasks" into a higher form of service to the sick and to the suffering in hospitals—and thus touch, at least for a time, the aspirations of the "right kind" of middle-class woman. In Philadelphia, to continue this case study, Ann Preston saw the number of appropriate applicants to her training school rise slowly but steadily through the 1870s as the romantic image of nursing strangers in hospitals, an image fed by the popular literature, meshed with some women's need for respectable, paid work. For the early 1870s graduates of the Woman's Hospital Training School, seeking to reconcile their need and desire for paid work with their society's rhetoric about appropriate roles for women, it was the Nightingale *image,* not the substance of her reform, that provided the essential respectability. Nightingale forged the link with the world of the home. Nurses' work became a "calling," not a job; their family was all the sick, not just parents, brothers, and sisters. The difference between them and women nursing their families at home would reside not in the duties performed but in the location of such work. The Nightingale image allowed women who needed to work to keep body and soul together.[34]

The reformed vision of nursing's work and nursing's relationship to the physicians worked out a generation earlier by middle-class nursing women in the home more directly influenced the way in which the Ladies Visiting Committee went about setting up their own training school for nurses at the better-known Hospital of the University of Pennsylvania (HUP) in the early 1880s. Frustrated by the less than respectable showing of the hospital's domestic departments, the male managers and physicians at HUP turned to their wives, sisters, and mothers in 1874 for advice and sorely needed help. The newly formed Board of Lady Visitors took to their mandate with an enthusiasm borne of some middle- and upper-class women's need for meaningful and socially acceptable volunteer work. A "lady" may have had a primary moral obligation to her own home and family, but once these obligations were fulfilled, she could and did extend the scope of domesticity to schools, orphanages, and, of course, hospitals.

The Board of Lady Visitors left little of the HUP's domestic world untouched. They supervised the kitchen and tasted the food; they inspected the ventilation system and checked for odors; they visited the patients and provided them with clothes. Even the laundry did not escape their careful review. They described washing conditions as "immoral" and suggested stationary tubs and heated hot water to save the nurses time and energy. But the board members took on more than they either could or wanted to handle. Unable and unwilling to perform all the routine chores needed to re-create efficient domesticity at the institutional bedside, these women looked for someone to do the physical work of nursing. This "someone" would have to share these women's middle-class sense of domestic duty and responsibility, but not necessarily their social status. The Board of Lady Visitors saw this "someone" as a trained nurse. As early as 1878 they pushed for a nurses training school. They finally succeeded in 1885. Trained nursing came to HUP less as a professionalizing strategy and more as a means of producing "the help."[35]

At this point in the late nineteenth century, traditional histories of professional nursing in the United States usually begin. However, to begin modern nursing history at this time overshadows a more important story played out in an earlier time and in a different historical context. By the end of this earlier story, the framework that structured the development of nursing in the United States had already been established. In the late 1860s and early 1870s nursing still centered in the home, but the ways in which the actual work of nursing would be accomplished had been substantially reformed. Middle-class nursing women had gained a meaningful managerial role in the hierarchical ordering of relations with physicians, one which trained nurses themselves were able to draw on in the next generation. At HUP, in fact, trained nurses did not remain "the help." Some nurses—many of whom would later become leaders in the drive to professionalize modern nursing practice—themselves became managers of the domestic life both on the wards and in the school. In exchange for this domestic authority, the hierarchical ordering of relationships remained sacrosanct. In matters of clinical care of the patient, the physician had "absolute" command.[36]

This reform, like all reforms, had its costs. It came at the expense of middle-class women's traditional alliances with their professed nursing sisters and at the expense of the social value placed on physical nursing care. With the actual work of nursing split along class lines, prestige and status followed. This, too, became a theme throughout modern nursing practice. By 1900, as nursing became a more viable and accessible occupational option for working-class women, training schools became flooded with applicants that the nursing elite explicitly called the "wrong kind" of women: working-class women whose care had been devalued a generation earlier.[37] The legacy of this reform— the giving and the taking of the prerogatives of nursing on the basis of class, or its code word, education—resonates today. It can be heard in today's tension between the head-work and the hand-work in nursing and in the debate about what kinds of nurses should do what kinds of nursing work.

We can also find the legacy of early nineteenth-century reform in today's disciplinary tensions between nurses and physicians. As this study suggests, the patterns of the relationships that have arisen between nurses and physicians involve more than simple boundary disputes over clinical practice, or, as historians have suggested, mere economic self-interest. It also reflects an ongoing, tortuous groping toward new ways to care for the sick when older ways lose their validity and power.

More important, the reform of the early nineteenth century touched on a topic that has always been known and is now being rediscovered: the faith and trust that patients place in their caregivers. The shared belief among caregivers, patients, and families that what is being done is right, good, and necessary is as important to healing as the most sophisticated technology and the most powerful drug. Without the technologies and without the drugs, early nineteenth-century physicians and nursing women experimented with different ways to reassert the centrality of the therapeutic relationship. They did not leave us an unambiguous legacy; it is a part of the past we carry with us when we meet at the bedside of the patient—wherever it may be.

NOTES

1. This quote is in Susan Reverby, *Ordered to Care: The Dilemma of American Nursing,* 1850–1945 (New York: Cambridge University Press, 1987), 12. For a sensitive and sophisticated treatment of physician–nurse tensions after 1875, see Joan E. Lynaugh, "Narrow Passageways: Physicians and Nurses in Conflict and Concert Since 1875," in *The Physician as Captain of the Ship: A Critical Reappraisal,* ed. Nancy M. P. King, Larry Churchill, and Alan Cross (Boston: D. Reidel Publishing Company, 1988).

2. Charles Rosenberg, "The Therapeutic Revolution: Medicine, Meaning, and Social Change in Nineteenth Century America," in *The Therapeutic Revolution: Essays in the Social History of American Medicine,* ed. Morris Vogel and Charles Rosenberg (Philadelphia: University of Pennsylvania Press, 1979), 3–25. For overviews of nineteenth-century physicians, practices, and diseases that have particularly informed this work, see Paul Starr, *The Social Transformation of American Medicine* (New York: Basic Books, 1982); William G. Rothstein, *American Physicians in the Nineteenth Century* (Baltimore: Johns Hopkins University Press, 1972); and Joseph Kett, *The Formation of the American Medical Profession* (New Haven, Conn.: Yale University Press, 1968).

3. Rosenberg, "Therapeutic Revolution"; *Medicine Without Doctors: Home Health Care in American History,* ed. Guenter B. Risse, Ronald L. Numbers, and Judith Walzer Leavitt (New York: Science History Publications, 1977).

4. Anthony Todd Thomson, *The Domestic Management of the Sick Room, Necessary in Aid of Medical Treatment, for the Cure of Diseases,* with revisions and additions by R. E. Griffith, MD (Philadelphia: Lea and Blanchard, 1845), 312. Thomson was, in fact, a Fellow of the Royal College of Physicians in London, and his book was originally published in England. Griffith, an American, orchestrated the publication of the first American edition (1845). He carefully delineated his own revisions and additions; his contribution was primarily to underscore those sections that addressed the necessity for those nursing the sick to support the interventions of the physician.

5. J. W. Comfort, *Thomsonian Practice of Midwifery, and the Treatment of Complaints Peculiar to Women and Children* (Philadelphia: Aaron Comfort, 1845), 84. Comfort also published *The Practice of Medicine on Thomsonian Principles, Adapted as well to the Use of Families as to that of Practitioners* (Philadelphia: Lindsay and Blakiston, 1850). While this chapter emphasizes strands of similar attitudes between Thomsonian and allopathic practitioners with regard to nurses and midwives, it is also important to

note that important differences existed. In general, Thomsonian practitioners gave families more information about diseases, differential diagnoses, and treatments than their allopathic contemporaries.

6. See, e.g., Comfort, *Thomsonian Practice of Midwifery;* and Joseph Warrington, *The Nurses Guide* (Philadelphia: Thomas Cowperthwait, 1839), 23–24.

7. Comfort, *Thomsonian Practice of Midwifery,* 63–64.

8. Descriptions of midwives' practices are in Comfort, *Thomsonian Practice of Midwifery,* and Warrington, *The Nurses Guide.* For an overview of midwifery practices, particularly later in the nineteenth century, see Judy Barrett Litoff, *American Midwives: 1860 to the Present* (Westport, Conn.: Greenwood Press, 1978).

9. Rosenberg, "Therapeutic Revolution."

10. Comfort, *Thomsonian Practice of Midwifery,* 83; Warrington, *The Nurses Guide,* 62.

11. Warrington, *The Nurses Guide,* 14, 27.

12. Thomson, *Domestic Management,* 335; Comfort, *Thomsonian Practice of Midwifery,* 83.

13. Warrington, *The Nurses Guide,* iv. For an analysis of the influence of Warrington and his nurses school on the development of nursing in Philadelphia, see Patricia O'Brien, "All a Woman's Life Can Bring: The Domestic Roots of Nursing in Philadelphia," *Nursing Research* 36 (January/February 1987): 12–17.

14. Thomson, *Domestic Management,* 335. Despite the similarity in names, Thomson, it should be noted, was an allopathic, not a Thomsonian practitioner.

15. Thomson, *Domestic Management,* 42, 57, 110. Because this chapter locates the patient's bedside in the home, nuns are not included in the summary of who nursed. For an excellent description of the backgrounds and work imperatives of the "born" or "professed" nurses, as well as one of the best analyses of the development of nursing, see Reverby, *Ordered to Care.*

16. Harriet Martineau, *Life in the Sick Room: Essays by an Invalid* (London: Edward Moxon, 1845), 34–35.

17. Reverby, *Ordered to Care.*

18. Thomson, *Domestic Management,* 335–36.

19. Robert Wallace Johnson, *Friendly Cautions to the Heads of Families and Others Very Necessary to be Observed in Order to Preserve Health, and Long Life* (Philadelphia: James Humphreys, 1804), 137–38, 141. This was the first American edition of a book originally published in England. The American editor added careful footnotes calling attention to those sections that described specific instructions to those supervising nurses of the sick.

20. Compare, e.g., Johnson's straightforward commands (1804) with Thomson's (1845) more careful etiquette and rules (108, 335–38).

21. See Stephanie Coontz, *The Social Origins of Private Life: A History of American Families, 1600–1900* (London and New York: Verso Press, 1988); Mary Ryan, *Cradle of the Middle Class: The Family in Oneida County, New York, 1790–1865* (New York: Cambridge University Press, 1981); Gerda Lerner's "The Lady and the Mill Girl: Changes in the Status of Women in the Age of Jackson, 1800–1840," in *A Heritage of Her Own: Toward a New Social History of American Women,* ed. Nancy F. Cott and Elizabeth H. Pleck (New York: Simon and Schuster, 1979), 182–96; and Kathryn Kish Sklar, *Catherine Beecher: A Study in American Domesticity* (New York: W. W. Norton and Co., 1973).

22. For an analysis of women's roles in nineteenth-century health reform, see Regina Morantz, "Making Women Modern," *Journal of Social History* 10 (1977). For one description of the use of domestic medicine manuals, see Ronald L. Numbers, "Do-It-Yourself the Sectarian Way," in *Sickness and Health in America: Readings in the History of Medicine and Public Health,* ed. J. Leavitt and R. Numbers (Madison: University of Wisconsin Press, 1978).

23. Reverby, *Ordered to Care*, chap. 1.
24. For a specific reference to patients as "children," see Ann Preston, *Nursing the Sick and the Training of Nurses* (Philadelphia: King and Baird, 1863). For "vulnerability," see Thomson, *Domestic Management*, 105.
25. Thomson, *Domestic Management*, 104.
26. Ibid., 102.
27. Ibid., 103
28. Ibid., 100.
29. Minutes of the Board of Managers, Woman's Hospital of Philadelphia, March 1861, Women in Medicine Archives, Medical College of Pennsylvania, Philadelphia, Pennsylvania (hereafter cited as WMA/MCP). A straightforward history of Ann Preston and the Woman's Hospital can be found in Guliema Fill Alsop's *A History of the Woman's Medical College, 1850–1950* (Philadelphia: J. B. Lippincott, 1950).
30. Patricia O'Brien, "Nursing the Sick and the Training of Nurses at the Woman's Hospital of Philadelphia," *Collections: The Newsletter of the Archives and Special Collections on Women in Medicine* (1986), 1–2. Virginia Drachman's *Hospital with a Heart: Women Doctors and the Paradox of Separatism at the New England Hospital for Women and Children, 1867–1969* (Ithaca, NY: Cornell University Press, 1984) also suggests that women physicians and nurses in Boston maintained the same hierarchical configuration at the hospital bedside at the expense of an alternative reordering on the basis of gender.
31. Preston, *Nursing the Sick*, 3, 15; O'Brien, "Nursing the Sick." The few graduates of the Woman's Hospital Training School, however, were influential in the introduction of hospital training schools in the later nineteenth century. Amanda Judson (1871) became the head nurse on the newly formed training ward at Bellevue Hospital in New York. Emily Bayard (1872) became the first superintendent of nurses at the Connecticut Hospital Training School for Nurses in New Haven.
32. WMA/MCP, January 18, 1865.
33. WMA/MCP, September 1864.
34. O'Brien, "All a Woman's Life can Bring."
35. Julie Fairman, "Voluntarism, Upper Class Women and Nursing: The Nurses Training School at the Hospital of the University of Pennsylvania, 1874–1886" (paper presented at the Third Annual Meeting of the American Association for the History of Nursing, September 1986). I am grateful for Fairman's help in drawing this connection.
36. For the opinions of two prominent nursing leaders on this hierarchical quid pro quo, see Isabel Hampton, "Educational Standards for Nurses," and Lavinia Dock, "The Relation of Training Schools to Hospitals," in Nursing of the Sick (1893; reprinted, New York: McGraw-Hill Book Co., 1949), 1–24. See also Janet James's "Isabel Hampton and the Professionalization of Nursing," in *The Therapeutic Revolution*, 201–44.
37. Barbara Melosh, *"The Physician's Hand": Work, Culture and Conflict in American Nursing* (Philadelphia: Temple University Press, 1982), and Susan Armeny's "Resolute Enthusiasts: The Effort to Professionalize American Nursing, 1880–1915" (Ph.D. dissertation, University of Missouri–Columbia, 1983).

CHAPTER 3

Unheralded Nurses: Male Caregivers in the Nineteenth-Century South

Linda E. Sabin

Accounts of nursing in the South during the last century portray women caring for the ill in times of war or epidemic, but this picture is incomplete. This chapter focuses on the practice of nineteenth-century men who worked as nurses in selected communities in Mississippi and Florida.[1] These men provided family-centered services in times of illness or community-oriented good deeds in times of public crisis. While men never provided the bulk of nursing services in any of the communities studied, they did answer the call to meet community needs in times of crisis. They also practiced nursing in small numbers after the Civil War in order to earn a living during hard economic times. The historical record of these men may be local in focus, fragmentary, and anecdotal, but it expands our understanding of how nursing was practiced in the South before the modern profession developed early in the twentieth century.[2]

THE WORLD IN WHICH THEY PRACTICED

The epidemiological, socioeconomic, and cultural environments in Southern communities came together to thrust the men into what is usually thought of as a typically feminine role, nursing the sick. The male nurses

This chapter was originally published in the *Nursing History Review*, 1997; 5:131–148. Copyright American Association for the History of Nursing. Reprinted with permission.

discussed here lived in a region well documented as a culturally unique and socially enduring area in nineteenth-century America. Characteristics of the Deep South significant to nurses' practice included slavery, recurring infectious diseases, poverty, and rural isolation. These traits shaped the personal and community lives of the men drawn into nursing work.[3]

The most distinctive characteristic of the region was the evolution of slavery. Growth of labor-intensive crops such as cotton linked with the spread of slavery early in the century. Although slavery officially ended after the Civil War, labor arrangements changed to sharecropping and tenancy, which locked men into work and community roles similar to those of antebellum times. Social and economic realities of slavery changed Southern society permanently.[4]

A cultural value system developed in response to the presence of slavery that was a mixture of religious and white supremacy beliefs. This system rationalized the race/class structure in slave states as an economic necessity for the community and a means to bring Christianity to Africans. The result was a caste-conscious culture that structured the roles of all men after the 1820s. Although many Southerners never owned slaves, the social structure of slavery affected how persons in communities could relate to one another. For example, only white, landowning males in communities could vote, hold office, or lead community institutions like churches. Thus, white male leaders developed special roles that mixed patriarchal power and religious obligation during community crises.[5]

In addition to slavery, disease profoundly affected the practice environment of male nurses in this era. The climate promoted many deadly communicable diseases. In addition, slavery stimulated the importation of African forms of several diseases, including malaria and yellow fever. People from both races sickened and died in outbreaks of these diseases.[6] Entire communities experienced periodic outbreaks of typhoid, dysentery, malaria, smallpox, yellow fever, and dengue fever. The rates of infectious diseases rose above antebellum rates for all races following the deprivations of the Civil War. Chronic diseases related to poverty and ignorance, such as hookworm and tuberculosis, debilitated thousands each year.[7]

African Americans suffered most in this disease-ridden environment. As slaves, they had received a modicum of medical attention because of their intrinsic value as property. But after emancipation, many freed slaves became impoverished and lived in squalor. Soon after the war there were successive outbreaks of cholera and typhoid. Public health reports of the period also indicate excess death rates among blacks from consumption, smallpox, and typhoid. In terms of diet and health care, some freedmen believed they had been better off in the old system.[8]

Southern historians have cited the chronic drain on human resources from disease and premature death as a major reason for delayed economic development.[9] With so many people of all races coping with acute and chronic health problems, personal productivity remained low. One indicator of the effect of prevalent illness was that life insurance cost more in the South than in the North as a result of excess death rates.[10]

Another aspect of nineteenth-century Southern society affecting nursing was its historic and prevailing poverty, later exacerbated by the Civil War and Reconstruction. In spite of the persistent plantation myth of large homes and a workforce of slaves, most people in the communities studied for this article lived in a culture of rustic subsistence.[11] After the Civil War, the loss of slaves who had been considered property further impoverished many planters and surrounding towns. Shortages of household goods and equipment lasted for years following the Civil War. Poor white citizens attempted to keep up old patterns of living but with little hope for improvement in the future. At the same time, many freed slaves faced disease, starvation, and destitution. A pattern of poverty became established in this period, and progress for common working people remained slow for the rest of the century.[12]

Economic woes, coupled with slow population growth and the absence of immigration, contributed to the persistent rural nature of the communities studied. These conditions also stimulated a strong sense of place and family.[13] Antebellum values insulated families from what many felt had become an alien world where old economic practices had died and new social structures were unsatisfactory.[14] Many of these communities responded to changes in their socioeconomic condition with episodes of racial segregation and violence, a longing for the return of a lost world, and a strong resistance to change. In addition, communities tightened restrictions on the roles of all freed slaves and women in an attempt to cope with postwar anxieties about race and loss of power. The men in Southern communities responded to emancipation and military defeat by overcontrolling their families and communities in daily life.[15]

Patterns of home management, health care, and community services established during the antebellum period persisted through the century. The traditional family, church, racial segregation, and economic system survived the loss of the Confederacy. This domestic continuity in Southern communities in the midst of change in the larger society is the background for looking at Southern men in nursing.[16]

Rural isolation and poverty in many communities limited development of health care services until late in the century. The numbers of doctors and hospitals remained small. Home remedies, patent medicines, local midwives (who also provided cures), and self-help manuals were all used to augment local medical care. By the end of the century, both

Mississippi and Florida were just beginning to develop private and public hospitals to augment pesthouses and poorhouses. Most illness care was given in the home, and nursing needs were met there. Nursing practice was an expression of cultural norms and values within highly structured communities. Caring for those in need outside one's family regardless of sexual or racial limitations was a complex social process stimulated by dire need.[17]

THE MEN WHO PRACTICED NURSING

The men who practiced nursing in this world had to mix cultural expectations with human needs in times of illness. White males in the patriarchal, segregated system were expected to be protectors and leaders. They were the only politically and practically empowered members of most communities. African American males had to provide similar leadership in their families and segregated communities while coping with the extra burdens of slavery or freedom in a white-dominated culture. Studies on the lives of Southern women during this era show that women's roles expanded somewhat during the war but then constricted after Reconstruction.[18]

Community roles based on race and sex were strictly defined during this time. Slavery divided communities racially, and then postwar codes restructured how persons should behave in each social circumstance. For example, throughout the century during yellow fever outbreaks, white male leaders would remove as many white women and children as possible from epidemic areas by train, riverboat, or cart before quarantines were announced. They then remained behind to protect investments and supervise the care of victims.[19] During the final yellow fever epidemic in Mississippi, Miss Caroline Benoist, her siblings, and her mother were sent to Cincinnati on a sealed evacuation train from Natchez to avoid the epidemic. Her father, a store owner, remained behind to help with relief.[20]

In addition to protecting their families, white men also took on special community roles determined by their status in the culture. Organizations such as the Howard Association were led by white males throughout the South from the 1830s onward. Members of the Howard Association came forward in each epidemic to organize relief, hire nurses, and in many cases give temporary nursing care themselves. They viewed this service as a Christian duty expected of able-bodied white men who were obligated to help those in need.[21] African American men served from a very different position in the community. Their roles were strictly defined as subservient. They followed directions of white male or female leaders whenever caring for persons outside of their homes or communities.

Small numbers of doctors, clergy, and teachers held leadership roles within the African American communities, but their relations with the white community remained subservient.

Two distinct roles for men emerge from the historical record. Domestic nurses provided the less visible, home-based, bedside care within the family unit during episodes of acute and chronic illness. Community nurses provided visible, recognized nursing care during community epidemics. The work of men in either of these roles reflected the expectations of their communities.

Domestic Nurses

Domestic nurses cared for loved ones and neighbors or earned wages serving in homes as specialized servants. Men responded to epidemics and provided bedside care to close friends or family members in need. For example, John Estey was living in Port Gibson, Mississippi, in 1822 when the town experienced a yellow fever outbreak. He wrote to his family in New York, explaining how sickly the town had gotten and how his friend had died the previous week. He reported that since he was a "stout, athletic man," he had felt "compelled to wait upon the sick." He did this for many days until his friend died. He then evacuated to northeastern Mississippi.[22]

Men also provided nursing care within their own families during chronic or acute illness. Sally McMillen described the activities of antebellum fathers who were active participants in the care of their families when acute illness would strike. McMillen's data came from diaries and correspondence of Southern males, revealing the concern and involvement of men in the nursing care of their sick children.[23] Henry Ball, from Greenville, Mississippi, served as a nurse for his physician father who suffered from a chronic heart condition. He also described his nursing duties during a typical outbreak of typhoid fever:

> I seem to have lost the ability to sleep. Everybody is sick. A perfect epidemic of typhoid fever and Hematuria . . . Mrs. War ill—Boarding house perfectly demoralized—Miss Whitley in charge and trying to stem the tide, and I nursing from sick room to sick room all night long, night, after night.[24]

Despite the hardships he endured, Henry Ball recorded numerous occasions of fulfilling the obligation he felt to his family and close friends when illness occurred. During a severe yellow fever epidemic in 1878, Frank Walter returned home from government duties in Jackson in order to help his father, H. W. Walter, care for family members sick with yellow fever in Holly Springs, Mississippi. Both men lost their lives in the epidemic.[25]

Male slave house servants provided domestic nursing services in the traditional plantation household, such as the care of the master in times of illness or other trouble.[26] Some servants who had labored in this role during slavery remained after their emancipation and continued to serve families with whom they had long-standing relationships. For example, Rinna Brown, a former slave, remembered that her father stayed with the Lea family in Franklin County, Mississippi, after he was freed. "Pappy" Brown nursed his former master during a terminal episode of consumption, which lasted for months.[27]

Advertisements for male domestic nurses appeared in the pages of business directories and local newspapers late in the century. For example, Vance's Jacksonville directory of 1898 listed Wm. H. Crawford as a nurse for hire along with four female domestic nurses.[28] Also, a private directory printed for physicians in Florida at about the same time listed one man, Leon H. Parker, as a domestic nurse for the sick.[29]

Men earning a living as domestic nurses appeared in manuscript census reports for 1880 and 1900. These census reports have serious limitations, but they provide skeletal data that offer a glimpse of nursing activities in Southern communities.[30] For example, a survey of the 1880 and 1900 manuscript census reports for 25 Mississippi counties indicates several male nurses in each report. There were 8 men working as domestic nurses in 1880. By 1900, 28 males were listed; 12 of them worked in hospitals or insane asylums. The other 16 were domestic nurses for hire. In 1880, 2% of the nurses were black, and by 1900, 50% were white.[31] The 1900 census of Jacksonville and surrounding counties in Florida lists 6 men as nurses, 5 of whom were white.[32] The increased number of white males involved in domestic nursing late in the century may reflect the chronic economic problems in the communities studied for this article.

A small number of domestic nurses worked for institutions instead of families. The 12 male hospital nurses employed in 1900 in Mississippi worked in four state-funded charity hospitals and one insane asylum. Five of these men were white and seven were black.[33] Historian John Hughes found that minority men and women made up a significant number of hospital nurses before the Civil War. After the war the number of white males working in the Alabama state asylum began to climb until the numbers became almost equal racially.[34]

Community Nurses

Men stayed to nurse in communities in spite of panic, evacuation, and quarantine when an outbreak of disease occurred. Yellow fever is a prime example of the epidemics that occurred with regularity in all the Southern states. This fever was most dreaded because its cause and cure remained a mystery throughout the period. In 1823, a deadly outbreak in Natchez caused panic and evacuation of the town, including all of its doctors. City leaders who remained called for organized relief efforts and opened the city hospital for victims. Most of the men who stayed in the city had to take turns caring for patients in the hospital because of a shortage of nurses. This is an example of how men had to assume nursing duties in order to meet a community need.[35]

In 1843, Rodney, Mississippi, was a thriving river town located just north of Natchez. Horace Fulkerson remembered the summer when yellow fever broke out in the town. Many residents panicked and fled, leaving behind only a small number of men led by John McGinly. McGinly had nursed Fulkerson during an earlier illness, so Fulkerson traveled to Rodney to help.[36] John McGinly was recognized as a community leader and nurse in the district and taught others how to care for victims of the fever. He organized a group of nurses and demonstrated how to maintain a hopeful, effective attitude in spite of fear. He cared for victims for more than one month before becoming ill with the fever himself. Unfortunately, once it was learned that McGinly was ill, the news seemed to "paralyze the whole town and a panic was the result, causing many of the well ones to take flight, a few shamelessly abandoning sick friends."[37]

Fulkerson cared for his friend day and night for a full week until friends arrived from a neighboring town to help. He also ventured out into Rodney to assist those suffering without any nursing care. On the day McGinly began to improve, Fulkerson became sick. Both men were then cared for by another nurse, John Coleman. All three volunteer nurses survived the fever.[38]

Yellow fever continued to plague the region after the Civil War, costing communities in human and economic resources. The last two major outbreaks that affected the studied communities were deadly and disabling. In 1878, the fever spread from New Orleans up river throughout the Mississippi Valley. The entire region from Memphis to New Orleans came to a halt under quarantine for months. The records of this epidemic provide a clear picture of how community responses to the fever had changed since the war. The Howard Association had grown since the 1830s. Most towns of any size had a group of white male leaders who organized all relief and nursing activities.[39]

J. L. Holland, a newspaper publisher in Holly Springs, Mississippi, is an example of the Howard volunteer nurses who served in this epidemic. He served as secretary and later chairman of the relief committee. He traveled with a friend to Grenada, Mississippi, where the fever occurred first, and helped victims evacuate to nearby Holly Springs, where they could receive care. He gave up his own room for a victim, caring for him at night after long days of directing relief activities. He continued publishing a small newspaper and communicating with cities outside the quarantine area until late in the epidemic. Unfortunately, Holland contracted yellow fever and died shortly before the end of the crisis.[40]

Racial segregation eased a bit when communities faced disease and death. A local physician recorded the efforts of Bob Reed, an African American male nurse who cared for many of the residents of both races sick with the fever in Water Valley, Mississippi.[41] In Friars Point, Mississippi, every white person was struck with the fever. The African American residents nursed the victims though the crisis. A local white resident noted: "The nurses cared for the sick, buried the dead and comforted the bereaved."[42]

Another example of a community nurse who volunteered throughout the century to assist people in need during yellow fever outbreaks was Charles Kimball Marshall. He moved to Mississippi in the 1830s to serve as a local Methodist minister. He cared for victims during 13 outbreaks of yellow fever, including the 1878 experience. In his younger years he provided bedside care, and as he grew older he coordinated relief efforts for the Howard Association in Vicksburg, Mississippi.[43] He kept written records of goods distributed and nurses hired by the association during the epidemic. He also took notes and wrote about alternative treatments for the fever and the significance of nursing: "A faithful nurse, who does not mind hard work [continuous cold sponging], will in a few hours bring the temperature down two or three degrees."[44] Charles K. Marshall's portrait now hangs in the Old Capitol in Jackson, Mississippi, as a member of the state's hall of fame.

One written report of the 1878 yellow fever epidemic listed 74 male volunteer nurses who served in Mississippi communities. Of those who served, 20 men died in the epidemic.[45] This figure does not include the other 126 male volunteers who were not listed as nurses but who assisted the nurses and gave direct care in the epidemic. All of these men provided a significant portion of community care for victims during the regional crisis.

The final disastrous outbreak of yellow fever identified in the studied communities was more localized but devastating for the city of Jacksonville, Florida. During this outbreak in the summer of 1888, normal community life stopped for more than five months. The city lay crippled economically and physically behind a tight quarantine. The environment, sanitation problems, and the introduction of an infected traveler all collided, leading to an outbreak that sickened thousands and killed hundreds.[46] With the public announcement of the epidemic, city leaders established the Jacksonville Auxiliary Sanitary Association. The men in this organization set up relief efforts for the city and provided leadership during the emergency. A committee on nurses distributed supplies and hired nurses for those needing help.[47]

In a report following the epidemic, the committee on nurses concluded: "The value of good nursing in the treatment of yellow fever is too well appreciated by all persons familiar with the disease to need argument."[48] Unfortunately, the minutes of the committee on nurses also reported several nurses' drunkenness, poor care, and sexual/racial etiquette problems. For example, African American nurses were sent to families demanding white nurses or male nurses were sent to female victims. In addition, the report indicated that many nurses volunteered to help and received payment through government relief revenues. The majority—440 out of 837 nurses—were black, and one-third of all nurses were male.[49]

More men volunteered than were actually needed in this disaster. The high wages being offered by the relief committee and the national publicity about the epidemic may explain why males responded in such large numbers. Also, men may have been freer to travel to an epidemic. For example, Harry Minor, a wealthy industrialist from New York, sent volunteer nurses to serve in the epidemic. The group consisted of eight men and one woman, Lavinia Dock.[50] The list of victims also indicates that more male patients needed help. By late September, newspapers were calling for more female volunteers, and males were being turned away at quarantine checkpoints. The Auxiliary Sanitary Association announced: "We want all the female nurses we can get, and we will not only pay them well for their services, but will furnish them with free transportation . . . of male nurses we have an abundance."[51]

The Reverend J. P. Sharpe, pastor of the St. Paul's Methodist Church in Jacksonville, died on September 9, 1888, after losing his battle with the fever. He had received medical attention from a local doctor, medicine from a local pharmacy, and nursing care from a black male nurse named Matthew. The *New York Times* had a reporter in Jacksonville during the epidemic who wrote a lead story that announced that Reverend Sharpe died through the "neglect of nurses." Headlines accused the nurse of brutality and abuse. He was labeled in the press as a vicious person who deserved punishment.[52] Years later the pastor's daughter, Lucy Sharpe Alvarez, who had also experienced yellow fever that summer, wrote two letters to the Jacksonville Historical Society explaining what had actually happened to her family:

> The truth is that he [Pastor Sharpe] had an excellent nurse. The negro man and my mother lay by my father's side and directed care of him. My father had a Kidney complication, and really died of congestion of

the brain. His forehead was perfectly black as if it were bruised. . . .
The negro Matthew, who nursed father was faithful to come back and
massage his skinny little legs and feet—trying to make blood which
wasn't tone to circulate.[53] My father was too exhausted to stand the
ravages of yellow fever and I don't believe the best of nurses could have
saved him. I have always regretted the injustice done to Matthew.[54]

Matthew's service was misunderstood and judged incorrectly because
of the erroneous newspaper article and other problems associated with
nurses in the city. He did violate accepted behavior in this epidemic by
continuing to serve the family after the father died, leaving him alone in
the house with white females. Mrs. Alvarez's letters, however, give clues
about the dedication nurses needed and difficulties that African American
male nurses faced.

Men stepped forward in this era to meet community nursing needs
during epidemics and thus fulfilled culturally accepted roles as providers,
protectors, and leaders of local society. The traditional female domestic
role of caring for the sick was transferred to the public male domain
when entire communities, commerce, and property were at stake. What
began before the war as a practice of male honor and paternalism continued in the difficult postwar years as an accepted cultural responsibility
of men who led communities.

THE NATURE OF CLINICAL PRACTICE

The practice of fever nursing depended on the treatment selected by the
physician and the condition of the patient. There were many types of
fever-related illnesses in addition to yellow fever, such as typhoid fever,
malaria, and smallpox. Nurses might watch and wait with a patient,
giving sips of lemonade until the fever broke, or participate in the
"heroic" interventions of medical therapeutics of the time. Bedside care
included giving mustard baths and removing excreta. Nurses had to offer
fluids and manage fever-induced delirium. The yellow fever patients often
developed black vomit (stomach hemorrhage). The illness could go on
for days, and nurses had to work with little rest. Some victims died
quickly, while others lingered for weeks. Survivors had to convalesce for
months; Horace Fulkerson described weakness and yellow skin and eyes
for six months after his fever.[55]

Antebellum medical therapy was harsh on the patient and exhausting for the nurse. Horace Fulkerson gave details of his own care in 1843.
When he got the chill, he was given a hot mustard bath. The doctor then
gave him "merciless cupping of the spine," since he had pain there.

Cupping was a process of applying red-hot glass cups to the skin, allowing a suction to form, and then lancing the reddened skin to promote bleeding. After blood was drawn, freshly heated cups were then applied. In less than an hour after the chill, he became delirious. It was a struggle to keep covers on, and after the fever broke he was prescribed alcohol spirits as a stimulant.[56]

Another antebellum physician in the area urged the heavy use of calomel, a strong laxative, and he endorsed the new drug mixture of quinine and opium to treat fever delirium. He stressed the value of the nurse providing continuous cold sponging during the fever period. He also warned against removing any covers during this period until the fever broke in five to six days.[57]

By the 1878 and 1888 yellow fever epidemics, the treatment of fevers had changed considerably. While the heroic approach was still practiced by some, alternative methods like homeopathy and hydropathy had become more popular.[58] Purges of calomel and castor oil were still given to stimulate the liver. Brandy and champagne were thought to be stimulants. The back and kidney area were rubbed with turpentine. Nurses were warned not to change the patient's clothing or bed linen for five to six days to prevent the patient from getting a chill. After purging, a hot mustard footbath was given. Tepid water enemas were given for the first four to five days.[59] One practitioner stated, "I generally keep them, the bowels full. Some water must be absorbed and it relieves kidney trouble."[60]

Nursing practice changed during the later epidemics, but bedside care was no less demanding. The heat, chronic shortages of ice, and lack of assistance made nursing difficult physically and emotionally. Patients died in spite of efforts to care for them, and many male nurses died because of the exhaustion from the work, poor nutrition, and exposure to contagion.[61]

WHY DID THESE NURSES PRACTICE?

There were several motivations acting on Southern men caring for the sick at the bedside. First, for white males the Southern code of honor demanded service to dependent females, children, and those considered inferior. The protection of property and business interests during community crises also required the service of white male leaders during epidemics. Duty to family during illness also fell to the male heads of households regardless of race. In rural settings, men had to help wives and children coping with illness without adequate services.

A practical impetus to serve as nurses during epidemics was the offer of premium pay. Fever-ridden communities like Natchez, Vicksburg, and Jacksonville offered daily rates that began at $2 per day early in the century and grew to $4 per day in the 1880s. The average daily wage in Mississippi in the 1870s was $1 a day.[62] These inflated salaries were subsidized by donations. Several weeks of fever duty could help a poor working family.

Men never represented more than 5% of the employed nurses identified in census and other public documents in Mississippi. In the Florida survey, less than 1% of the nurses identified were men. Thus, nursing was not a significant occupational choice of men in this era. Nursing as a field of employment for white males seems to have become more acceptable during the hard times after the war as indicated by the increase of workers in public hospitals, but it was not a popular vocational option.

Epidemics and chronic endemic diseases created family and community crises that made nursing an acceptable if not a preferred activity for men. They practiced as needed and provided nursing care to families and communities until the crises were over. With the demise of epidemics after 1900 and the development of nurses' training schools, Southern men readily relinquished nursing activities to Southern women. The images identified in this chapter give only a glimpse of patterns that may have been present in other sections of the South. Much of the story of men who contributed to nursing before 1900 is yet to be explored.

ACKNOWLEDGMENTS

The author wishes to thank Drs. James Crooks, Frank Moak, and Joanne V. Hawks for their assistance in completing the research that made this chapter possible. My special thanks also go to the research librarians at the Mississippi Department of Archives and History and at the Mississippi College Library for the many hours they devoted to assisting me in this project.

NOTES

1. The primary research for this chapter is drawn from my two studies: "Nursing and Health Care in Jacksonville, Florida, 1900–1930" (master's thesis, University of Florida, 1988) and "From the Home to the Community: Nursing in Mississippi, 1870–1940" (PhD diss., University of Mississippi, 1994).
2. St. Luke's Hospital in Jacksonville, Florida, established the first school in Florida in 1885, but regular classes were not admitted until the late 1890s. The first training school in Mississippi opened in 1898 at the Charity Hospital in Natchez. Although a

few urban centers in the South had established schools of nursing before 1900, the majority of communities in the study area did not develop trained nursing programs until after 1900.

3. Edward Ayers, *The Promise of the New South: Life After Reconstruction* (New York: Oxford University Press, 1992), vii–xi; John Boles and Evelyn Nolen, eds., *Interpreting Southern History* (Baton Rouge: Louisiana State University Press, 1987), vi–ix; C. Vann Woodward, *The Future of the Past* (New York: Oxford University Press, 1989), viii–xii, 53–72; William J. Cooper and Thomas Terrill, *The American South: A History* (New York: McGraw-Hill, 1991), xv-xvi.

4. Todd L. Savitt, "Black Health on the Plantation: Masters, Slaves and Physicians," in *Science and Medicine in the Old South,* ed. Ronald L. Numbers and Todd L. Savitt (Baton Rouge: Louisiana State University Press, 1989), 332; Edward Akin, *Mississippi: An Illustrated History* (Northridge, Calif.: Mississippi Historical Society, 1987), 22, 24, 50; William Scarborough, "Heartland of the Cotton Kingdom," in *History of Mississippi,* ed. Richard A. McLemore (Jackson: University and College Press of Mississippi, 1976), 1: 331–32; Charlton W. Tebeau, *A History of Florida* (Coral Gables, Fla.: University of Miami Press, 1971), 181.

5. Francis Butler Simkins, *The Everlasting South* (Baton Rouge: Louisiana State University Press, 1963), 37; Sam Hill, *Religion in the Solid South* (Nashville: Abingdon, 1972), 39–40; Jean Friedman, *The Enclosed Garden: Women and Community in the Evangelical South, 1830–1900* (Chapel Hill: University of North Carolina Press, 1985), 6; Donald Mathews, *Religion in the Old South* (Chicago: University of Chicago Press, 1977), 75–80; Charles Reagan Wilson, *Baptized in the Blood: The Religion of the Lost Cause, 1865–1920* (Athens: University of Georgia Press, 1980), 3, 7, 11; Akin, *Mississippi,* 51; Scarborough, "Heartland," 350; Lucy Robertson Bridgforth, "Medicine in Antebellum Mississippi," *Journal of Mississippi History* (hereafter cited as *JMH*) 56 (May 1984): 104.

6. James Breedon, "Disease as a Factor in Southern Distinctiveness," in *Disease and Distinctiveness in the American South,* ed. Todd L. Savitt and James Harvey Young (Knoxville: University of Tennessee Press, 1988), 1, 8, 9; Richard Shyrock, "Medical Practice in the Old South," in *American Historical Essays* (Baltimore: Johns Hopkins University Press, 1966), 49; K. David Patterson, "Disease Environments of the Antebellum South," in Numbers and Savitt, eds., *Science and Medicine in the Old South,* 152–53; A. Cash Koeniger, "Climate and Southern Distinctiveness," *Journal of Southern History* (hereafter cited as *JSH*) 54 (February 1988): 30–35.

7. Breedon, "Disease as a Factor," 11, 12; Patterson, "Disease Environments," 153; Bridgforth, "Medicine in Antebellum Mississippi," 85–87; Mary Stovall, "To Be, To Do and To Suffer in the Nineteenth Century South," *JMH* 52 (May 1900): 96–99.

8. Marshall Scott Legan, "Disease and the Freedmen in Mississippi During Reconstruction," *Journal of the History of Medicine* 28 (July 1973): 258–61, 263; *Biennial Report of the Mississippi State Board of Health: 1894–1895* (Jackson: Clarion Ledger, 1895), 32.

9. Breedon, "Disease as a Factor," 1–2; C. Vann Woodward, *Origins of the New South* (Baton Rouge: Louisiana State University Press, 1971), 227–28; Cooper and Terrill, *The American South,* 587.

10. Woodward, *Origins,* 227–28; Cooper and Terrill, *The American South,* 587; Breedon, "Disease as a Factor," 1–2, 9; Shyrock, "Medical Practice," 63–64.

11. Akin, *Mississippi,* 51; James C. Cobb, *The Most Southern Place on Earth* (New York: Oxford University Press, 1992), 58–60; Ayers, *The Promise of the New South,* 195–200, 150–51.

12. George Rable, *But There Was No Peace: The Role of Violence in the Politics of Reconstruction in the South, 1865–1867* (Athens: University of Georgia Press, 1984),

145, Cooper and Terrill, *The American South*, 507–9; William Harris, *Days of the Carpetbagger: Republican Reconstruction in Mississippi* (Baton Rouge: Louisiana State University Press, 1979), 20–21; Legan, "Disease and the Freedmen," 259–60; Dan T. Carter, *When the War Was Over: The Failure of Reconstruction in the South, 1865–1867* (Baton Rouge: Louisiana State University Press, 1985), 3; Woodward, *Origins*, 175–80.

13. Rowland Berthoff, "Southern Attitudes Toward Immigration," *JSH* 17 (September 1951): 331–33; Marie Hemphill, *Fevers, Floods and Faith: A History of Sunflower County, Mississippi, 1844–1976* (Indianola, Miss.: Sunflower Historical Society, 1976), 4–5.

14. Paul Buck, *The Road to Reunion, 1865–1900* (Boston: Little, Brown and Company, 1938), 301, 302, 306.

15. Warren Ellem, "The Overthrow of Reconstruction in Mississippi," *JMH* 54 (May 1992):176–79; Gaines Foster, *Ghosts of the Confederacy* (New York: Oxford University Press, 1987), 6–7; Rable, *But There Was No Peace*, 3; Woodward, *Origins*, 340; Jean Friedman, "Women's History and the Revision of Southern History," in *Sex, Race and the Role of Women in the South*, ed. Joanne V. Hawks and Sheila Skemp (Jackson: University Press of Mississippi, 1983), II.

16. Joanne V. Hawks, "Nancy McDougall Robinson (1808–1873): A Personal Story," *JMH* 55 (February, 1993): 23, 28; Ann Firor Scott, *The Southern Lady: From Pedestal to Politics, 1830–1930* (Chicago: University of Chicago Press, 1970), 41–44, 144–60; Jacqueline Jones, *Labor of Love, Labor of Sorrow: Black Women, Work and the Family from Slavery to the Present* (New York: Vintage Books, 1985), 58–68; Patricia O'Brien D'Antonio, "The Legacy of Domesticity: Nursing in Early Nineteenth-Century America," *Nursing History Review* (hereafter cited as *NHR*) 1 (1993): 229–30; Linda Hughes, "Professionalizing Domesticity: A Synthesis of Selected Nursing Historiography," *Advances in Nursing Science* 12 (July 1990): 26.

17. Derrell Roberts, "Social Legislation in Reconstruction Florida," *Florida Historical Quarterly* 43 (March 1965): 349–51, 356–57; Richard Martin, *A Century of Service: St. Luke's Hospital* (Jacksonville, Fla.: St. Luke's Hospital, 1973), 2–11; Webster Merritt, *A Century of Medicine in Jacksonville and Duval County* (Gainesville: University of Florida Press, 1949), 32, 66, 149–50; Daniel Vogt, "Poor Relief in Frontier Mississippi, 1798–1832," *JMH* 54, no. 3 (August 1989): 192–93; Laura Harrell, "Medical Services in Mississippi, 1860–1970," in *A History of Mississippi,* ed. Richard A. McLemore (Jackson, Miss.: University and College Press, 1973), 2: 516–22. A survey of newspapers in 25 towns and cities of Mississippi between 1865 and 1900 and in Jacksonville, Florida, from 1865 to 1900 revealed personal columns and news reports about the ill and injured being treated by local physicians at home; Karen Buhler-Wilkinson, "Guarded by Standards and Directed by Strangers," *NHR* 1 (1993): 143, 144, 149.

18. Anne Firor Scott, "Historians Reconstruct the Southern Woman," in Boles and Nolen, *Interpreting Southern History,* 97; Delores Janiewski, "Sisters Under the Skin: Southern Working Women," in *Sex, Race and the Role of Women in the South,* ed. Joanne V. Hawks and Sheila Skemp (Jackson: University Press of Mississippi, 1983), 13, 33; Jones, 46–52, 80–86.

19. James Ward, *Old Hickory's Town: An Illustrated History of Jacksonville* (Jacksonville: Florida Publishing Co., 1982), 167; John H. Ellis, *Yellow Fever and Public Health in the New South* (Lexington: University Press of Kentucky, 1992), 31, 45–47.

20. Caroline Benoist, interview by author, August 22, 1994, Natchez, Mississippi.

21. William Robinson, *Diary of a Samaritan by a Member of the Howard Association of New Orleans* (New York: Harper and Brothers, 1860), 14, 16–18; John Duffy, *Sword of Pestilence: New Orleans Yellow Fever Epidemic of 1853* (Baton Rouge: Louisiana State University Press, 1966), 56.

22. John Estey to his brother Joseph Estey, October 19, 1822, from Choctaw Agency, near Monroe County, Mississippi, John Estey Papers, Mississippi Department of Archives and History, Jackson (hereafter cited as MDAH).

23. Sally G. McMillen, "Antebellum Fathers and the Health Care of Children," *JSH* 60, no. 3 (August 1994), 514–15, 519–21.

24. Henry Waring Ball Papers, Diary Series 1, October 5, 1886, MDAH.

25. J. L. Power, *The Epidemic of 1878 in Mississippi: Report of the Yellow Fever Relief Work* (Jackson, Miss.: Clarion Ledger, 1879), 173, 233.

26. Eugene D. Genovese, *Roll, Jordan, Roll: The World the Slaves Made* (New York: Vintage Books, 1976), 343–48.

27. Rinna Brown, autobiography, in *The American Slave: A Composite Autobiography*, ed. George Rawick, supplement series 1, vol. 6 (Westport, Conn.: Greenwood Press, 1977), 273.

28. *Jacksonville, Florida, City Directory* (Jacksonville, Fla.: Vance's Printing Co., 1898), 283.

29. *Directory for Physicians' Convenience* (Jacksonville, Fla.: Drew Printing Co., 1901), District 2, Florida Nurses' Association Historical Collection, University of North Florida, Jacksonville.

30. David E. Kyvig and Myron M. Marty, *Nearby History: Exploring the Past Around You* (Nashville, Tenn.: American Association for State and Local History, 1982), 96–l00.

31. U.S. Bureau of the Census, manuscript census reports for Mississippi, Tenth and Twelfth Census Reports (Washington, D.C., 1880 and 1900). The survey included the 25 selected cities and towns, and the counties in which these communities were located in 1880 and 1900.

32. Ibid., manuscript census report for Florida (Duval, Clay, and Nassau Counties), Twelfth Census Report (Washington, D.C., 1900).

33. Ibid., manuscript census report for Mississippi (1900).

34. John Hughes, "'Country Boys Make the Best Nurses': Nursing the Insane in Alabama, 1861–1910," *Journal of the History of Medicine and Allied Sciences* 49, no. 1 (January 1994): 85–86.

35. Henry Wooley, *History of Yellow Fever at the City of Natchez, August, September, October, 1823* (Washington, Miss.: Author, 1824), 2–3; Works Progress Administration Papers, "Adams County," Record Group 60, vol. 233, MDAH, 11–13.

36. P. L. Rainwater, "Notes and Documents: Notes on Southern Personalities," *JSH* 2 (May 1938): 209–10; Horace Fulkerson, *Random Recollections of Early Days in Mississippi* (Baton Rouge: Otto Clator, 1937), 34–40.

37. Fulkerson, *Random Recollections*, 37.

38. Ibid., 37–41.

39. Ellis, *Yellow Fever and Public Health*, 43–44; Power, *The Epidemic of 1878*, 175–76, 206.

40. Olga Reed Pruit, *It Happened Here: True Stories of Holly Springs* (Holly Springs, Miss.: South Reporter Printing Co., 1950), 76–79; Helen Anderson, "A Chapter in the Yellow Fever Epidemic of 1878," *Papers of the Mississippi Historical Society* (Oxford, Miss.) 10 (1909): 225–26, 228.

41. Dr. H. H. Gant, "The Yellow Fever Epidemic," in *Yalobusha County History*, ed. Yalobusha Heritage Committee (Dallas, Tex.: National Share Graphics, 1982), 162.

42. Linton Weeks, *Clarksdale and Coahoma County: A History* (Clarksdale, Miss.: Carnegie Public Library, 1982), 57.

43. "Personal Autobiography," Charles Kimball Marshall Papers, MDAH, Jackson; Charles Bettes Galloway, "The Reverend C. K. Marshall, D. D.," *Quarterly Review*, July 1891, 385.

44. J. M. Keating, *History of the Yellow Fever Epidemic, 1878* (Memphis, Tenn.: Howard Association, 1879), 51.

45. T. J. Dromgoogle, *Yellow Fever: Heroes, Heroines and Horrors of 1878* (Louisville, Ky.: John Morton Co., 1879), 161–70.

46. Ward, *Old Hickory's Town,* 167–70; Martin, *A Century of Service,* 84; Richard Martin, *The City Makers* (Jacksonville, Fla.: Convention Press, 1972), 224–29.

47. Martin, *A Century of Service,* 69; Martin, *The City Makers,* 26; Charles Adams, *Report of the Jacksonville Auxiliary Sanitary Association* (Jacksonville, Fla.: Times Union Printers, 1889), 134–35, 138–41.

48. Adams, *Report of the Jacksonville Auxiliary,* 139.

49. Ibid., 139, 140, 149.

50. Ibid., 146–47.

51. *New York Times,* September 29, 1888, 8.

52. *New York Times,* September 11, 1888, 1.

53. Lucy Sharpe Alvarez to Mr. Daniels, Jacksonville Historical Society, January 20, 1936, 3–5, Jacksonville Historical Society Archives, Jacksonville University, Jacksonville, Florida.

54. Lucy Sharpe Alvarez to Colonel Gibb, Jacksonville Historical Society, April 20, 1936, 3–4, Jacksonville Historical Society Archives, Jacksonville University, Jacksonville, Florida.

55. Fulkerson, *Random Recollections,* 41.

56. Ibid., 37–41; John Duffy, "Medical Practice in the Ante-Bellum South," *JSH* 25, no. 1 (February 1959): 70.

57. Andrew Kilpatrick, "An Account of Yellow Fever Which Prevailed in Woodville, Mississippi, 1844," *New Orleans Medical Journal* 2 (July 1845): 44–48.

58. Jo Ann Carrigan, "Yellow Fever in New Orleans, 1853: Abstractions and Realities," *JSH* 25 (August 1959): 351–52.

59. Merritt, *A Century of Medicine,* 155; John C. Gunn, *Gunn's New Family Physician, or Home Book of Health* (New York: Moore, Wilstach and Baldwin,1865), 416.

60. Dr. Austin, "Letter from Dr. Austin to His Daughter on the Care of Yellow Fever Victims," *New Orleans Christian Advocate* 10 (October 1878): 1.

61. Keating, 52, 54, 57, 63; Joel Shew, *The Hydropathic Family Physician* (New York: Samuel Well, 1874), 42–43, 83–88, 741–91.

62. *Annual Report of the Mississippi State Board of Health, 1878* (Jackson: Clarion Press, 1879), 52.

CHAPTER 4

Satisfied to Carry the Bag: Three Black Community Health Nurses' Contributions to Health Care Reform, 1900–1937

Marie O. Pitts Mosley

Since the early twentieth century, community health agencies and visiting nursing organizations in New York City have employed a number of outstanding black nurses. Among these exceptional women were three pioneers: Jessie Sleet, the first paid district black nurse in New York City[1] and the first black public health nurse in the United States[2]; Elizabeth Tyler, the first black nurse hired as a visiting nurse by the Henry Street Settlement Visiting Nursing Service[3]; and Edith Carter, a senior nurse at Henry Street for 28 years.[4]

This chapter shows that these three black community health nurse pioneers made significant contributions to the development of New York City's community health nursing by providing much-needed health care to hundreds of unserved members of the black community, providing strong leadership in their roles as supervisors, administrators, and educators in patients' homes, babies' health stations, settlement houses, and clinics.

This chapter was originally published in the *Nursing History Review*, 1996; 4:65–82. Copyright American Association for the History of Nursing. Reprinted with permission.

A SUCCESSFUL EXPERIMENT: JESSIE SLEET, FIRST
BLACK PUBLIC HEALTH NURSE

In October 1900, Dr. Edward T. Devine, general secretary of the Charity Organization Society's (COS) tuberculosis committee, met with members of his committee to discuss the spiraling death rates from tuberculosis in the city and the high incidence of tuberculosis among the city's black population. Prior to this, Dr. Devine had studied the health crisis among the city's blacks and tried to come up with possible solutions to help eliminate the problem.

Knowing that tuberculosis was a preventable disease born from lack of knowledge, he determined that in order to alleviate the poor health that seemed to be embedded in the black community's life, a district nurse who was of the same race should be hired. This nurse would go into the black communities both to do district visiting and to persuade the people to accept treatment.[5] Having never had any black person in their organization, the COS's tuberculosis committee was disinclined to change their policies. Dr. Devine was finally able to convince the committee members of the benefits of having a black nurse on the staff, but their consent came with a number of conditions. First, they would not be responsible for her salary; this was to be the responsibility of Mr. Herbert Parsons, a white philanthropist interested in blacks' health. And, second, she was to be hired on an experimental basis, for two months only.

The nurse they chose was Jessie Sleet, who had been trained at the Provident Hospital in Chicago, a hospital for black patients, with a nurses' training school for black women.[6] Having been told that the tuberculosis committee had not wanted to hire her and that her employment was temporary, Jessie Sleet accepted, with reservations, the position of district nurse with the COS on October 3, 1900.

"A Successful Experiment" was a news item that appeared in the first volume of the *American Journal of Nursing* in 1901. This article was unusual, especially for this time period, and contained a report written by Sleet for the COS describing her community health work among black immigrants in New York:

> I beg to render to you a report of the work done by me as district nurse among the colored people of New York City during the months of October and November. I have endeavored to search out families in which there was sickness and destitution. But I have never hesitated to visit anyone when I have felt that a word of advice or a friendly warning was all they needed.
>
> I have visited forty-one sick families and made one hundred and fifty-six calls in connection with these families, caring for nine cases

of consumption, four cases of peritonitis, two cases of chicken pox, two cases of cancer, one case of diphtheria, two cases of heart disease, two cases of tumor, one case of gastric catarrh, two cases of pneumonia, four cases of rheumatism, and two cases of scalp-wound.

I have given baths, applied poultices, dressed wounds, washed and dressed new-born babes, cared for mothers. When there has been an intelligent member of the family on whom I could depend, I have instructed them how to care for the sick one. When there was not one, as was often the case, I have made daily visits if the case required it, caring for them until they were able to care for themselves. Whenever I have felt it advisable, I have urged them to go into hospitals.

Sleet then describes in detail two cases that interested her greatly and for which she obtained good results. The following excerpt is from the second case:

B—S—, a consumptive, twenty-seven years of age, with no means of support, a little girl of three years, and a mother sixty-five, lived in three small rooms. . . . The three persons occupied the one room and slept in the same bed, the sick woman refusing to be separated from her child for a few hours. After I had visited the family a few times I succeeded in convincing the mother that she was endangering the life of her child. On my advice, she agreed to occupy the room alone, permitting the others to sleep in another apartment. A marked improvement was noticeable in other directions. The sputum was always carefully covered and a window lowered from the top whenever the weather permitted. The mother of the sick girl did not ask for relief, but that assistance be given her in obtaining work. I was successful in finding her work for ten days to do house-cleaning. The lady became interested in the family, and procured for the daughter the services of a specialist, who gave her every attention. The mother earned sufficient to pay a month's rent which was overdue, thus keeping her little home together, which was on the verge of going to pieces. The daughter, who passed away a few days ago, was made comfortable up to the day of her death.[7]

Jessie Sleet performed her duties so well that after a year she was given a permanent position with the organization.[8] Sleet became a legendary figure in the field of community health nursing and paved the way for black nurses to practice in the community health nursing field. She is credited with providing district nursing care to hundreds and was instrumental in persuading more black patients to seek nursing and medical care.

ELIZABETH TYLER: INNOVATOR AND COMMUNITY NURSING HEALTH CARE REFORMER

In 1906, Lillian D. Wald, founder and director of the Henry Street Settlement Visiting Nursing Service, heard of Sleet's success at the COS and asked her to recommend a black nurse for her organization. Jessie Sleet recommended Miss Elizabeth Tyler, a schoolmate and graduate of Freedmen's Hospital Training School for Nurses in Washington, D.C.[9] Freedmen's[10] was established in 1894 for the sole purpose of training black women who were interested in becoming nurses. Applicants had first to work under the supervision of the superintendent of nurses at Freedmen's Hospital, who determined if applicants were physically and psychologically suited for the profession. After working for an undetermined amount of time and obtaining the superintendent's approval, the young women were tentatively accepted into the training school and served a probation period of one month, during which all applicants were also given pretests in reading, penmanship, English diction, and arithmetic. After completion of all of the screening procedures, applicants were then officially admitted into the program; admission took place at any time during the year, whenever there was a vacancy.

On November 15, 1894, Freedmen's received its first students, and 37 young women, including Elizabeth Tyler, embarked upon lifelong and rewarding careers. The course of study at Freedmen's was not easy. As was the case in so many other nurses' training schools in the country at the time, student nurses constituted Freedmen's primary labor force. During the first nine months of training, Tyler and her classmates served as assistants on the wards of Freedmen's Hospital. Along with providing care to assigned patients, their duties included cleaning, meal preparations, and staff relief. They worked around the clock with very little free time for recreation. When they were not actively involved in practical work on the wards, the students had to attend lectures and recitations. During the second nine months of their training, the students were required to perform any duties assigned them by the superintendent of nurses. These assignments covered the full range of responsibilities usually assumed by nurses who had already graduated. Ward work, charge nurse assignments, staffing and relief responsibilities, and private duty nursing assignments were just a few of the types of jobs performed by Tyler and her classmates. When assigned as private duty nurses, these students, although unsupervised, were responsible for providing total care for patients, be they rich or poor, in their homes throughout the Washington area.

After graduating from Freedmen's, Tyler left Washington and sought employment in the surrounding states. The only job offered her was in private duty nursing. Tyler, like the other black nurses of her time, was primarily confined to providing care to members of her own race and a limited number of white patients. The best assignments, however, usually went to white nurses who worked through hospital registries. Since few black people could afford the fees for private duty nurses, little work was available for black nurses. The only other positions available for black nurses were those in general duty nursing for blacks in hospitals that admitted prescribed quotas of black patients. These positions were also scarce, since much of the hospital care was given by pupil nurses. Tyler settled for employment as a private duty nurse in Northampton, Massachusetts.[11] Here her patient caseload was limited mainly to students enrolled at Smith College,[12] and after two years Tyler decided that this experience was neither financially nor professionally rewarding. Hearing of job possibilities in Alabama through other black nurses, she left Massachusetts and went south.

After her arrival in Alabama, Tyler initially appeared to be in another job maze, and she was not quite sure what she wanted to do; but she was relatively sure she no longer wanted to work as a private duty nurse. When the opening for a resident nurse at A&M College in Normal, Alabama, was announced, Tyler immediately applied and was hired. In addition to her responsibilities as resident nurse at A&M, Tyler taught physiology and hygiene.[13] She so thoroughly enjoyed this kind of nursing that when an opening of the same type was offered in Virginia, she resigned her position at A&M and assumed the same responsibilities at St. Paul Normal and Industrial School in Lawrenceville, where she worked for two years. Although she was very happy with this job, she wanted to continue her education and experience in other areas of nursing. When she heard about the postgraduate course offered at Lincoln School for Nurses in New York City (which had been inspired by Adah B. Thorns, a Lincoln graduate and the school's only black nursing supervisor), she resigned her position in Lawrenceville and moved to New York.

Shortly after her arrival in New York City, Tyler learned of the possibility for employment in the area of community health nursing. In need of employment as well as desiring an education, she applied to the Henry Street Settlement for a position as a visiting health nurse and, in addition, enrolled in the postgraduate course in general nursing at Lincoln. In 1906, Tyler became the first black Henry Street Settlement visiting nurse.

Tyler's job as a Henry Street nurse would not be as rewarding as she had at first believed, nor would it be an easy one. Because there were no black patients at Henry Street, Tyler began to ask apartment house janitors if they knew of any cases of illness among the black tenants in their buildings. Although she had a difficult time at first convincing the janitors that she did not have anything to sell and was not an intruder, she finally gained their confidence and was permitted to go through the buildings to make friendly visits to the tenants. After three months, she had acquired enough patients to require the assistance of a second nurse.[14] Tyler reported her progress among the black people in her district to Lillian Wald and informed her that she would need another nurse to assist her. The nurse sent to help Tyler was Edith Carter, the second black nurse hired by Henry Street. (Carter's life and career will be described in more detail below.)[15]

Stillman House: A Settlement House for Blacks

A news item in the September 1906 issue of the *American Journal of Nursing* reported:

> From Miss Dock we learn that the Nurses' Settlement in New York is happy in several important additions to its work. A most gratifying and needed extension in the Visiting Nursing Service has been made in an upper west side region where the colored people live. Salaries have been given for two nurses who are also colored and who have settled in their district in a flat. The work is fortunate indeed in the rare ability and devotion of these two women, Miss Tyler and Miss Carter. . . . Beside being excellent nurses, they are both especially alive to social movement organized preventive work.[16]

In December 1906, Elizabeth Tyler established the Stillman House Branch of the Henry Street Settlement for Colored People in a small store on West 61st Street. Stillman House was one of several outreach houses throughout the city under the Henry Street Settlement organization. Tyler hoped that this work would grow and become as important to San Juan Hill as the work of Henry Street Settlement was to the Lower East Side.[17]

San Juan Hill

Located in the borough of Manhattan on the west side of New York City, San Juan Hill (now known as Columbus Hill) was the most congested, disease-ridden community in the city. Bounded by 54th Street on the south, 70th Street on the north, Central Park West and Eighth Avenue on the east, and the Hudson River on the west, this teeming community encompassed 55 city blocks and housed thousands of native whites, Jews, Irish, Italians, and blacks. San Juan Hill, like other communities in the city, had quiet and attractive neighborhoods, but the section where blacks lived was the most severely congested section of the area. Large numbers of blacks lived mostly on one street: West 61st Street.

On the lower end of West 61st Street was an area of two and a half acres that contained 1,641 blacks. West 61st Street and the areas surrounding it were so heavily populated that the New York Department of Health divided it in half and designated it as Sanitary Areas 47 and 51.[18] Eighty percent of the entire San Juan Hill black population lived in these areas; more than half were foreign born. In 1922, 5,861 blacks hailed from the West Indies, while the remaining 2,048 came from Central America, Cuba, and South America. Each of these groups of foreign blacks strove to maintain their cultural heritage and ethnic beliefs, as did their Jewish, Italian, and Irish neighbors.

The settlement of foreign-born blacks in San Juan Hill added another complication to existing racial problems in this ethnically diverse and divided community. For years, San Juan Hill had been known for infighting among blacks and whites; now it was also known as a community where blacks were pitted against blacks. There were regular clashes between one group or another (in fact, the district was satirically called San Juan Hill because fighting among all of the races was so common); however, conflicts between blacks and the Irish were the most frequent. The antagonism between these two groups was undoubtedly one of the harshest intergroup hatreds in American history. Blacks born in the United States often expressed their dislike of foreigners, black or white, and of the Irish in particular.

Such statements as "In this land of Bibles where the outcasts—the scum of European society—can come and enjoy the fullest social and political privileges, the Native Born American with wooly hair and dark complexion is made the victim . . . of Social Ostracism"; "Tens of thousand of aliens are being landed on these shores and freely given the employment which is denied the Negro citizens"; and "The time is upon us when some of the restriction will have to be placed upon the volume and character of European immigration" could be read in *The New York Age, The Crisis, and The New York Freeman.*[19] Throughout the nineteenth century, this mutual antipathy erupted into violence many times, leading to numerous deaths among Irish and blacks.

Notwithstanding the racial and ethnic conflict, the growing numbers of deaths among blacks in San Juan Hill were also a result of the relative lack of medical care offered by the medical establishment and ineffective responses to the all-too-frequent epidemics of disease. In the second decade of the twentieth century, the death rate per 100,000 blacks of all ages in the San Juan Hill district was 5,255. The most prevalent causes of death were tuberculosis (544 per 100,000), pneumonia (561 per 100,000), heart disease (412 per 100,000), and diarrhea (168 per 100,000). The infant mortality rate in the district stood at 255 per 100,000, and the most prevalent causes of death were diarrhea, congenital debility, and respiratory disease.[20]

Initially, the opportunity for black community health nurses to serve this heretofore unserved population was made possible entirely through the generosity of Mrs. Edward Harkness and her sister, Miss Charlotte Stillman, who provided funds for nurses' salaries, office rents, supplies, and, later, rent for nurses' apartments in the neighborhood. Mrs. Harkness and Miss Stillman's act of kindness to the blacks on New York's west side, it is said, was an expression of gratitude to a black nanny who had cared for them throughout most of their childhood.

When Tyler and Carter requested assignment to the San Juan Hill district, they assumed the responsibility for the care of all the black people residing on Manhattan's west side.[21] Their district included several other black neighborhoods in addition to San Juan Hill. Realizing the vastness of their work, the two nurses decided to divide the district in half, with Tyler covering the area from 62nd Street to Harlem and Carter covering the area from 61st Street to the Battery. The nurses were not immediately well received by the black people in their district. Despite the fact that they too were black, Tyler and Carter's presence represented an unrequested intrusion by the white establishment, and they were therefore viewed with fear and mistrust. Tyler and Carter visited doctors' offices to seek their assistance and visited churches to look at the "tablets" to see who was sick in the congregation; they followed people who were obviously ill to their homes and tried to convince them to accept help. Much persuasion was needed to gain entry into blacks' homes. However, once these patients and potential patients accepted the two nurses, they were treated as friends and were graciously received into their homes.

Faced with rampant disease, neglect, ignorance, and the prevailing racial tension, Tyler and Carter confronted a tremendous amount of work. They spent their days in unsafe, dirty, disease-ridden, and congested neighborhoods. Moving purposefully in and out of dingy, overcrowded houses described as "human hives, honeycombed with rooms thick with human beings,"[22] these courageous, self-assured women assumed the monumental task of providing physical comfort, psychological support, health education, and bedside care to thousands of black infants, children, men, and women.

Tyler and Carter not only concerned themselves with the social, economic, and political environment, which bore directly on high mortality rates among blacks in their district, they also contended with a multitude of traditional cures, including potions, deliverance, exorcism, physical healing, herbs and roots, and superstitions associated with each of the different groups of blacks they served. So many different beliefs about illness and other social and health-related issues in such close proximity greatly affected the population's health and posed a major problem for public officials.

In addition, the two nurses often had to compete with local quacks who guaranteed they could purge their patients of every imaginable ailment.[23] Reliance on quackery and medical superstition played a more harmful role in black social life than it did for any other minority group.[24] Determined to serve and save as many people as they could, Tyler and Carter were on a mission that, given its scope and complexity, was a distinct work of faith.

The Work Continues: More Contributions
by Elizabeth Tyler

In 1914, nine years after her career as a Henry Street nurse began, Tyler, confident that the work at Stillman House was well established, resigned and moved to Philadelphia. The Henry Phipps Institute was the primary treatment facility in Philadelphia for blacks who were afflicted with tuberculosis. It was located in the center of the city's black community. Despite the fact that Phipps was in a convenient location and that large numbers of blacks in this area were infected with the disease, few availed themselves of the services offered. Prior to Tyler's employment at Phipps, the facility treated fewer than 100 patients annually. Blacks in Philadelphia, like those in New York, feared and distrusted the medical establishment and all those affiliated with it, be they black or white. Tyler set in motion a patient recruitment campaign similar to the one she and Carter used when they established Stillman House. So successful was she that by the time she left the institute in 1921, the number of patients treated annually had grown from 100 to 3,000.

After Tyler resigned from Phipps, she became the first black nurse to be employed by the State Health and Welfare Commission of Delaware. Her responsibilities at this agency were to organize and take charge of the child hygiene work for the state. Under Tyler's leadership, well-baby and tuberculosis clinics were established. After her work in Delaware was well established and a permanent and competent staff in place, Tyler resigned her position and went to New Jersey, where she accepted a job in Newark with the New Jersey Tuberculosis League (a position very similar to the one she had held in Delaware). Tyler was the first black nurse to be employed there. For the next three and a half years, she developed educational programs geared to the health needs of blacks at the local and state levels. When she left this position, Tyler next moved to the Essex County Tuberculosis League in Newark, where she continued to provide health education for New Jersey's black population. So successful was her work that the state closed the state black health education department and transferred its work to the Essex County Tuberculosis League.

EDITH M. CARTER: SATISFIED TO CARRY THE BAG

Edith M. Carter was born on April 17, 1865, in New Rochelle, New York.[25] Growing up there, Carter, like most young women of any race, was taught to be a homemaker. She was expected to remain with or close to her family and was never encouraged to go off into the world to become a professional worker. She was also expected to find a suitable young man, marry, have children, and settle into a life much like that of her mother. Following the social norms, Carter did remain at home, close to her family; however, she never married or had any children.

It is not known if caring for her ailing mother for so many years was her motivation to choose nursing as a career; but what is known is that after the death of her mother and after consulting her minister,[26] Carter, at the age of thirty-one, entered nurses' training at Freedmen's Hospital School of Nursing in 1896. In 1898, she earned her nursing diploma and returned to her family in New Rochelle. During the next eight years she worked in a hospital owned by one of the most prominent physicians in town, who had known her since childhood.

In the spring of 1906, Carter went to the Henry Street Settlement for a job interview, and on May 6 of the same year she was hired. She left New Rochelle and her work in the hospital when she heard of the work being done by Lillian Wald and her staff at the Settlement House on Henry Street. The Henry Street Settlement Visiting Nurse Service hired her and assigned her to work with Elizabeth Tyler in San Juan Hill.

Being a dedicated nurse and truly caring about the people she served, Carter fought for them, believed in them, and nursed them when others had given them up. In one case, a doctor had done all that he could for a patient, and still she showed no progress. He felt that the patient was beyond help, and so gave Carter permission to do whatever she wished to provide the patient comfort. Under her care, the patient's ulcers, which were the cause of her poor prognosis, healed and she recovered. Another patient, who had been in the hospital for weeks fighting what appeared to be a losing battle against pneumonia, had become emaciated and had developed such huge infected decubitus ulcers that she was sent home to die. When Carter arrived at her home, the neighbors were standing helplessly outside her door. Again, under the nurse's care the ulcers were healed and the patient not only recovered, she later gave birth to two babies.[27]

Carter describes a third successful intervention in a summary of patients she cared for in November 1916:

> I have been interested in the care of Jessie N—. . . . This poor woman had two children ages 3 years—18 mo. and the baby of three mo. who had never gained an ounce since birth, died in Oct. The family was supported

by her aged mother as the husband was worthless, and living away from home. When the mother could spare a dollar she would stop on her way home from work and ask the Dr. to come and see Jessie. The last time he called, he told her not to send for him again until she had six dollars, when he would bring an assistant and tap the Pt. This was the second Dr. called to the case—the first gave a diagnosis of uterine cancer and Pul T.B. He afterward said the sputum was neg. The sec. physician gave Brights. Had tried to persuade Pt. to call a Dr. from Van. Clinic, but they feared that he would only send her to Bellevue where she had been during the month of Sept. and came home rather than be transferred to the Island.[28]

Carter continued to work with Jessie despite the fact that the medical establishment considered her noncompliant and had given up on her. According to Carter's progress notes, she finally convinced Jessie to accept medical care and convinced an institution to accept her. Jessie was referred to Vanderbilt Clinic, where she received free medical treatment. Having taken care of Jessie's immediate problem, Carter informed the Social Service Department at Vanderbilt about the family's situation. Through Carter's persistent efforts, Jessie and her family were able to receive groceries and bed linens free of charge. The mother was given $4.50 per week so that she might spend more time at home with her daughter. The husband was given work temporarily and he was made to contribute to the family. In addition, Dr. Schulman of the Vanderbilt Clinic visited Jessie on an outpatient basis every other day, and her medicine was furnished free from the dispensary. Because of Carter's commitment to her patient's well-being, Jessie recovered from her illness and was discharged, cured by Vanderbilt and Henry Street. In addition to the care provided to Jessie and her family during November of 1916, Carter made 185 nursing visits, 51 substitution visits, and 8 social service visits.[29]

Edith Carter gained much notoriety among the patients she served in San Juan Hill. According to Dorothy Cooper, supervisor of the Longacre Office of the Henry Street Visiting Nurse Service:

To the people in this area Miss Carter *is* Henry Street. She is a welcome friend to all who live there and to walk through this district with her makes you wonder how she ever gets to the homes to visit cases, for she is stopped every other step to give advice to some mother, talk to a child, or to pass the time of day with some old friend who is so glad to see her nurse. Families wait on their doorsteps to see Miss Carter as she comes down the block so they can ask her to call on a sick friend or member of their family. . . .

To Miss Carter the area is just one large family she is happy to serve as their nurse. To the families Miss Carter is "Their Henry Street

Nurse" and the friend to whom they can take all their problems knowing that she will somehow help them find a satisfactory solution. . . .

Miss Carter's twenty-eight years [*sic*] experience give to one a picture of the development of Visiting Nursing. When she came to the organization, she was given her bag and appointed to the area in which she was to work and instructed to visit Doctors, Ministers, Clinics, and the Janitors to find out who was ill in the homes and needed her care. She lived in the district so that families could come to her apartment for consultation. Once a week down to Henry Street Settlement to have her records supervised and to discuss the families she was visiting. To the nurse who comes to Henry Street today for experience her introduction to our field is carefully planned and supervised and Miss Carter is always a help to the younger nurse. To have seen and to have been a part of the growth of this organization from one to twenty-one offices and from about twenty-five nurses to two hundred nurses is an experience we all envy. [Emphasis in original] [30]

CONCLUSION

Jessie Sleet, Elizabeth Tyler, and Edith Carter, pioneers in community health nursing in New York City, began their work during a period of industrialization, immigration, and great population growth in the midst of teeming slums, disease, and death. For blacks, it was a time of change, turmoil, deplorable living and health conditions, and extremely high death rates among individuals of all ages. For community health nursing, it was a time of establishment, activism, expansion, and development. And for these black community health nurse pioneers, it was a time of tremendous challenges and growth.

Confronted with pervasive ignorance and superstitions among culturally diverse blacks, black community health nurses serving in New York City had to struggle unrelentingly to correct harmful and deadly practices while attempting to render health care to their patients. Hindered also by educational, professional, and racial barriers, and confronted with increasing mortality among people of their race, Sleet, Tyler, and Carter found creative ways to transcend these barriers and overcome the circumstances that restricted their practices and destroyed their patients' lives.

NOTES

1. Mabel Keaton Staupers, *No Time for Prejudice: A Story of the Integration of Negroes in Nursing in the United States* (New York: Macmillan, 1961), 7; Adah B. Thorns, *Pathfinders: A History of the Progress of Colored Graduate Nurses* (New York: Kay Printing House, 1929), 9; Mary Roberts, *American Nursing: History and Interpretation* (New York: Macmillan, 1955), 56.

2. Mary Elizabeth Carnegie, *The Path We Tread: Blacks in Nursing, 1854–1984* (New York: J. B. Lippincott, 1986), 146.

3. "Nurses' Settlement News," *American Journal of Nursing* 6 (September 1906): 832–33 (hereafter cited as *AJN*); Lavinia L. Dock, *A History of Nursing from the Earliest Time to the Present Day with Special Reference to the Work of the Past Thirty Years* (New York: G. P Putnam's Sons, 1912), 3: 104.

4. "Nurses' Settlement News," *AJN*, 832–33.

5. Staupers, *No Time for Prejudice*, 7.

6. Ulysses Grant Dailey, "Daniel Hale Williams: Pioneer Surgeon and Father of Negro Hospitals" (paper delivered at meeting of the National Hospital Association, Chicago, August 18, 1941, mimeographed at Providence Hospital and Training School), 1.

7. Lucy L. Drown, "A Successful Experiment," *AJN* 1, no. 10 (July 1901): 729–31.

8. Ibid. For additional discussion relative to Miss Sleet's employment as a district nurse in New York City, see Marie O. Pitts Mosley, "Jessie Sleet Scales: First Black Public Health Nurse," *ABNF Journal* 5, no. 2 (March/April 1994): 45–51; Mosley, "A History of Black Leaders in Nursing: The Influence of Four Black Community Health Nurses on the Establishment, Growth, and Practice of Public Health Nursing in New York City, 1906–1930" (PhD diss., Teachers College, Columbia University, 1992), 72–98; Anna B. Coles, "The Howard University School of Nursing in Historical Perspective," *Journal of the National Medical Association* 61, no. 2 (March 1969): 105; Joyce Ann Elmore, "Black Nurses: Their Service and Their Struggle," *AJN* 76, no. 3 (March 1976): 436; Staupers, *No Time for Prejudice*, 47; Thorns, *Pathfinders*, 15–17.

9. Carnegie, *The Path We Tread*, 146.

10. For additional information on the Freedmen's Hospital Training School for Nurses, see Elmore, "A History of Freedmen's Hospital Training School for Nursing in Washington, D.C., 1894–1901" (master's thesis, Catholic University, 1965).

11. Thorns, *Pathfinders*, 40.

12. Ibid.

13. Ibid.

14. Ibid., 41.

15. Minutes of Semiannual Meeting of the Board of Directors, May 1, 1907, Visiting Nurse Service Archives; "Nurses' Settlement News" *AJN*, 832; Coles, "Howard University School of Nursing," 107; Carnegie, *The Path We Tread*, 149; Thorns, *Pathfinders*, 44.

16. "Nurses' Settlement News" *AJN*, 832.

17. Thorns, *Pathfinders*, 41.

18. During the late nineteenth and early twentieth centuries, in order to provide the most accurate illness and disease statistical information to New York City health officials, Dr. Walter Laidlaw, a statistician, developed a disease inventory system designed to allow health officials to plan for the provision of health services, both under public and private leadership in all branches of health work. The Laidlaw system divided and sub-divided already existing health districts into smaller, more contained health districts called *sanitary areas*. Using statistical information such as that provided by Dr. Laidlaw, health officials could pinpoint conditions that were peculiar to particular areas in order to dictate the types and amounts of health care resources needed.

19. For more discussions on the interracial conflicts between blacks and the Irish in New York City, see *The Crisis* 12 (August 1917): 166–67; *The New York Freeman*, May 15, 1886; and *The New York Age*, May 25, 1905, and October 5, 1916.

20. *Summary of Negro Population in Columbus Hill and Vicinity, 1910 and 1920*, Lillian D. Wald Collection, Rare Books and Manuscript Library, Butler Library, Columbia University, New York, box 45, folder: "Summary of Negro Population." Information found in this document discusses the population, racial classes, housing, and mortality statistics in the Columbus Hill District for 1910 and 1920. For additional health statistical

information on this district, see also *Report of Dependent Negro Families Under A.I.C.P Care, Fiscal Year 1926–1927,* Community Service Society, Rare Books and Manuscript Library, Butler Library, box 36, folder: "Study of 336 Dependent Negro Families"; General Director to Mr. Franklin B. Kirkbride, January 13, 1917, April 11, 1917, and February 5, 1918, Butler Library; and L. Hollingworth Wood of the National League on Urban Conditions among Negroes to Mr. Franklin P Kirkbride, March 7, 1917, Butler Library.

21. The nursing care provided by Tyler and Carter was primarily for blacks residing in their district. They did provide care to whites in the district, but only in cases of emergency. The reason for this segregated nursing care was related to the special interest of the Stillman family. Additionally, Tyler and Carter, wishing to work with members of their own race, requested a health district with large numbers of unserved blacks, an area whose numbers would keep them extremely busy. Additional discussion about the racial background of patients cared for by Tyler and Carter in their district can be found in Lillian D. Wald's Report of the Henry Street (Nurses') Settlement, March 17, 1909, Visiting Nurse Service of New York Archives.

22. Mary White Ovington, *Half a Man: The Status of the Negro in New York* (New York: Hill and Wang, 1969), 22.

23. *New York Globe,* February 16, 1884.

24. Gilbert Osofsky, *Harlem: The Making of a Ghetto* (New York: Harper & Row, 1966), 9.

25. Date and place of birth are contained in file letters located at the Visiting Nursing Service of New York Archives.

26. Information extracted from "File Letter," Visiting Nursing Service of New York Archives.

27. Dorothy Elizabeth Jensen, "The Henry Street Settlement: A Response to the Needs of the Sick Poor, 1893–1913" (PhD diss., Teachers College, Columbia University, 1979), 130.

28. The "Island" referred to in this document was Ward's Island, located on New York City's East River adjacent to Manhattan. Patients infected with tuberculosis were sent there for treatment and cure. Black patients, however, were particularly afraid of being sent there because it was viewed as a place where one went to die; they would only consent to admission when home remedies, religious interventions, or culturally derived approaches failed to provide cures, or when health officials forced them to go. From Edith M. Carter's summary of Stillman for the month of November 1916 (entry dated December 10, 1916), addressed to Bessie Ely Amerman, RN, superintendent of nurses at the Henry Street Settlement, document located at Visiting Nursing Service of New York Archives.

29. Carter, summary of Stillman for the month of November 1916.

30. Dorothy Cooper, supervisor of the Longacre Office of the Henry Street Settlement Visiting Nurse Service, "Longacre," Visiting Nursing Service of New York Archives.

SECTION 2

Nursing's Ambivalent Relationship With Money

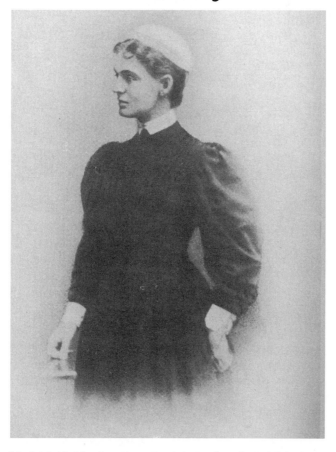

M. Adelaide Nutting. From Lavinia Dock and M. Adelaide
Nutting's *A History of Nursing From the Earliest Times to the
Present Day With Special Reference to the Work of the Past
Thirty Years*, volume 3 (1912).

Introduction

Ellen D. Baer

> The root of all the main problems in nursing will be found, I believe, if carefully studied, to be economic in nature.[1]

At the end of her illustrious career as superintendent of the Johns Hopkins Hospital School for Nurses (1894 to 1907) and head of Teachers College graduate program for nurses (1907 to 1925), M. Adelaide Nutting introduced a book of her papers with the words quoted above. She elaborated further:

> At the time that Miss Nightingale was evolving this system of training, the economic conditions of the day made long hours of work and low wages, particularly for women, accepted conditions. The traditions of the free service of the religious orders which hospitals had long enjoyed strengthened this attitude and made it difficult for them to get a correct point of view on the value of nurses' work.[2]

It probably would not surprise Miss Nutting to learn that we have not solved these economic problems in the 100-plus years since she began to speak and write about them. Habitually, nursing authors blame the system and other professions for most of this economic travail. But nursing historians and women's studies researchers make a different argument. They argue that nursing has a complicated identity, in which philanthropic and altruistic ideals conflict with professional self-determination.[3]

Economics is the area in which this conflict is most evident. Philanthropic and altruistic agents do not usually seek economic gain or even parity for their efforts. But, professionals who have spent years developing a particular expertise do expect to be paid for their work and recognized in other ways as well. This section on the economic issues of clinical nursing practice will address the early years of nursing in hopes of providing readers with insight into the beginnings of nursing's long struggle with appropriate economic recognition.

PRIVATE WORK IN A PUBLIC DOMAIN

In its beginning and formative years, "nursing was seen as an innate and loving responsibility of women and mothers."[4] It was work that began in the home and moved to the workplace (hospitals and patients' homes) carrying with it, for good or ill, the status and obligations of its origin. "Nurses [were] the ones who have been able to make a home of the hospital, to personalize an increasingly impersonal environment."[5] One could argue that nursing always has occupied a place between the private and public lives of people, caught between and within two domains. And in that space between two worlds, economic rewards foundered. Although nurses entered the marketplace of health care, most of them did not initially seek the rewards of the market. They sought training, room and board, and preparation for a life of family service or private duty nursing.

Nurses entered the public domain to provide the caring and nurturing services associated with the private domain and sought the rewards they saw as relevant. Nurses occupied hospital positions that carried major marketplace decision-making powers at the same time that they articulated and maintained the values of the nonmarket or private environment. As Miss Nutting elaborated:

> The whole situation can, I think, be traced back to the economic position of woman in the home in which nursing arose and in which, notwithstanding our many hospitals, most nursing is still carried on, and to her position in the monastic orders, in which for centuries the care of the sick was a main activity, a voluntary service, with poverty as the rule rule of life.[6]

NURSING AS A FREE SERVICE

In the first chapter reprinted here, "A Sound Economic Basis for Schools of Nursing,"[7] M. Adelaide Nutting synopsizes another basis of the problem. This address to the New York State Nurses Association in October 1916 reminds us that, almost until World War II, training schools of nursing *were* the nursing departments of hospitals. When students entered the schools for training, they began immediately to deliver the nursing services of the institution. The only paid nurses were the very few who supervised and taught the students. As a consequence, from the outset of hospital usage in this country, everyone from administrator to trustee to patient to doctor and even nurse expected that nursing care would be free. And, in fact, all gave periodic complaint that the hospital had even the expense of providing room or board or educational materials to the training school. Thus embedded in hospital culture from the outset, this expectation of no-cost nursing has proved very difficult to dislodge.

As nurses realized that they had to fight for their own resources in their work environments, they strove to distance themselves from their domestic and no-cost roots, finding instead that attachment to professional and scientific roots carried greater weight among the arbiters of power and money. In viewing American society in general, feminists Ehrenreich and English described this dilemma as a "fatal moral compromise" within marketplace capitalism, wherein:

> The inanimate things of the marketplace—money and the commodities which represent money—are alive and possessed of almost sacred significance. Conversely, things truly alive are, from a strictly "rational" point of view, worthless except as they impinge on the market and affect one's economic self-interest.[8]

Problems developed because protections that existed for caregivers in the domestic world did not exist in the public sphere. In a family, women who provided unpaid family services were often protected and supported by male family members. Such paternalistic providers did not exist in the public domain to buttress the nurses' life needs when sickness, old age, and episodes of unemployment occurred.

In fact, nurses often discovered the opposite. Rather than protecting them, nurses found that male hospital administrators, physicians, and trustees sometimes exploited them for hospital advantage. In Chapter 6, "Nursing's Divided Loyalties: An Historical Case Study,"[9] Ellen Baer describes the following situation. At the Presbyterian Hospital in Philadelphia in the early 1890s, nurses who graduated from the hospital's training school placed their names on the hospital's registry and earned fees doing private duty nursing in patients' homes. But the hospital trustees, seeking to gain income from the training school, sent pupil nurses into private homes, charged a fee equal to that charged by the graduate nurses, and kept the fees for the hospital's use. The hospital trustees thereby managed a trifecta of exploitation: They deprived graduate nurses of employment, set pupil-nurses up as competitors to the graduate nurses, and kept the money for the hospital's use.

Baer further demonstrates how, even in that effort, nurses hamstrung their own purposes in several ways, such as creating rules that disenfranchised members who could have been helpful and distancing nursing groups from women's and professional groups that might have accorded them some power. In essence, nurses hesitantly saw that they had to create a commodity out of personal care in order to make it economically viable for them to engage in the practice of nursing. But such terms seemed antithetical to what nurses wished to do—give compassion and care—and, in consequence, they didn't fully or successfully engage in the process.

PERSONAL CARE AS A BUSINESS COMMODITY

The next two chapters in this section demonstrate the ways in which nurses attempted to make their work adhere to business principles. In Chapter 7, "'A Necessity in the Nursing World': The Chicago Nurses Professional Registry, 1913–1950,"[10] Jean Whelan documents the rising and falling fortunes of nursing registries for private duty nurses. Whelan discusses dilemmas faced by private duty nurses from the outset, such as one presented by Katherine DeWitt in her 1913 book *Private Duty Nursing*.[11] DeWitt described the difficulty of nurses awaiting a baby's delivery in an obstetric case. The nurse could not accept other cases, in case the baby arrived while she was otherwise employed. Yet, while waiting, the nurse earned no income. DeWitt suggested:

> If she explains that her time is, in a way, her capital, and that weeks lost can never be regained, the patient will see that it is not fair to expect her to wait for an indefinite period of time without compensation, even though she is not at work. If the patient is unable to pay for waiting time, she may agree that the nurse can take other cases until called to her. These other cases are taken with the understanding that the nurse may be called away. It is not a thoroughly comfortable arrangement for either patient, or for the nurse, but it is sometimes necessary, and is better and more honest than to present the obstetrical patient with a bill for waiting time which she did not expect. Sometimes a patient is able to pay a nurse one-half her usual rates while waiting, and this seems fair, if she is allowed to stay at home and rest.[12]

In "The Cost of Caring: The Metropolitan Life Insurance Company's Visiting Nurse Service, 1909–1953,"[13] Diane Hamilton analyzes the arrangement whereby the Metropolitan Life Insurance Company paid visiting nurse associations across the nation to deliver home health services to their immigrant clients in order to prolong their lives and build greater premium income for the company.

In the chapters in this section, nurses wind up with the shorter end of the stick when business interests slight and trump professional values. For in both the Registry and Metropolitan cases, although nurses saw that they could sell their services as a commodity, they did not understand that once they agreed to buy into business methods, their commodity had to conform to business rules rather than professional values. As Hamilton reports elsewhere on the arrangement, one of the Met Life administrators "maintained that nurses did not understand business practices because they believed their skills were acts of charity, not business."[14] Nurses also did not appreciate the enormous impact on nursing that was brought by two world wars and the Great Depression. Once again focusing on "a little world of our own,"[15] nurses missed the importance of context: What happens in the world outside of nursing and hospitals changes what can and must occur within nursing and hospitals.

It has taken almost 150 years for nursing to evolve from an assumed part of the private role of women in their homes to a paid work of educated professional people in public institutions. This evolution has occurred haltingly, awkwardly, and with difficulty and dismay on the parts of many who preferred to view the role romantically as the loving acts of caring people unattached to fees. Beyond our interest in these events for their content, they also serve as excellent examples of the way history happens. It is not the neat series of events that it often appears to be from a future vantage point. In consequence, for the purposes of this book, this section serves a double purpose: an example of how history happens, and an example of nursing's ambivalent relationship with money.

NOTES

1. Mary Adelaide Nutting, *A Sound Economic Basis for Schools of Nursing and Other Addresses* (New York: G. P. Putnam's Sons, 1926), vi. This book is in the collection of the Barbara Bates Center for the Study of the History of Nursing, University of Pennsylvania School of Nursing, Philadelphia. It also has been reprinted by Garland Publishing in its series *The History of American Nursing*, edited by Susan Reverby.
2. Nutting, *Sound Economic Basis*, 268.
3. Susan Reverby, *Ordered to Care: The Dilemma of American Nursing* (New York: Cambridge University Press, 1987).
4. Patricia O'Brien [D'Antonio], "'All a Woman's Life Can Bring': The Domestic Roots of Nursing in Philadelphia, 1830–1885," *Nursing Research* 36 (Jan/Feb 1987): 12.
5. O'Brien, "All a Woman's Life," 16.
6. Nutting, *Sound Economic Basis*, vi.

7. Ibid., 3–17.

8. Barbara Ehrenreich and Deidre English, *For Her Own Good: 150 Years of the Experts Advice to Women* (New York: Anchor Press, 1978), 17, 283.

9. A reprint of Ellen D. Baer, "Nursing's Divided Loyalties: An Historical Case Study," *Nursing Research* 38 (1989): 3.

10. A reprint of Jean Whelan, "'A Necessity in the Nursing World': The Chicago Nurses Professional Registry, 1913–1950," *Nursing History Review* 13 (2005).

11. Katharine DeWitt, *Private Duty Nursing* (Philadelphia and London: J. B. Lippincott Co., 1913), 44–45. This book is in the collection of the Barbara Bates Center for the Study of the History of Nursing, University of Pennsylvania School of Nursing, Philadelphia. It also has been reprinted by Garland Publishing in its series *The History of American Nursing*, edited by Susan Reverby.

12. DeWitt, *Private Duty Nursing*, 45.

13. Diane Hamilton, "The Cost of Caring: The Metropolitan Life Insurance Company's Visiting Nurse Service, 1909–1953," *Bulletin of the History of Medicine* 63 (1989).

14. Diane Hamilton, "Faith and Finance," *Image: Journal of Nursing Scholarship* 20 (1988): 125.

15. Nancy Tomes, "'Little World of Our Own': The Pennsylvania Hospital Training School for Nurses," *Journal of the History of Medicine and Allied Science* 33 (1978): 507–30.

CHAPTER 5

A Sound Economic Basis for Schools of Nursing[1]

Mary Adelaide Nutting

The clear implication in the title of this chapter is that training schools for nurses do not at present rest upon an entirely sound economic foundation. It is advisable, therefore, I suppose, at the outset to try to show upon what kind of a basis such schools for nurses do actually rest, and to see how it compares with that of other schools and colleges.

The ordinary school or college with which we are familiar has three main ways of securing support. These are through public funds derived from taxation, through private funds by gifts, and through fees from students. The older of our great universities were founded by public moneys; the younger, such as Johns Hopkins, Stanford, and Chicago Universities, by private benevolence. Women's colleges have almost without exception arisen through private gifts, individual or collective. Both universities and women's colleges are largely maintained by private philanthropy, and all of them are perpetually seeking additional funds.

The alumnae of Vassar, Smith, Wellesley, and others labor assiduously to gather contributions for their several colleges, either to increase existing endowments, to add new buildings, or to establish some new branch of instruction. Smith College, which just reports the admission of 1,700 students, has quite recently closed a successful campaign for a million dollars[2]; Wellesley has in an astonishingly brief time secured a much larger sum to restore her buildings lost by her disastrous fire. Bryn Mawr has recently had about three-quarters of a million given her by one alumna for the establishment and development of a particular line of work. Barnard has within the last month received from Jacob Schiff the splendid gift of over half a million for a new building. Within the space of two or three days, recently, there were announced in the daily press gifts to a few of our eastern colleges within a comparatively small area which, in the aggregate, amount to over a million and a half of dollars. These gifts may be devoted to the field of general education or to the support and advancement of technical or professional schools. Our great professional schools of medicine, law, and theology, and also of applied science and of art, have rejoiced in splendid gifts for buildings, for endowment, for special developments. The School of Journalism at Columbia is a recent instance of such a foundation, given for the creation of a new form of professional training. Our schools of philanthropy are richly endowed. These, together with such institutes as Stevens, Pratt, Drexel, Carnegie, all proclaim the beneficence of many individuals who believe in the higher and specialized education and training of men and women.

I know of few things more impressive, to me, indeed, more profoundly moving, than to survey the field of education and to note the richness of the gifts which have been there poured forth with such lavish hand in so many directions, and to perceive the ways through which men and women are striving to put into the hands of their fellows the supreme weapon of knowledge. These enormous private contributions made to education are the wonder and glory of our age.

Of the variety of institutions supported or aided by public funds our state systems of education show an interesting picture. Here we see support which reaches through the whole public school system and culminates in universities, colleges, and in professional and technical schools. Looking upon it, one is inclined to believe that the need for training, in almost any direction promising useful service to the community, has only to be recognized to ensure it a place in the concern of the state, or to bring it definitely within the scope of state responsibility. It is of special interest to us to note the number and variety of private institutions to which the state finds itself able to lend support. The wide availability of such public funds for the aid of already established schools giving instruction which is needed, suggests the advisability of bringing the financial condition of training schools for nurses to the attention of the educational authorities of the state.

We now come to students' fees as a source of income. In the conduct of such educational work as we have been considering in colleges and universities, they do not ordinarily play a large part, since usually not more than one-third of the annual expenses are met in this way.

Under exceptionally able administration they may cover a slightly larger proportion, and since there seems to be a tendency toward increasing them, they may in future play a considerably larger part. But ordinarily, in any genuine educational work, tuition fees go a very small way toward meeting the expense. This fact makes it clear that the students from great colleges and professional schools are in one sense receivers of charity, since what they pay for their education is far below its actual cost; and, indeed, it is this great sense of obligation, this conviction that some adequate return is due to society for benefits received, that impels the alumnae from schools and colleges to such continuous efforts for the financial strengthening and upbuilding of these institutions.

The most casual study of these matters brings forth strikingly the cost of modern education. "Present educational demands, upon even a modest college," says Mr. Furst, secretary of the Carnegie Foundation, "require resources of approximately a million dollars."[3] The endowment per student in colleges like Bryn Mawr, Smith, Vassar, is $1,600; in certain colleges for men, it is $4,000 per student. Good teaching, he urges, is not only expensive, but absolutely not to be had below a certain minimum of expenditure, and financial resources constitute the fundamental problem. In other words, any institution which proposes to educate must depend upon appropriate, definite, and permanent sources of income.

In all this long list of great gifts for education, in all this imposing array of colleges and schools supported by such gifts, I am astonished to realize that no reference whatever is made anywhere to one of the most fundamentally important branches of professional education now in existence—schools for the training of nurses, of which there are about eleven hundred in this country alone. I suppose if Mr. Abraham Flexner were here, he would take issue with me on the use of the word "professional" in its usually accepted sense as applied to nursing, and I hope to take up that point at some later time, but is it not strange that, search as you will from one end of the country (I had almost said the world) to the other, you will not find one single gift of any appreciable amount, not one endowment placed at the disposal of a training school for nurses for the proper conduct of its educational work. There have been in history two important gifts made for the education of nurses. Florence Nightingale gave the first, in providing, a half century ago, $200,000 for the founding of the Nightingale School at St. Thomas Hospital, London. The first training school in history was, therefore, established and has been maintained by an endowment. A half century later, Mrs. Helen Hartley Jenkins of New York gave a second considerable gift, in endowing the Department for Graduate Nurses at the College for Teachers of Columbia University, and these two large gifts complete the list. There is literally nothing to add: so far as my knowledge goes there is no training school for nurses supported anywhere in this country by private endowment; there are none maintained by public funds, and public treasuries and private philanthropy alike seem to be innocent of any recognition of the fact that there are between thirty and forty thousand student nurses in training in the eleven hundred schools recorded, and that every one of these schools is carrying on its work with difficulty and at a disadvantage because of lack of resources.

There remain for consideration, among the usual sources of income for educational Institutions, tuition fees. These, in so far as training schools for nurses are concerned, may be summarily disposed of. There are four or five schools in this country charging small fees for the special instruction given in the few months of the preliminary course and one school, only, charging tuition for its entire course. Thus it is clear that every one of the usual sources of income must be eliminated in the case of training schools for nurses, and some way which is not the common way of meeting the legitimate expenses of a school must be looked for. Such a way appears to be found as one studies the relationship existing between training schools and the hospitals in which they have arisen. It is a most unusual form of relationship and nothing at all like it exists in connection with any other school of the present day. It is universal, in so far as training schools are concerned.

Through this relationship the training school for nurses becomes an institution established by the hospital with one large main purpose and what we might call one subsidiary purpose in mind. The first purpose is clear-cut and imperative. The nursing work of the hospital, its most important task, must be done: the training school, through its students, can do it. The primary function of all training schools is that of carrying on the regular nursing work of the hospital. It is not anywhere the education of the nurse. That education is the subsidiary, secondary purpose of the hospital in establishing a training school, and it follows, as a matter of course, that it can be carried out only in so far as is compatible with the main purpose of nursing the patients through the students of the school.

The most casual glance at this situation would therefore show that the expense of maintaining training schools under such conditions would probably be slight, and a second glance would lead one to the conclusion that, whatever it is, it is really met by the students themselves.

That their services cover the expense of instruction is formally recognized in the announcements of training schools, where it is usually explicitly stated that the services of the pupil are considered as an equivalent for tuition. The expenses of actual instruction, therefore, are met by the pupils themselves, and, placing the minimum estimate upon the value of their services, it is unquestionable that they pay larger tuition fees than are exacted of students in any college in the country.

In considering this aspect of affairs, two points must be kept in mind. One is, that pupil nurses are from the beginning given necessary tasks, which somebody would otherwise have to be paid to do. This principle is so well maintained throughout all hospital work that the staff of students in a hospital ward is no larger than would be needed if such a staff were composed of paid workers. Students are preferred, indeed, because of the fact that they do more work than graduate nurses will do under similar conditions. Even the roughest estimate of the cost of any form of paid service to replace students shows that maintenance of an approximately similar number of workers would be required, and wages or salaries ranging from those of the unskilled household employee up to those of the highly skilled nurse would have to be paid. Anyone wishing to obtain a recent estimate of the value of pupil nurses' services to hospitals should study the records of the efforts made last year in California to repeal the eight-hour law required there for pupil nurses in hospitals. The additional expense and injury to the hospital of maintaining shorter hours were urged with emphasis from many such institutions, while one exceedingly indiscreet superintendent of a hospital declared that, in order to live up to the law, he would be obliged to increase the number of students by 50 per cent. Further light on this matter may be had by noting the charges made by hospitals for the services of student nurses when on special duty with private patients.

It is entirely clear that large expenses for service, which the hospitals would have to incur under any other system whatever, are avoided by the establishment of a training school for nurses, and a very considerable sum is thus set free for the instruction and training for which the labor of pupils is asked and is so freely given. Not very long ago I saw a statement in some hospital or nursing journal to the effect that it cost the hospital between three and four hundred dollars a year for the education of each pupil. This, of course, may be literally correct, but it is essentially incorrect, since it fails to estimate in any way the value to the hospital of the returns which the student always makes. There appears to me to be no way of getting around the actual economic value of the student's services.

Let us consider these expenses which hospitals have to meet, taking first the administration of the school of nursing. Here there can be little question of expense, because those who manage the school are in reality officers of the nursing department of the hospital who would have to be there in about the same numbers and grades to direct and supervise the nursing if there were no school and the work were done by a staff of paid workers. And, of course, there are many schools, the majority, in fact, in which most of these official supervisory positions are filled by senior students, thus adding another item to the contributions made by students to their own education.

Actual instruction comes next for consideration, and this is of two kinds: theoretical teaching in the classroom; practical teaching in the wards.

Here again the hospital has been released from any appreciable additional expense since the bulk of the teaching has always been done by the officers of the nursing department, in addition to their regular executive and supervising duties. Until within the last few years, no training school for nurses had even one regular instructor on its staff, and the great majority of schools are still in this position. In all the larger schools of the better grade one regular instructor is now provided and in some cases there are two. As yet, however, no considerable expense for such instruction is incurred. Lectures are still in the majority of schools given by physicians without payment, though, again, in some of the larger schools part of these lectures are paid for, and all of them are, in a few schools. As, however, the number of lectures is small, not more than two or three a week at the utmost, the expense thus incurred is slight. For libraries and teaching material and equipment it can be truthfully said that few hospitals have even attempted to make respectable provision. In providing suitable housing and living conditions for students, hospitals are doing more to meet their obligations to them than in any other aspect of their work, but it is, of course, pertinent here to mention that such expense cannot be charged to the maintenance of a training school, since suitable quarters would be required equally for any kind of a staff the hospital might employ.

Moreover there are still hundreds of hospitals in which the quarters and the food provided for student nurses are a scandal to their communities. As for hours of work, notwithstanding some improvements, they are still a burning question and are such as to make it very difficult and frequently impossible for pupils to take their theoretical work seriously. Yet hospitals do not find themselves able or willing to meet the expense involved in providing the larger staff of paid workers of various grades which would admit of shorter hours for students. One would suppose that any institution thus miraculously supplied with a body of pupils whom it could at will translate into an entire working force, would not question the justice and wisdom of adjusting its hours of work in such a way that the educational needs of the students would be satisfied. Yet tonight, as I read this to you, hundreds of young student nurses are at work on night duty in the hospitals of this city and country and this night of work will be twelve hours long. Service of this kind will usually be made to occupy about six months out of a three years' training. Yet from any conceivable educational standpoint, one month of such service would usually be ample.

We were impressed, a little while ago, in reviewing briefly the field of education with its great, and apparently unavoidable, cost. The more carefully I study the work of training schools for nurses, the more I am convinced that failure to recognize this elementary fact, as applying to their conduct, is at the root of many of the troubles in the present training school situation. What is needed now in our hospitals is a truer conception of the responsibilities which are inevitably assumed in attempting to direct, control, and develop in any adequate way this large, complicated, and most vital branch of professional education, and ability to face the situation squarely and recognize that adequate funds are just as necessary for the proper maintenance of training schools for nurses as they are for medical, engineering, or any other professional schools.

No equitable and stable adjustment can ever be made between hospital and training schools until this fact is understood, accepted, and made to bear upon the whole scheme of training. In thinking this whole problem over, I have been impressed with the fact that though hospitals are constantly and properly making the public acquainted with their needs, I do not remember ever hearing of any instances of hospitals asking for funds for the maintenance of their training schools for nurses. Yet I can hardly imagine any branch of their work for the maintenance of which they could with better grace turn to the public. There are literally thousands of men and women who owe their health or their lives to the skill, knowledge, and devotion of nurses. There are those among them who have given liberally to other forms of education and would, I am confident, willingly contribute to the education of nurses were they but made aware of the need. It is not because of any lack of appreciation of the valuable and indeed indispensable services which nurses are rendering to society that nothing is given to help forward their education and training, but because of a prevalent conviction that this is wholly the business of hospitals, which are believed to be quite able to do all that is necessary. There is much need of a really correct understanding of what hospitals can and cannot do. They cannot, for instance, on funds which are seldom if ever sufficient for actual hospital needs, maintain training schools as they should be maintained. They cannot unaided carry forward the important educational work which has been entrusted to them. They could, however, make some effort to secure the necessary aid.

Certain it is that from some source, either from private gifts for endowment, from public funds for maintenance, or even partly from tuition fees (but under different conditions of service), training schools must be enabled to command adequate funds.

I have been asked what an endowment could do for a training school. It might do any, or all, of the following things:

It might provide a sufficient body of trained and expert lecturers and teachers to give appropriate and adequate instruction in all of the necessary and desirable subjects included in any adequate scheme for the education of nurses, and this would apply to practical instruction at the bed-side as well as to theory in the classroom.

It might provide suitably for such teaching equipment and material as is commonly found in all schools having any scientific or technical subjects to handle.

It might provide teaching buildings which would have libraries, both professional and general, lecture and class-rooms, and laboratories and offices. It should also provide suitable living and recreation rooms. Cheerful surroundings and a chance for wholesome diversion are particularly important for those whose work lies entirely among the sick. These it might do quite directly. Indirectly by assisting in providing a larger staff, it might aid in securing for students shorter hours both for day and night work, and proper vacations and holidays. For the hospital, openly relieved from any expense whatever in connection with the training school, could turn its attention and its funds to the provision of a regular salaried staff of nurses and other workers for much of the routine work now done by students.

This, in increasing the number of workers, would logically bring about the shorter hours. And these, in connection with improvements in the amount and character of instruction, would attract the better qualified candidate who is so urgently needed. Such measures have brought this result in every instance where they have been established and steadily and intelligently applied.

I firmly believe that generous financial help would flow into our training schools from private sources were the need fully recognized, and I see no reason whatever why schools rendering an important public service should not also secure substantial aid from public funds. The problem of the poor, ill-equipped training schools connected with struggling hospitals in the small communities might be in a measure solved through such aid.

From whatever source funds may come, they are necessary to place schools on a secure and dignified foundation, and to release them from their present helpless and somewhat ignominious position, due very largely to an entirely unsound economic status.

This chapter merely touches the subject, which needs, and doubtless will eventually get, careful and searching inquiry. But in the meantime those nurses who are genuinely interested in improving their own profession can do so in no more effective way than by helping their training schools up to a higher and freer plane of work which suitable financial resources alone can ensure. Already the alumni of the Johns Hopkins Training School, and of the Massachusetts General, have taken up the question of the endowments of their schools, and committees are being formed to consider ways and means. Nurses may with courage and confidence take up this question of proper support for their training schools since, in the last analysis, it is the concern, and the grave concern, of the whole community. The public cannot longer leave entirely to hospitals, or to the labors of student nurses, the maintenance of so essential a branch of modern education.

Let me repeat. There have been in history but two large gifts for the education of nurses. The first, by Florence Nightingale, created and set in motion the whole modern system of training schools and of nursing; the second, by Mrs. Helen Hartley Jenkins, has established in a great university a department for the special professional training of graduate nurses, and has made possible the opening up of some entirely new avenues of work, such, for instance, as education for public health nursing and training for public school work. The next great service to be rendered is to place all training schools for nurses upon a sounder economic foundation.

(Author's note to the December 1920 reprint.)

Since this pamphlet was written in January, 1916, the question of education has taken on new and acute importance. Provision for it in about every accepted form and in many new branches is being made with a lavishness that is beyond any dreams of the past. Where a few years ago a college sought one million dollars, it would now as readily seek ten million, and the alumni of most of the great colleges in the country, Harvard, Princeton, Cornell, Smith, Wellesley, and Bryn Mawr, have of late carried on vigorous campaigns for very large increases in their endowments which they have been splendidly successful in obtaining.

Quite untouched, however, by this great tide of generosity our Schools of Nursing still remain. They lie seemingly wholly outside of its reach or even interest. Meanwhile the trained women who are the products of these schools are entering more deeply and vitally into every level of human society, as the importance and value of their services are more fully recognized and understood. With the developments in public health work and preventive medicine and the highly creditable record which the nurses who have entered this field have already established, fresh demands are made upon our Schools of Nursing which they cannot meet.

The poverty of their educational resources is indescribable. It would have to be seen to be realized, and little in the way of further growth or progress can be looked for until these schools are rescued from their economic helplessness and provided with the financial resources upon which all worthy educational work must rest. A. N.

NOTES

1. Copyright (c) 1926 from the Center for the Study of the History of Nursing, School of Nursing, University of Pennsylvania, by Nutting MA. Reproduced by permission of Routledge/Taylor & Francis Group, LLC.
2. And another following closely for four millions.
3. Clyde Furst, "Ideals of Women's Colleges." Paper presented at the 12th Annual Meeting of the Southern Association of College Women, Atlanta, Ga., April 1915.

CHAPTER 6

Nursing's Divided Loyalties: An Historical Case Study

Ellen D. Baer

Reform-minded philanthropic women, concerned about the poor quality of sick-care in nineteenth-century American hospitals, initiated Nightingale-like systems of organized nursing to solve institutions' problems. From the outset, the nurses found that to provide proper care for the sick, they needed to reorganize the institutions' methods of management by: creating orderly systems to accomplish needed services; establishing hierarchical lines of discipline to maintain accountability; and teaching the methods of care-giving and systematic management to the untrained pupil-nurses who were to provide these services. These competing responsibilities created conflict within the nursing profession and caused division among nurses. Initially, nurses tried to perform all three roles simultaneously. As size and numbers grew, however, they divided into subgroups (practice, management, education) that competed for status, students' time, and their piece of the meager pie assigned to nursing by the institutions.[1]

   In the present study, a variation on the theme of nurses' conflicted loyalties was explored using the historical version of the case study

This chapter was originally published in *Nursing Research*, 1989, 38(3): 166–171. Copyright Lippincott Williams & Wilkins. Reprinted with permission.

method, in which one relatively typical situation is presented to reflect patterns apparent in many other instances. Nurses' alumnae associations provided good examples of nurses' conflicting loyalties at the turn of the twentieth century. The specific case examined here is the Alumnae Association of the Training School for Nurses of the Presbyterian Hospital in Philadelphia, 1897–1922. The purpose of the study was to examine the formation events and protective, socioeducative, and political activities of the association during its first 25 years. The argument put forth is that though the organization fulfilled certain tacit purposes by providing a supportive community to single working women seeking life satisfaction in nineteenth-century America, it ultimately compromised its stated goals due to conflicts between its desire to recruit all graduates into its ranks and its insistence on stringent eligibility requirements, its commitment to the nurses and its loyalty to the hospital, and its attention to local rather than national nursing concerns.

SINGLE WOMEN IN NINETEENTH-CENTURY AMERICA

Small communities of single working women became common in industrialized nineteenth-century America. Women's newly found passion for work outside the home provided the companionships, security, and the means out of the garden, out of idleness, out of ignorance, and into wisdom, service, and adventure.[2]

When women left their homes to take up nursing in the last quarter of the nineteenth century, they left the certainty of family protection and support as well. Youngish (aged 21–26) single or widowed women from farms, clergy homes, small towns, and "middling" class American families detached themselves from their roots in pursuit of self-sufficiency, independence, and "the better understanding of my fellowman in every walk of life."[3] The hospital nursing schools provided for their needs during the three years of their training. But after completing their programs, graduate nurses supported themselves. As historian Susan Reverby points out, nurses worked primarily in private duty prior to the Great Depression, going from case to case, living in the home of their charge for the duration of their responsibility and living between cases in boarding houses, graduate nurses clubs, or other such arrangements.[4] In times of sickness, economic recession, or sporadic unemployment, the nurses had no alternative means of support. Ultimately they looked to their colleagues for assistance, forming alumnae associations for financial, social, and political protection.

Alumnae associations were created by many groups during the late nineteenth century when America's passion for forming societies grew strong. As Lavinia Dock wrote from the Henry Street Settlement House: "Congresses were as numerous as blades of grass, and the association idea was in the air."[5] At the 1893 World's Fair, Hopkins Nursing Superintendent Isabel Hampton identified alumnae associations as the grassroots base for nursing's organizational master plan that would link schools into districts, districts into states, states into a national association, and national groups into a world federation of nursing.[6] This scheme typified the major social shifts occurring in post-Civil War America. In order to cope with rising pressures of industrialization, immigration, and urbanization, America built a bureaucratic-minded middle class that organized, administered, regularized, and nationalized various aspects of its social life. Hampton envisioned this structure as the professional framework within which nurses would establish and maintain standards of practice and education for nursing and communicate those standards to the world at large. Although Hampton's agenda was not fully successful,[7] it encouraged the proliferation of alumnae associations in training schools that collectively became the Nurses' Associated Alumnae of the United States and Canada in 1896 with Mrs. Robb (formerly Hampton) as its first president. The group divided into two entities in 1911 and the U.S. half became the American Nurses' Association.[8]

The nurses' professional goals thus merged with their more personal needs within the associational context. It might have been possible to handle this dichotomy between members' personal and professional interests, but the additional conflict regarding institutional loyalty made matters insolvable. Though founded by the independent graduates of particular training schools, the schools themselves were not independent of hospitals. When the graduates required certain services for the association, such as meeting rooms, kitchens, clerical records, doctors and hospital nurses to deliver homilies at the meetings, and other trappings that gave their society its identity, they were forced to turn to their "home" hospital and its board, whose primary concern lay elsewhere.

FOUNDING IDEALS OF THE PRESBYTERIAN HOSPITAL

An 1869 alliance of two branches of the Presbyterian Church "combine[d] the interests and energies of Presbyterians" to found hospitals and homes for the care of the sick and needy.[9] Rev. E. D. Saunders, who wished to provide care "irrespective of creed, color or country," contributed property, and in 1872 the Presbyterian Hospital of Philadelphia opened, "built, endowed, and supported entirely by private contributions, largely Presbyterian, although other generous friends have helped."[10] The Ladies Aid Society, formed in 1873 and reputed to have initiated one of America's earliest efforts in social work, began its "Benevolent work" in 1880 with visits by its members to sick patients in the hospital and to their families at home. In 1887 the Ladies Aid hired Caroline Farnum, a Philadelphia [General] Hospital trained nurse, to be in charge of the visits and who they later called upon to take charge when "the Training School began work" on October 1, 1889.[11]

Interest in an alumnae association began during the school's early years[12] and came to fruition in 1897 when Directress Caroline Milne and 13 alumnae founded the association for purposes of: (1) promoting unity and good feelings among the alumnae of the training school; (2) advancing in every way the professional standing of trained nurses; (3) promoting social intercourse and good fellowship among the said alumnae; (4) extending aid to those in trouble; (5) establishing a fund for the benefit of any sick among the members.[13]

To be eligible, alumnae had to be "in good standing in the profession and possess other qualifications and privileges as [were] . . . provided in the bylaws."[14] There were two classes of membership, *full* for active and *associate* for inactive nurses. Restrictive eligibility requirements caused difficulty from the outset.

ELIGIBILITY, DUES, AND "CONDUCT UNBECOMING A NURSE"

Though the initiation fee of $5 and annual full membership charge of $5 seemed modest, a private duty nurse made $15 per week in 1904, from which all her own expenses were paid and on which she could depend only for an average of 33–35 weeks of work per year.[15] Some simply could not afford the fees. Others, who lived so far away they could not use the benefits to which the dues entitled them, chose to resign and use those funds for more pressing personal needs. When members were in arrears with their dues for two years (later 3), they were dropped from membership.[16] Yet it was often the case that they were in arrears because of need and once dropped from membership, they were, ironically, ineligible for assistance.

Active nurses who married changed to associate status because social custom dictated that married women did not work, and the eligibility requirement identified full members as those in active work. Associate members paid only the initiation fee, but were ineligible to hold office before 1904, seek benefits until 1919, often could not make the evening meetings due to family responsibilities, and gradually many drifted away.[17] The loss of women who married successful men included lost potential finances and prestige as well as the participation of the particular alumnae. Thus, the membership never grew significantly in number, power, or funds. The number of new members each graduation garnered was offset by the attrition of those no longer eligible or able to pay. In modern parlance, the association did not build a "critical mass" of active, contributing members in its early years.[18] In 1916 bylaws changes enabled alumnae to choose full or associate status regardless of work activity.[19] State registration became an additional eligibility requirement in 1918. As a result, new graduates could not join at graduation because they were not yet registered. By the time they were registered and became eligible, as much as a year could have passed and their interest waned. In addition, early graduates whose course of study had not included the number of hours in each clinical specialty area required by registration, or who resided outside of Pennsylvania without reciprocal registration options, could not obtain registration.[20]

The second problematic eligibility issue involved definitions of conduct "unbecoming a nurse" that jeopardized one's "good standing." The terrible nature of hospital care before the reforms of the 1860s and '70s

accustomed people to regard paid nurses as self-seeking menials engaged in something far lower than domestic work, and whose only object was to benefit by others' misfortune at the least expenditure of care or trouble on their own part.[21]

This Dickensian perception and society's general suspicions regarding single working women made early trained nurses particularly sensitive to accusations of misconduct and led the alumnae association to establish "appropriate behavior" as a criterion for membership. The association encouraged reports concerning graduates who had erred so that investigations might be made and the school's honor protected.[22] Examples included one reported by Miss Milne in which "a graduate nurse of our own alumnae who wanted to leave a case . . . had caused a telegram to be sent to her calling her home immediately." The Hospital Board removed her name from the registry. She defended herself, stating her action to be a "customary thing to do." The subsequent investigation bore out the nurse's story that "the practice of having fictitious telegrams sent seemed to be prevalent amongst members of the association especially the more recent graduates."[23] These events were viewed as a "charge made against the Alumnae" which called for resolutions and greater vigilance to uphold the honor of nursing.

Justifying the worst fears of the day, 1906 graduate Mrs. Katherine Field Barr drew accusations that went to the heart of society's concerns about women in general and nurses in particular. Association member Mrs. Sloan met with the 1919 Executive Committee:

> to present to the committee what she had heard concerning Mrs. Katharine Field Barr. . . . Mrs. Barr had nursed Mr. Barr's first wife at the birth of her child. That when the child was four months old Mr. Barr started to call on the present Mrs. Barr and that she had broken up the home. That a Mrs. Mansfield had requested Miss Field and her mother to vacate the apartment they had in her house and that they found Mrs. Barr could see from her apartment Mr. Barr spending his evenings with Miss Field. It was understood that Miss Field announced her engagement to a gentleman without mentioning his name before Mr. Barr obtained his divorce.

Within a week Mrs. Barr met with the executive committee to:

> answer Mrs. Sloan's charges. . . . Mrs. Barr said she had nursed Mrs. Barr, the 1st, twelve months and for two years after leaving, she and the first Mrs. Barr were good friends. That Mr. Barr had obtained his divorce in May of 1918 instead of November 1918 as had been quoted by Mrs. Sloan. That Mrs. Hitch, Mrs. Barr 1st's mother, had tried to get Miss Field into the divorce court but her name was cleared absolutely. . . . Mrs. Sloan begged Mrs. Barr to accept her apology and said she wanted to take back everything she had said at the last executive meeting and that she accepted the court's decision. . . . Mrs. Barr [was thereby] cleared.[24]

Emerging from this tangled web of restrictive and stringent eligibility requirements was an aura of exclusion, abandonment, and nonprotection of members not fitting narrow norms. Some of the aura reflected nineteenth century society's demand that women lead exemplary lives. But many internal matters decided by the association, such as dues and state registration, contributed greatly to this sense of exclusion. It appears the association used membership in its group as a carrot to entice members to conform to certain desired behaviors, such as becoming registered as nurses. But in the long run, the association lost out because fewer graduates chose or were able to join. Thus, these eligibility demands did not advance the stated purposes and supportive intentions of the association, but set up a conflict of loyalty between individual members' needs and the association's needs.

HOSPITAL AS COMPETITOR AND EMPLOYER

Problems about money plagued all nurses of this era and compromised their lives. Whether working through referrals in private duty or specials on a case in the hospitals' private pavilions, which became more common as hospital use increased following World War I,[25] most graduate nurses found their fees subject to hospital scrutiny. Time and again Presbyterian Hospital's graduate nurses sought support from the alumnae association in their negotiations with the hospital. The hospital trustees, seeking to gain income from the training school, sent pupil-nurses into private homes and charged a fee equal to that of the graduate nurses of $15/week, thus setting up the pupil-nurses as competitors, though the hospital kept the public-nurses' fees.[26] In 1902 it took the graduate nurses two years to obtain a $6/week raise.[27] In 1912 they formed a committee to gain a bathroom.[28] By 1919 the nurses petitioned the hospital board for "$32/week without extra charges when nursing a case in the hospital,"[29] and in 1920 the nurses asked that their pay be added to the patient's bill and collected by the registry officer because they had such difficulty collecting their fees.[30]

As an institution in which 90% of its patients obtained free care, as its mission intended, at a cost of $1.40/day in 1891, the hospital's Board of Trustees engaged in an endless battle with the budget.[31] For example, in 1892 the hospital ran over a $10,000 deficit, a substantial figure for that time.[32] Engaging a "force of nurses" to maintain care levels without extending costs required a delicate balance. Private patients provided an important source of income, which could be compromised if these patients had to double their costs by paying private nurses in addition to their hospital rate. Ironically, the nurses found themselves in competition with the hospital, which, at the same time, controlled the nurses' rates. The tension heightened between the nurses seeking self-support and the hospital trustees wanting to do for patients "the least of these my brethren."[33]

The association trod a hesitant path. Unwilling to anger the board, the nurses' representatives postponed action, accepted long periods between petitions to the board and its answers, and ultimately agreed to "nurse a patient at a reduced rate if the hospital deemed it necessary" and to "never ask of their patients in the hospital a higher rate than that asked by the Board."[34] In other words, the association representing the nurses experienced repeated instances of conflict between their commitment to members and their institutional loyalty.

TO NURSE THE NURSES

Two of the association's five founding purposes concerned attending to members who were sick or "in trouble." To meet those goals, the alumnae association's charter asserted that "all moneys from dues and contributions shall constitute the benefit and general expense fund. This fund shall be used toward endowing a bed for sick members in the Presbyterian Hospital in Philadelphia."[35]

In November 1900, the Magee brothers donated one endowed bed and partly endowed a second bed in the alumnae's name, on condition that the alumnae contribute $4,000. The association looked primarily for funds from the constituents it intended to help. The members believed it to be "our own burden and responsibility . . . [to] raise the money through the society instead of asking outsiders."[36] Seeking sources for money led to "entertainments" such as fairs, bazaars, sales of dolls in various hospital training school uniforms and caps, and the like, as well as creating the dues structure described earlier. The second bed-fund reached its goal in October 1902 and provided the core of the association's benefits for its members.

Similarly the Visiting Committee formed at the outset of the association visited "sick members, [to] ascertain their needs and see that they are properly cared for."[37] The illness of Mary S. Young (Class of 1908) represented a case of the fulfillment of this mission.[38] The Visiting Committee first reported her sick in "the form of Tuberculosis" and in the hospital in November 1915. The executive board and Finance Committee sent a nurse with her to Bell's Camp, Pennsylvania, and paid their transportation and board at the sanitarium for the first four weeks.[39] Entries in the association's minutes over a three-year-period trace Miss Young's declining health and the association's help through visits, loans, and gifts. In April 1919 the visitors reported her as "very ill" and in June recorded her death.[40] But married members, members with dues in arrears, and graduates ineligible for membership were not allowed access to these major benefits.

The association's endeavors corresponded to the purposes of fraternal organizations representing many laboring groups in early industrial America and arose from the founding philosophy of the nurses' organization to respond to the needs, illnesses, or death of its members. But, by insisting that the group be its own major source for funds, the association placed itself in a bind. To raise funds from its constituents, it required dues, imposed penalties for dues in arrears, and used members' private time running bazaars and other fund-raisers. The gradual assumption of general welfare responsibilities by the American Nurses' Association (ANA), through its National Nurses Relief Fund and Nurses' Sick Benefit Society in the century's second decade, reduced the individual alumnae associations' major role in "nursing the nurses." As the ANA grew, it attempted to refocus the attention of nurses beyond their local associations to the pressing issues of nursing in the larger world: World War I, seeking rank in the military, establishing licensure, and participating in the newly won vote for women.

POLITICAL ENDEAVORS

The association's founding purposes placed it firmly within the professionalization movement in nursing. It joined the newly formed Nurses Associated Alumnae of the United States and Canada, sending delegates to the annual convention, contributing to the financial support of the national organization and participating in establishing the Pennsylvania State and Philadelphia District derivative groups.[41]

Cooperative efforts began in February 1900 when "a special meeting of the officers of the Pennsylvania, University and Presbyterian Hospital's 'Nurses' Alumnae' [was] held in Pennsylvania Hospital . . . [to discuss] the course of studies suggested by the Associated Alumnae." The three groups decided to share topics and expenses, with the University Hospital Alumnae "taking up English literature [on] 2nd and 4th Mondays. The Pennsylvania Hospital [group]—Parliamentary Law 2nd and 4th Thursdays. Presbyterian Hospital—Current Topic—1st and 3rd Thursday in the month." They printed cards to announce the lectures and the Presbyterian Association empowered its president to hire a teacher.[42]

In subsequent years arrangements varied and other schools joined. Special people were invited to speak on particular topics: Mrs. Bedford Fenwick (nee Ethel Manson) President, International Council of Nurses, came from England in 1901; in 1904, Sophia Palmer, editor of the *American Journal of Nursing*, spoke about the National Associated Alumnae's planned purchase of all the journal stock; Miss Thornton, Secretary of the Associated Alumnae, visited in 1905 and M. Adelaide Nutting, head of the Teachers College program for graduate nurses, addressed the group in 1908.

As collective educational events increased among the Philadelphia Alumnae groups, so did political and organizational efforts. In 1901 the groups met at the College of Physicians to organize and, by year's end, the Committee for Philadelphia Association of Trained Nurses developed a constitution and bylaws and elected officers.[43]

Yet even as the Philadelphia County Association met each Wednesday, worked toward state registration and offered support to a Navy Nurse Bill in Congress, the Presbyterian Alumnae Association voted against affiliation with women's suffrage and rejected membership in the Philadelphia Graduate Nurses' Club.[44] Rather, it turned its attention back to more local, inward concerns: negotiating private nurses schedules and fees with the hospital, giving receptions for new graduates, announcing who was ill, married, had a baby or died, and raising money for charities such as missions in India and China, sister alumnae associations' sick bed funds, San Francisco nurses in need (after the fire), and the purchase of dishes and silver for alumnae receptions.

When the State Registration bill failed to pass the state legislature in 1907, Miss Milne chastised the group, declaring the "failure of the bill being due to two causes, 1st the indifference of the nurses themselves, 2nd the failure of the nurses to care for patients of moderate means."[45] Though individual Presbyterian Alumnae continued important work in the state and national associations (Miss Dunlop was elected President of the state association in 1920), the focus of the group as a whole remained what historian Nancy Tomes reported from the Pennsylvania Hospital Training School as a self-proclaimed "little world of their own."[46]

GOOD FELLOWSHIP

From its inception, the promotion of unity, good feeling, social inter-course, and good fellowship formed a core motivation and the most last-ing function of this alumnae association and many other small American ethnic, religious and/or occupationally relevant groups of the early twen-tieth century. As larger organizations assumed responsibility for the health, welfare, and political activity of American citizens, including eventually the federalization of some protective endeavors, the social functions of associations became more and more their predominant theme and activity.

In its early years, for example, the Presbyterian Alumnae Association meetings always featured a speaker and topics of professional or edu-cational interest. In 1897, Miss Lantz spoke on "Small Hospitals" and Dr. John Swan on "Antitoxin." In 1898–9, a series of talks reminded the nurses of their "Responsibility to the Public," "to the Patient and Physician," and "to her sister nurses." By 1907 the topics expanded to "District Work," "Progress and Benefits of State Registration," "History of Nursing," "General Hints on Private Nursing," "Traveling with a Patient," and the practical demonstration of how to manage an "Operation in a private house."[47]

Not forgotten were the eight members "in the field" of the Spanish-American War or, later, the over 50 members nursing in World War I camps at home and bases abroad. Miss Milne's reading of "letters from our nurses in the war zone" became a regular meeting feature even before America's 1917 entry into the war.[48] As the war effort increased, the asso-ciation's business became preoccupied with related activities: raising money to purchase dressings for the Red Cross Division of Emergency Aid, responding to Miss Dunlop's request from Paris for volunteers, lis-tening to a Mrs. Martin from the Pennsylvania Women's Division for National Preparedness on "the nursing side of the subject" and Miss Jane Delano on the National Red Cross. A roll of honor was started to hang in the nurses' home to honor the more than fifty nurses serving their country by 1918.[49] Nonetheless, the lectures continued (such as on "Eugenics and Heredity"), members visited (such as Miss Young in this period), and reports were made of marriages, births, and deaths.

UNRESOLVED CONFLICTS

Though formed to extend benefits to needy members, the association imposed eligibility requirements, such as up-to-date dues payments, that often blocked access of the most needy. Though an original journal stockholder (later American Journal of Nursing Company), and founding member of the Nurses' Associated Alumnae (later American Nurses' Association) and Superintendents' Society (later National League for Nursing), the association voted against affiliation with women's suffrage, rejected membership in the Philadelphia Graduate Nurses' Club, and equivocated in graduate nursing salary negotiations with the hospital board. Focused on their home hospital and its local concerns, the nurses opted time and again to preserve the hospital as a "little world of our own" creating and protecting their particular domestic sphere. Unwilling or unable to marry, living distant from their families and bonding to each other as sisters, many of these early nurses concentrated their attention, affection, and loyalty on the hospital as the focus of their meaningful work and, arguably, a substitute domestic center. As historian Vicinus points out: turn-of-the-century women "could not easily escape stereotypes of behavior and expectation. Immersed in old ideologies and patterns, women replicated [domestic] relationships"and engaged in "the continuing struggle to build a new family."[50]

As a result, the protection of graduate nurses was not the single motive, value, or focus of the alumnae association. Maintenance of the hospital asserted an equal claim. It seems that the nurses, as prototypical members of their nineteenth-century culture, were acting out the female social roles of nurturance, self-sacrifice, and commitment to the good of others. In such a context, they exchanged the private sphere of the home for the public institution of the hospital as niches in which to exercise their roles and apply their values. Believing that their new "family" would protect their interests in compensation for their efforts, they relied upon the hospital board for financial and legal advice even as the board restricted their salaries and living conditions in order to balance the hospital's books.

Alumnae who married or moved beyond the hospital sphere either through distance or more independent practice lost contact and power within the association, which met always at the hospital at times convenient to hospital schedules. As the bigger world asserted its charms, many talented alumnae went on to other things—larger nursing associations, jobs in other places, the military, missions, public health, marriage and families. Through its exclusionary eligibility policies, the association ensured that the alumnae who left the "home" hospital sphere had smaller voices. The gradual falling away of these more worldly members restricted the association's access to their ideas, experiences, and purses, and reinforced the parochial, domestic course set by the association within the hospital walls.

Nurses such as those whose story is told in this paper were firstly women. At the time these events occurred they were without franchise as citizens and without domestic base as women: They did not control any base so their conversion of what base they had in the workplace into the only one that carried power for women, a domestic sphere with related domestic-like loyalties, seems in retrospect neither surprising nor misguided. But their assumption that the hospital was analogous to the domestic sphere in which they could comfortably associate was mistaken and their loyalty sometimes unappreciated. Their identification with an institution (local) to the exclusion of a profession (national) hindered their achievement of their own goals and as a result of multiple divided loyalties, the nurses did not meet the organizational goals they set for themselves.

ACKNOWLEDGMENTS

Research for this chapter was supported by a National Research Service Award from the National Center for Nursing Research, National Institutes of Health, Professor Charles E. Rosenberg, Sponsor; and, by a Small Projects Grant, Center for Nursing Research, University of Pennsylvania School of Nursing.

The author wishes to acknowledge the assistance of Joan Lynaugh in preparation of this work.

NOTES

1. Ellen D. Baer "Nursings Divided House—An Historical View," *Nursing Research* 34(1), pp. 32–38; Ellen D. Baer "'A Cooperative Venture' in Search of Professional Status: A Research Journal for Nursing," *Nursing Research,* 36(1), pp. 18–25.
2. Martha Vicinus, *Independent Women Work and Community for Single Women, 1850–1920* (Chicago: University of Chicago Press, 1985), p. 1.
3. Mary Williams Brinton, *My Cap and My Cape An Autobiography* (Philadelphia: Dorrance & Co., 1950), foreword.
4. Susan Reverby, *Ordered to Care: The Dilemma of American Nursing, 1850–1945* (New York: Cambridge University Press, 1987).
5. Lavinia L. Dock, *A History of Nursing,* Vol. III (New York: G. P. Putnam's Sons, 1912) p. 125.

6. Isabel A. Hampton and others, *Nursing of the Sick, 1893* (New York: McGraw Hill Book Co., 1949) p. 157–158.

7. Ellen D. Baer "Nursings Divided House-An Historical View," Nursing Research, 34(1), p. 32–38.

8. Arlowayne Swort, "The ANA: The Formative Years, 1875–1922," Unpublished Doctoral Dissertation (New York: Teachers College, 1973) pp. 84–86 identifies six alumnae associations before the 1893 Fair and rapid growth thereafter.

9. James E. Talley, M. D. "The Presbyterian Hospital in Philadelphia" In Frederick P. Henry, A. M., M. D. (Ed), *Founders Week Memorial Volume* (Philadelphia: F. A. Davis, 1909) p. 690. Minutes of Board of Trustees, Presbyterian Hospital, December, 1889, p. 81, describe the demise of the Alliance. Presbyterian Hospital Health Science Library Archives.

10. Talley, "The Presbyterian Hospital," 695, 702.

11. Caroline I. Farnum, Directress, First Report of the Training School of the Presbyterian Hospital, reprint in the 37th Annual Report of the Alumnae Association, 1939, Presbyterian Hospital Nursing Education Building, Director's Office Archives. Miss Caroline Farnum (a Philadelphia Hospital 1889 graduate) was Directress until 1891. Subsequent directresses included Alice Brownlee (Royal Victoria Hospital, Belfast) for one year, Lucy Walker (St. Bartholomews, London) for two years, Caroline Milne (St. Bartholomews, London) for twenty-five years, Mary Close Eden (Presbyterian Hospital, '01) 1920–1936, Helen Leader (Protestant Episcopal), 1936–1952, Mary Ellen Brown (Presbyterian Hospital, '40) 1952–1966, Dorothy Richards (Presbyterian Hospital, '37), 1966–1977, Doris Zell Wardell (Chestnut Hill Hospital, '60) 1977–1978, Florence Crawford (Presbyterian Hospital, '63) 1978–1979, Mary Ann Morgan (Presbyterian Hospital, '52) 1979–1984, and Josephine Cantone (Fitzgerald-Mercy, '71) 1984–1987. Mary Beth Byrnes "Celebrating 100 Years of Excellence in Nursing Education," Commemorative Pamphlet, Philadelphia: Presbyterian School of Nursing at Presbyterian-University of Pennsylvania Medical Center, May 1, 1987.

12. Lucy Walker-Donnell letter to Lilian Lavelle with notes by Margaret Dunlop, August 1939, scrapbook, Director's Office, Presbyterian Hospital School of Nursing Archives. In these notes, Miss Walker who adopted a family name Donnell with hyphen after her 1907 retirement from The Pennsylvania Hospital Training School for Nurses, asserted that she started the alumnae association in 1894 and wrote the bylaws "personally, without aid." Corroboration of this assertion is not available, though the plan was proposed to the first Superintendents' Society meetings in 1893 and 1894 which Miss Walker attended.

13. Ledger I of Alumnae Association Minutes, June 3, 1897, pp. 3–4. Alumnae named Davenport, Ambler, Trout, Foster, Stuart, Lisle, Howard, Zanet, Neeke, Manly, Brown, Dunlop and Cope.

14. Ledger I of Alumnae Association Minutes, June 3, 1897, p. 4.

15. Reverby, *op cit*, p. 102.

16. Ledger I of Alumnae Association Charter, Fees, p. 11 and May 23, 1898, p. 18. January, 1905, p. 85, executive committee decided arrears dues must be paid before alumna can use endowed sick bed. November 17, 1915, p. 287, executive committee decided that members three years in arrears be dropped from association.

17. Ledger I of Alumnae Association Minutes, May 1904, p. 73. Ledger II of Alumnae Association Minutes, March 12, 1919, p. 40.

18. Ledger I of Alumnae Association Minutes, May 1906, p. 113, 103 active and 26 associate members, provided a 4:1 ratio of fees paid to not paid; In May 1910, p. 184, 137 active and 36 associate members yielded 3.8:1 ratio of fees paid to not paid; In May 1913, p. 244, 157 active and 50 associate members yielded a 3:1 ratio; and, In May 1916, p. 296, there were 169 active and 65 associate members, a 2.6:1 ratio of fee paying vs. non-paying members.

19. Ledger I of Alumnae Association Minutes, February 1916, p. 291, recorded the attempt of the association to change its name to "Graduate Nurses of Presbyterian Hospital" with two classes of membership offered to members who could choose their level of membership so that distance and marriage need not limit participation. Hospital board lawyer Bedford advised against the change. At the annual meeting in May 1916, pp. 299-300, they voted in reinstatement of members dropped for dues or poor conduct and other changes except non-resident membership status which might have retained greater participation by distant members. Subsequently, married members did choose to remain active, for example 4 of 8 members who married in 1917, Ledger-II, p. 11.

20. Ledger II of Alumnae Association Minutes, pp. 32, 135. See also letters on registration difficulties across states, alumnae Etta L. Gile, Ledger entitled *Epitome of Training School Candidates,* p. 587. The registration requirements were initiated by ANA, not the individual association.

21. Isabel Hampton Robb, *Nursing Ethics for Hospital and Private Use* (Cleveland: E. C. Koeckert, 1916, Copyright 1900 to Mrs. Robb) p. 28.

22. Ledger I of Alumnae Association Minutes, October 11, 1910, p. 201 and February 1911, p. 201, report on such a case in which "Miss Muffly" who was dropped from the membership for "undesirable conduct" after a communication requesting "an explanation of her conduct" brought an unsatisfactory and unreported response.

23. Ledger I of Alumnae Association Minutes, January 12, 1909, p. 158 and February 9, 1909, p. 159.

24. Ledger I of Alumnae Association Minutes, April 9, 1919, pp. 40–41.

25. Reverby, *op cit,* 103.

26. Minutes of Board of Trustees of Presbyterian Hospital, Volume 5, 1891, pp. 153, 193 and 1892, p. 219. Presbyterian Hospital Health Science Library Archives.

27. Ledger I of Alumnae Association, February 24, 1902, p. 53, first notations of discussions. May 12, 1902, p. 57, noted petition to Board for an "increase in Graduate Nurses pay"; June 3, 1902, p. 59, petition recorded and sent. October 14, 1902, p. 61, Household Committee of Board referred problem to executive committee of hospital. November 1903, pp. 67–68, discussed what to do again at alumnae association meeting and postponed decision to next meeting. January 1904, pp. 69–70, discussed again and new petition sent to Household Committee of Board requesting a "reconsideration" and reporting that the "other important hospitals in Philadelphia" pay nurses their "full fee, usually $21.00 per week" when the nurse is nursing a patient in the hospital. In March 1904, p. 71, the Board granted the request for graduate nurses to charge their usual fee when nursing in hospital provided that "graduates should nurse a patient at a reduced rate if the hospital deemed it necessary" and "graduates should never ask of their patients in the hospital a higher rate than that asked by the Board."

28. Ledger I of Alumnae Association Minutes, April 1912, p. 221.

29. Ledger II of Alumnae Association Minutes, October 1919, p. 53.

30. Ibid., November 1920, p. 72.

31. Minutes of Board of Trustees of Presbyterian Hospital, Volume 5, 1891, pp. 170 and 182–83. Presbyterian Hospital Health Science Library Archives.

32. Ibid., p. 266.

33. *The Presbyterian Hospital in Philadelphia, History, Charter and By Laws* (Philadelphia: Alfred Martien, 1871) p. 21 in quoting the New Testament as the guide for the institution's mission.

34. Ledger I of Alumnae Association Minutes, March 1904, p. 71.

35. Ledger I of Alumnae Association Minutes, p. 11. The use of the endowed beds was subsequently reported annually by number of days per year, 150–200 range common.

36. Ledger II of Alumnae Association Minutes, p. 86.

37. Ledger II of Alumnae Association Minutes, p. 10.

38. School entry notes and Ledger entitled *Epitome of Training School candidates as they are admitted on probation and are accepted or rejected with brief synopsis of character and work in the Presbyterian Hospital,* Book II, 1904, p. 309 records that Miss Young, born January 13, 1883 and living in Bradford, Pennsylvania, "entered into probation" (as Miss Milne always called it) in 1904. After a 1908 graduation, delayed due to illness during training, she became a private nurse for four years and a Philadelphia school nurse until her January 1916 resignation due to ill health.

39. Ledger I of Alumnae Association Minutes, November 1915, p. 287 and December 1915, 288–89, and May 1916, p. 297.

40. Ledger II of Alumnae Association Minutes, pp. 2, 9–10,17–18, 37–38, 44–48.

41. Ledger I of Alumnae Association Minutes, November 1897, p. 13; March 1898, p. 16; May 1898, p. 17 reported the earliest efforts. Philadelphia Association efforts took formal shape from October–December 1901, pp. 47–51. Philadelphia County, forerunner to a state association, formed April 1903, p. 64.

42. Ibid., February 1900, pp. 27–29.

43. Cf. 35, President, Miss Walker of Pennsylvania Hospital; Vice Presidents, Miss Smith of Philadelphia Hospital, Miss Ramsden of University Hospital, and Miss Harris of Episcopal Hospital; Secretary, Miss Anders of Presbyterian; Treasurer, Miss Fulum of Pennsylvania and five councillors, one from each alumnae group.

44. Ledger I of Alumnae Association Minutes, October 9, 1906, p. 119: "Papers were read from Miss Dock and The National American Women's Suffrage Association, asking us to act as a society and as individuals for the Women's Suffrage bill." It was moved "that as an association we take no part in the Women's Suffrage question." No further discussion or action is noted, though speeches were given from time to time to the group. Ledger I of Alumnae Association Minutes, June 6, 1905, p. 97, discussed "advisability of concurring with local associations to establish a private registry for nurses." Full discussion postponed. On October 10, 1905 (p. 100), local alumnae associations join to start a Graduate Nurses Club House in Philadelphia with a Directory at 13th and Locust Streets. On December 12, 1905 (p. 102), was discussed an idea for a club room or house in which nurses could rent rooms, belong to the association, and pay dues. On January 9, 1906, the costs of the house were discussed ($55–65/month for a room in a 13–14-room house, a furnished house at $75/month, and a suite of rooms at $45–50, including light and heat); p. 105, voted not to join other city alumnae in forming a stock cornpany. May 2, 1906, p. 113, annual meeting voted not to enter city club house as a group, only as individuals. February 9, 1909, p. 160, the Graduate Nurses Club sought new members and the association sent $100 to help. In February 1910 (p. 181), the club asked Presbyterian to give up its own registry to join the club and the alumnae voted no again.

45. Ledger I of Alumnae Association Minutes, p. 137.

46. Nancy Tomes, "'Little World of Our Own': The Pennsylvania Hospital Training School for Nurses, 1895–1907," *Journal of the History of Medicine and Allied Sciences* 33 (1978):507–530.

47. Ledger I of Alumnae Association Minutes, pp. 21–25, 122. Unfortunately, the texts have not been found so the titles are our guides as to content.

48. Ibid., November 1914, p. 269; January 1915, p. 273.

49. Ibid., April 1915, p. 277; January 1916, p. 289; February 1916, p. 291. In January 1918, a hospital unit from Presbyterian Hospital sailed to Europe, Ledger II, p. 20; p. 22.

50. Martha Vicinus, *Independent Women*: work and community for single women 1850–1920. (Chicago: University of Chicago Press, 1985) p. 161.

CHAPTER 7

"A Necessity in the Nursing World": The Chicago Nurses Professional Registry, 1913–1950

Jean C. Whelan

In 1923, Lucy Van Frank, head registrar of the Chicago-based Nurses Professional Registry, addressed the annual meeting of the Illinois State Nurses Association (ISNA).[1] The main topic of her talk centered on the problems encountered in administering a private duty registry. However, Van Frank seized the opportunity to emphasize the importance of the establishment of nurse-owned and -operated central registries. Central registries were agencies that placed private duty nurses with patients and provided a source of jobs for nurses in a particular locality. Van Frank's remarks focused specifically on central registries owned and operated either by or in close affiliation with a professional association of nurses, the formation of which was a growing movement among nurses in the early twentieth century.[2] Van Frank's comments left no doubt in the audience's mind of the value she placed on central registries. She declared: "They are now considered as much a necessity in the nursing world as are commercial bureaus in the business world, and as essential a part of the

This chapter was originally published in the *Nursing History Review*, 2005; 13:49–75. Copyright Springer Publishing Company. Reprinted with permission.

great plan of caring for the sick, as is the system of Training Schools in the hospitals."[3]

Van Frank's position as head of one of the largest and fastest-growing central registries in the United States most likely influenced her view of central registries. But many in the professional nursing world of the 1920s agreed absolutely with her assessment.[4] Private duty registries offered early twentieth-century nurses a convenient means of obtaining work, and professional registries, run specifically by and for nurses, were a vehicle through which nurses could achieve a degree of independent practice and autonomy. Contemporary nursing leaders urged nurses to align with professional registries and forecast the future of nursing as centering around these organizations.

Yet by the mid-twentieth century the vision Van Frank and other nurse leaders held for private duty registries owned and operated by nurses remained unfulfilled. The radical changes in the ways nurses were employed, created by the demands of an acute care-centered modern hospital system, would render professional private duty registries obsolete.

This chapter records the rise and demise of professional private duty registries as demonstrated by the experience of the Chicago Nurses Professional Registry during the years 1913–1950. I examine the origins of the private duty system, describe how private nurses were distributed to patients, and analyze patterns of supply and demand for nursing services. My perspective differs from previous interpretations, which generally attribute the demise of private duty to the circumstances surrounding the Great Depression.[5] I argue that the private duty nurse market remained viable and very important until sometime after World War II. Private duty nursing declined, not as a direct result of changes taking place in the 1930s, but rather several years later as a consequence of the inability of the labor market to supply sufficient numbers of nurses to meet heightened demand for their services. This examination recognizes the significance of changes during the 1930s but stresses the importance of fluctuating patterns of supply and demand as a major factor in nurse employment arrangements and how they affected the nurse labor market and created vast changes in the ways nurses were employed.

Highlighting the importance of how supply and demand functions in the nurse labor market refines our understanding of the transformation of nurses from independent private practitioners to hospital employees. Examining this intriguing nurse job market offers a unique view of nurses' work and illuminates the foundations on which the contemporary labor market for nurses was formed.

BEGINNINGS: BUSINESSES OWNED AND OPERATED
BY NURSES

The genesis of private duty nursing lies in the peculiar system of hospital-based nursing education that began in the nineteenth century and combined education with employment in the same body of workers. By 1900, 432 hospital schools of nursing were operating in the United States, using what has been called an apprenticeship type of training.[6] Students worked in the hospital, learning whatever nursing procedures the particular institution provided for its patients. After 3 years, they were given a diploma and sent out to find employment.

As hospitals did not hire their own graduates, the majority of nurses sought work in the private duty sector. Private duty nursing meant the direct employment of an individual nurse by a patient. A patient or family hired a nurse either upon the advice of the attending physician or when the family's ability to care for ill members was insufficient. Late nineteenth-century private duty nurses, typically employed for the duration of an illness, generally provided care to patients in their own homes on a 24-hour, 7-day-a-week basis.[7] When middle-class patients began to seek hospital care, private duty nurses followed their patients into the hospital. The setting changed, but the work arrangement remained the same. Nurses were hired by patients, who assumed full responsibility for paying them. The nurse delivered whatever nursing services the patient required.

The success of nursing schools in establishing professional nursing as a necessary requisite for care of the ill ensured a demand for private duty services, and nurses eagerly took on the job of setting up the conventions of the work. How to connect easily with patients, however, was a perplexing problem for early private duty nurses. Chronicles of private duty nursing in the late nineteenth century indicate that physicians or patients requiring the services of a graduate nurse relied on local knowledge of which nurses were competent and available for taking patients.[8] This word-of-mouth method of securing a nurse was sufficient for rural or low-population areas, but large cities or towns required a more systematic method of hiring nurses. Nurses needed a reliable way to seek cases; patients and physicians needed an easy means of obtaining nurses and verifying their capabilities.

Several options for connecting with patients existed for nurses. For many the most familiar way involved a private duty registry affiliated with a specific hospital. Hospital-based registries, often operated by alumnae associations of the hospital nursing school, listed nurses, referred to as registrants, who were available for private duty.[9] By 1896, approximately 40 alumnae associations existed across the country, several of which operated private duty registries.[10] Persons who wanted a nurse contacted the registry, which then sent out a suitable candidate. By sending only nurses who held a diploma from the specific hospital's school, the registry verified that the nurse met school standards, however high or low those standards might be. The registry thus served as a rudimentary credentialing system.

Hospital-based registries were convenient for nurses who lived close to the hospital from which they graduated. Nurses who moved away from their home hospital, however, lost the benefit of the registry, as these registries usually served only a local area. Furthermore, patients who resided some distance from a hospital and those in hospitals without a school of nursing had difficulty obtaining nurses. The idea that private duty nurse services could be centralized for a locality began to gain favor from nurses in the last decades of the nineteenth century.[11]

Centralized registries were intended to enroll nurses who did not belong to a local hospital-based registry or who were willing to accept cases in a number of different hospitals. Physicians and patients who needed a nurse could contact a central registry, which would assume responsibility for locating the nurse and sending her to the patient. The benefits of a centralized registry seemed obvious. The need for only one contact to one agency meant less time spent trying to locate a nurse. The registry assumed responsibility for checking the credentials of the nurses enrolled on it, lessening the possibility that an unqualified nurse would be sent to a patient. Presumably, a centralized registry serving an entire city or region would receive a greater volume of calls for nurses, thus ensuring steady employment for the nurse registrants.

By the turn of the century, a number of different types of centralized registries existed and were available to nurses seeking work. Commercial employment bureaus often placed nurses with patients, serving as one means through which nurses could obtain patient cases. In Chicago, by 1923, 25 commercial registries placing nurses were in business.[12] Contemporary nurse leaders, however, viewed commercial agencies with suspicion. Articles in professional nursing journals frequently referred to commercial agencies in disparaging terms, citing their profit motives, the high fees charged nurses for placement, and their practice of sending out untrained workers as nurses. Nurse leaders, such as Lavinia Dock, cautioned nurses to avoid such agencies when seeking employment. Dock claimed commercial agencies were run by unfit lay people who not only charged nurses a fee for services but took a portion of their earnings as well.[13]

In some cities, medical societies and libraries operated revenue-generating centralized registries. These registries, many of which were established in the late nineteenth century, operated as a convenience for physician members and had the added advantage of providing a source of income for the sponsoring organization. In 1879, the Medical Library

Association of Boston established the Boston Medical Library Directory for Nurses, considered to be the first of its kind.[14] Philadelphia physicians, frustrated by difficulties in obtaining the services of trained nurses for their patients, founded the Directory for Nurses of the College of Physicians in 1882. This registry remained in business for 54 years.[15]

As was the case with commercial employment agencies, registries operated by medical groups often came under criticism from nursing groups. Dock, a relentless critic of registries operated by those outside the nursing profession, claimed that medical society registries created local monopolies and often intimidated nurses into accepting physician-set rules.[16] Yet the success of physician-controlled and other commercial nurse placement ventures also convinced nurse leaders that establishing nurse-run centralized registries was an achievable goal. By the end of the nineteenth century, the idea that centralized registries should be nurse owned, nurse operated, and nurse controlled had become popular in organized nursing.[17] And whereas the convenience of using one agency to provide nursing service was a prime driving force behind the establishment of many of the original registries, the central registry movement was more than just a handy way for nurses to acquire jobs.

The benefits of nurse-owned and -operated private duty registries were evident to early nurse leaders such as Isabel Hampton Robb and Lavinia L. Dock. Both Robb and Dock recognized the potential for nurses to control their own practice via nurse-controlled registries and spoke to the issue in professional meetings. Dock addressed the subject in a paper presented in 1895 at the Second Annual Convention of the American Society of Superintendents of Training Schools for Nurses. She strongly recommended the establishment of nurse-owned and -operated central registries as one means of strengthening a professional spirit among nurses. Robb echoed Dock's remarks, forcefully arguing that nurse-operated central registries were the best mechanism for controlling nursing practice in a city and keeping outside forces from interfering with nurses' work.[18]

Professional nurse leaders did not wish to limit the business of centralized registries to the private duty market. Registries were encouraged to serve as placement agencies for hospitals and other health-related agencies interested in filling positions for nurses.[19] By offering a complete line of nursing services, leaders hoped the central registry would become the prime distributor of nurses to all those who needed nursing services whether at home or in the hospital. Some envisioned statewide networks of central registries with one headquarters connected to smaller centers. Nurses enrolled on the registries could be moved about and distributed throughout the state as local needs required, promoting more efficient use of nursing services and providing greater opportunities for nurses to obtain cases.[20]

To achieve such a wide array of goals was a large undertaking. Nurse leaders believed that objectives could be met more easily by connecting the nurse-run central registry to a local professional nurse association.[21] An already organized nurse association offered a structure for readily establishing a registry. The perceived interest of a local nurse association in wider community affairs was, of course, considered an asset in providing systematic nursing services. Members of professional nurse associations included individuals who could give the benefits of their leadership experience to registry governance. Professional nursing journals in the initial years of the twentieth century reported enthusiastically on the establishment of a number of local nurse association–sponsored central registries.[22] These formed the nucleus of what would later be known as professional private duty registries, the type of registries to which Lucy Van Frank referred in her 1923 talk to the ISNA.[23] And it was Van Frank's Chicago Nurses Professional Registry that best exemplified the ideals of what a professional nurse registry was meant to be.

CHICAGO: THE GOLDEN YEARS FOR PROFESSIONAL REGISTRIES

Illinois had possessed all the necessary elements for operating a successful central registry. The ISNA, formed in 1901, was one of the earliest and best organized state nurse associations in the nation. In 1911, the state association, originally composed of nursing school alumnae associations, began a reorganization process that resulted in the establishment of local components called district nurse associations. Shortly thereafter, in 1912, nurses in Cook, DuPage, and Lake Counties formed the Chicago-area nurses association, named the First District of the Illinois State Nurses Association. Due to its location in the state's largest city and its ample nurse population, the Chicago district became the center of nursing activity in Illinois.[24]

Members of the new district association quickly went to work on achieving one of the main district objectives: to establish a centralized registry. They were aware that nurse-run central registries flourished in a number of other cities. Chicago offered a promising environment in which to open a registry. At the time, Chicago was the second largest city in the United States and well known for its fast pace and rapid growth.[25] Its large population promised a supply of patients in need of private care. It was home to many of the nation's leading medical facilities, which provided the necessary demand for professional nurse services.[26] By 1913 more than 32 schools of nursing were operating within and around the city, guaranteeing a sufficient number of nurses interested in working in the private duty market.[27]

The Central Registry, originally called the Central Directory and later renamed the Nurses Professional Registry (NPR), opened its doors for services in 1913.[28] Under the direction of Van Frank, who would serve as director for its first three decades, the registry was organized along lines similar to other professional registries of the day. Nurses meeting the qualifications of the registry—usually referred to as registrants—paid a fee to enroll as members. In return, they received all the privileges of membership. When a nurse decided she wanted to work, she placed her name on the list of nurses on call. Nurses were assigned to patients as the registry received requests. A nurse not wishing to take on patients simply did not place her name on the list, or removed it.[29]

The new registry met with immediate success in delivering private duty services and experienced tremendous growth in a very short period of time. One month after the NPR opened for business, it claimed 150 members and averaged eight nurse placements a day; it ended its first year of operation with over 500 members.[30] By its ten-year anniversary in 1923, registry membership hovered around 950 and received more than 11,000 yearly requests for nurses, a considerable number by professional registry standards.[31]

What accounted for this rapid expansion? The NPR was quickly able to mobilize and capitalize on considerable financial and moral support from the Chicago nursing community. The city had a well-organized group of active school-of-nursing alumnae associations, several of which were instrumental in forming the Chicago district and advancing the concept of a central registry. The relationship between these alumnae associations and the NPR was both cooperative and collegial. The associations donated substantial amounts of money to cover the initial expense of launching the NPR. Contributions amounting to $500 were received from the Illinois Training School for Nurses and St. Luke's Hospital alumnae associations. The Michael Reese Hospital alumnae association contributed in excess of $350, and others donated $100 or more each.[32]

In addition to financial support, several area alumnae associations agreed to turn over their own private duty registries to the NPR, thus enlarging its membership. The Illinois Training School for Nurses and Presbyterian Hospital registries were the first to join, bringing in a large number of nurse registrants. By the mid-1930s, twelve alumnae association registries would be listed as NPR members.[33]

The benefits accruing to the NPR from aligning with the alumnae associations were significant. The large number of registrants the alumnae associations brought into the registry, all paying registry fees, ensured financial solvency for the NPR. The arrangement benefited the alumnae associations as well. Joining the NPR spared the associations the expense and effort of running separate registries, while at the same time they received credit for providing means for members to obtain work. Nurses enrolled on the NPR but not aligned with a specific alumnae association (e.g., nurses who had graduated from schools outside the Chicago area) also gained. Tradition required that when an alumnae association registry joined the NPR, the registry would keep a separate list of affiliated alumnae association members. The hospital's own graduates received preference for calls received from the association's home hospital. When such a nurse was unavailable, a non–alumnae association nurse was sent. This improved work opportunities for all registrants, increased the chances of filling a request for a nurse, and resulted in more nurses finding employment.

A PREMIER PRIVATE DUTY REGISTRY

By the mid-1920s, the conventions of modern private duty nursing were well established. Nurses cared for patients primarily in acute care hospital settings, generally working twelve-hour shifts.[34] As the NPR entered its second decade of operation, the business affairs of the registry were extremely encouraging. Each year the NPR recorded more success than the year before. From 1923 to 1929, the average number of monthly patient assignments rose 178%, from 919 to 2,555, and membership doubled to almost 2,000 registrants.[35] The NPR's membership represented a significant portion of graduate nurses, not just from Chicago but from Illinois as a whole: 9% of the state nurses and 17% of the city area nurses in 1930.[36] The twelve affiliated alumnae associations represented some of the largest hospitals in Chicago and surrounding areas. Presbyterian, Mercy, and St. Luke's had more than 400 beds each; Augustana and West Surburban had more than 300 beds.[37] The NPR provided a stable number of registrants and served as a reliable source of patient calls in the Chicago area. Enough confidence existed in 1927 to permit a private duty fee increase from $6 to $7 for twelve-hour cases.[38] Registry records indicated a financially healthy enterprise. In 1929, the NPR recorded an impressive profit of almost $11,000.[39]

To manage the large numbers of members and patient requests for nurses, the NPR increased its staff, secured larger offices, and installed a switchboard service during the 1920s.[40] By 1930, the staff was composed of a registrar and five assistants, all registered nurses.[41] The NPR developed plans to expand services offered to patients, nurses, and health care agencies by providing hourly nursing services and institutional placement services.[42] First District took pride in the NPR, reporting on tributes it received, such as the warm appreciation expressed by Illinois Central

Hospital for the promptness with which NPR nurses responded to and cared for victims of a 1926 train wreck.[43]

Amid the many accomplishments achieved by the NPR it is well to keep in mind one serious limitation. The NPR, which intended to be the main distributor of all nurses for the Chicago area, simply was not. Reflecting the deplorable racist attitudes and common exclusionary practices of the times, the NPR was open to only a select population of nurses—those who were white. This situation did not change until the 1940s, when minority nurses first began appearing on the membership rolls. When asked about the placement of African American nurses, Minnie Aherns, executive secretary of the Chicago District, justified the segregated policy. Commenting on the reasons African American nurses were excluded by the registry, Aherns said, "We cannot place them, the social differences are too great."[44]

PRIVATE DUTY NURSING: A LABOR MARKET IN DISTRESS

The success of the NPR in placing private duty nurses, though impressive, took place in a labor market plagued by serious problems. Private duty nursing had always been an unreliable means of making a living, and by the end of the 1920s difficulties that had been identified at the beginning of the century were reaching crisis proportions.

The main issue was a substantial imbalance between supply of and demand for private duty nurse services. There were just too many nurses seeking work in a labor market in which jobs were few and employment uneven. During the 1920s, the number of schools nationwide increased substantially, from around 1,775 in 1920 to 2,286 in 1928, and the number of nurses doubled from 104,000 in 1920 to 214,000 in 1930.[45] Most of these nurses continued to seek work in the private duty field. While the percentage of nurses working as private duty nurses declined from 80% in 1920 to approximately 55% in 1930, the actual number of private duty nurses stabilized at a little over 100,000.[46] This would not have been a major concern except that demand for private duty services remained flat.

Private duty nursing was expensive. By the end of the 1920s, the average fee was around $6–7 dollars for a 12-hour shift. In a cash-based system, a patient needed to have a ready supply of money to pay the nurse. At a time when the average American could barely afford hospital or medical care, another $80 to $100 dollars a week for private nurses was out of reach for most.[47]

Studies carried out during the late 1920s validated the idea that the nursing education system had produced too many nurses for the amount of work available. The Committee on the Grading of Nursing Schools' (CGNS) study on private duty nursing, published in 1928 as *Nurses, Patients, and Pocketbooks,* recorded a dismal picture of the field, documenting dangerously low employment levels for private duty nurses and salaries that trailed considerably behind those for nurses employed in other fields.[48] Equally troubling was the revelation that private duty nurses were increasingly disenchanted with their work: 36% of private duty nurses surveyed indicated that they planned to leave the field in the near future.[49]

Private duty nurses were not alone in expressing discontent. Professional nurse leaders began to question the value of private duty nursing as a legitimate occupational field for the majority of nurses. In the early part of the century, it was commonly accepted that most nurses would spend part of their career in private duty. By the late 1920s, however, many saw a different future for nursing, one more closely tied to hospital employment. Private duty was described as an inefficient method of patient care delivery, one that wasted precious nurse resources on a limited number of patients.[50] The CGNS suggested sweeping changes, recommending that, whereas elements of the private system of nurse distribution should remain in place, the majority of nurses should seek employment in hospitals.[51]

Despite dissatisfaction expressed by private duty nurses and a growing consensus among nurse leaders that private duty as an occupational field was in decline, the private duty labor market continued to demonstrate significant resilience. The negative reports on private duty during the 1920s and the conviction of leaders that change was necessary may in fact have overstated nurse unhappiness with the field. If read from the opposite point of view, the CGNS findings reveal that the majority of the nurses surveyed, 55%, intended to remain private duty nurses.[52] Comments from nurses received by the CGNS also indicated that although private duty nurses identified many areas of complaints, particularly in relation to pay and working conditions, they clearly enjoyed bedside nursing. One nurse from Massachusetts succinctly described her feelings: "Personally, I like private duty even though it is harder; you come in close touch with your patient and see better the results of your work."[53] A New York nurse expressed similar thoughts but added a proviso, "I love my work. I don't regret that I have taken up nursing as a profession, but I do ask for a square deal."[54]

Van Frank observed a high degree of loyalty on the part of nurses to the field, noting that nurses would accept jobs in hospitals in slow periods when calls were scarce but would leave them as soon as the private duty market picked up.[55] Private duty may well have been a field with significant difficulties, but it was also one in which nurses experienced pride in their work and contentment with their practice.

THE GREAT DEPRESSION YEARS: BEGINNING THE TRANSFORMATION

The collapse of the economy in 1929 brought havoc and despair to the lives of all Americans. Over twelve million people, about 25% of the workforce, joined the ranks of the unemployed.[56] Workers in all fields searched for ways to endure the lean economic years. By 1930, nurses registered with the NPR were feeling the full effects of the Great Depression. The registry turned its attention to simple survival.

Van Frank reported the unemployment situation among private duty nurses as the worst she had ever encountered.[57] For 3 years, beginning in 1930, the situation deteriorated. The NPR recorded a 30% drop in patient assignments in 1931.[58] By 1932, nurses registered with the NPR averaged 8.75 days of work per month, or 80 days a year.[59] The NPR lost more than 700 members in one two-year period; membership dropped from 1,912 in 1929 to 1,149 in 1933.[60] The decline in membership resulted in a drop in registry profits. NPR income over expenses in 1932 was a meager $86.18, a decrease of about $4,000 from 1931.[61]

The NPR instituted a number of actions in an attempt to help its membership. A loan fund was established to provide small amounts of money to those in dire straits.[62] The NPR gave nurses in great need special consideration, calling them out of turn for cases.[63] The registry relaxed policies that required nurses to live in the Chicago area when on call, helping nurses to cut down on living expenses.[64] To preserve their spirits, nurses were encouraged to keep busy by maintaining an interest in professional affairs, studying new methods in medicine, pursuing higher education, and developing recreational interests in areas such as music and art.[65]

More ambitious programs aimed at increasing employment of graduate nurses by hospitals. The ISNA asked hospitals to hire only licensed nursing personnel.[66] In May 1932, the ISNA petitioned hospitals to limit the number of students admitted for the coming year.[67] Several hospitals in the Chicago area complied with this request; others closed their schools altogether.[68] Private duty nurses volunteered a month or more of free service to hospitals that promised to reduce student enrollments, an offer hospitals were quick to accept. Hospitals also offered nurses a variety of schemes that provided small amounts of remuneration, maintenance in the form of room and board, or a combination of both. Some hospitals offered compensation ranging from $1 a day to $20 a month with maintenance for 4 hours of work a day. In other cases, hospitals provided full or partial maintenance with no salary to nurses who were willing to work as staff nurses for a varying number of hours.[69] The NPR sought to decrease the number of nurses seeking private duty work. Nurses graduating from schools outside the Chicago area were first discouraged and then refused membership. Word went our that employment opportunities in Chicago were extremely poor.[70]

Traditionally the Depression years have been characterized as the period of the "Great Transformation" in nursing, the time when large numbers of private duty nurses deserted the field to seek employment as general duty nurses, the predecessors of our contemporary staff nurses.[71] This characterization is only partly true. For a number of reasons, hospitals during the 1930s did begin to turn away from the traditional student nurse–centered care and employ more graduate nurses in staff positions.[72] Technological changes created complex care requirements necessitating practitioners more expert than students. Middle-class patients unable to afford private duty nurses expected hospitals to provide personalized care. Private and semiprivate rooms replaced multiple-bed wards, creating a need for more nurses. Finally, the economic effects of the Depression made graduate nurses relatively cheaper workers, increasing their attractiveness as employees.[73] Hospital employment, even at very low wages, often offered nurses the only opportunity for work.

At the same time that hospitals were beginning to value graduate nurses as appropriate patient caregivers, they also demonstrated significant reluctance to employ registered nurses permanently. Rather, significant evidence exists that hospitals resorted to hiring private duty nurses on a per diem basis as temporary staff.[74] Many general duty nurses during this period were actually private duty nurses placed in temporary positions.

Using private duty nurses as general duty nurses, a movement that continued to grow as the 1930s ended, represented a tremendous economic boost for the private duty market. The additional work created an increased demand for private duty nurses that translated into more jobs. As the economy slowly stabilized during the late 1930s, professional nurse registries nationwide reported better employment conditions overall.[75] The NPR documented a steady increase in nurse assignments in the years 1934–1940, recording a rise in average monthly assignments from 1,265 to 2,758, an increase of approximately 1,500 patient cases.[76]

Hospitals found that employing private duty nurses, who could be hired and dismissed as patient occupancy rates rose and fell, was an easy way to temporarily supplement short staffs and save the expense of permanent employees.[77] But the practice was a double-edged sword for private duty nurses and did not enjoy universal appeal. Temporary general duty work did offer nurses a chance to make some money, but problems with determining rates of pay and hours of work and reprisals against private duty nurses who refused to comply with hospitals' requests for temporary help marred the relationship between the parties.[78]

The rate of pay was a major source of contention between hospitals and private duty nurses. Private duty nurses generally received a set fee per shift of work. In the late 1930s, in large cities this may have averaged around $5 a shift.[79] Hospitals hiring per diem nurses generally calculated a daily fee prorated from the monthly salary paid permanent general duty nurses. In most cases this meant that the private duty nurse might be earning a paltry $3–4 a shift.[80] To make matters worse, the nurse was also expected to do a great deal more work.

In Chicago, nurses registered with the NPR reluctantly filled calls for general duty, but complained bitterly over the treatment they received as per diem nurses.[81] They resented the lower fees and the conditions under which they were expected to work.[82] In most instances, when private duty nurses took on a general duty assignment they were required to work split shifts, two 4-hour periods separated by a 4-hour or longer break. In some hospitals nurses were required to give up their position on the registry list when on general duty service. This lessened their chances of obtaining private duty cases. Many NPR nurses reported that hospitals discriminated against them if they refused temporary general duty service. Even in hospitals that did not discriminate, nurses were warned that refusing requests for temporary service would not be regarded in a positive manner by hospital authorities.[83]

At the 1936 national convention of the American Nurses Association (ANA), private duty nurses voiced frustration at being asked to fill in as temporary general duty nurses. One Chicago nurse reported that private duty nurses sometimes did not even receive a salary. Some hospitals merely provided room and board and the privilege of taking a private case if one became available. In other instances, the nurse might earn a meager $2 a day. Yet, as this nurse noted, nurses' primary complaint was not their low salaries: "But of all of the nurses I asked why they did not wish to help out in hospitals, not one complained about the money, but she said in every case when she had gone in to do general duty the amount of work required of her was beyond the physical capacity of any person and she just could not go back under those conditions."[84]

Concerns about the use of private duty nurses as temporary general duty nurses emerged as a recurring topic of discussion at the leadership level of the ANA.[85] Acting on reports of trouble among working nurses and the difficulties hospitals encountered in obtaining sufficient numbers of general duty nurses, the ANA launched a study examining the working conditions of nurses. The 1936 *Study of Incomes, Salaries, and Employment Conditions Affecting Nurses* surveyed nurses in three different fields of nursing: private duty nurses, institutional staff, and office nurses.[86] Although the study was based on a small sample (only 11,432 nurses in 23 states participated), the ANA board of directors expressed confidence in the accuracy of the results.[87] The study findings confirmed private duty nurses' dissatisfaction with temporary general duty positions and exposed the widespread use of poor labor practices by hospitals. The board, faced with evidence that nurses were employed under dismal conditions, decided to use the results of the study to achieve reform.

The board carefully formulated a number of recommendations intended to improve working conditions for private duty nurses engaged in temporary general duty nursing jobs. Hospitals were asked not to require private duty nurses to work as general duty nurses in order to secure work as private duty nurses. The board recommended that private duty nurses employed as relief general duty nurses be paid based on prevailing private duty rates. Finally, they urged that nurses work straight, not split or broken-hour shifts.[88] Believing that hospitals would seriously consider adopting their recommendations, the board put significant thought into the ways hospitals would put them into practice, taking into account the feasibility and practicality of each recommendation. Board discussions indicated confidence that the study and its accompanying recommendations would receive careful consideration from hospitals.[89]

Wholesale acceptance of the ANA position on working conditions and action on the study's recommendations by hospital authorities proved to be an elusive goal. To publicize the results of the study among hospital groups, Alma Scott, director of ANA headquarters, presented a paper describing the study, its findings, and recommendations to the American Hospital Association (AHA) 1938 annual convention.[90] The paper failed to stimulate discussion. Exactly how many hospitals followed up on the ANA recommendations, or even reflected on the study's implications, is unknown. Continued complaints from private duty nurses indicated that hospitals demonstrated little interest in changing employment practices toward private duty nurses. In reality, the ANA occupied a weak position from which to convince hospital authorities to improve nurses' working conditions. The association had no actual bargaining power and relied primarily on the good intentions of hospitals to act.[91] In the late 1930s, this was an insufficient strategy to effect change.

WORLD WAR II YEARS: A FAILURE OF THE MARKET

As the country entered the war years, the nursing profession as a whole and the private duty field in particular faced considerable challenges. Although the future looked bright for the private duty field as the decade began, significant changes in the ways hospitals staffed their institutions disrupted the private system of nurse distribution and led to its eventual demise.

In 1940, the NPR reported its busiest year on record. Twenty-two hospitals used the NPR exclusively for private nursing services; another 40 institutions used the registry as needed.[92] NPR finances improved, showing the highest post-Depression profit.[93] Reports of registry effectiveness in meeting demand for nurses began to resemble those of the 1920s. The improved outlook for the NPR was directly tied to the changing need for nurses occurring nationwide.

During the 1940s, several factors came together to create an unprecedented demand for nurses. The most immediate need was for nurses to serve in the armed forces. About 70,000 nurses joined military service.[94] The unavailability of approximately 25% of the registered nurse population for civilian needs plunged the country into an immediate critical nurse shortage.[95] At the same time, an increase in hospital use (due to the availability of health insurance), a growing population, and wartime activities caused demand for nurses to soar.[96]

By 1942, the NPR was overwhelmed with requests for nurses. For the first time in its history, the registry, which only 10 years before had been unable to supply enough work for its nurses, was unable to supply enough nurses for all the work. Registry statistics documenting the number of calls filled per request reflected the seriousness of the situation. In the late 1930s, the NPR generally had a 98–99% fill rate. Between 1942 and 1945, this rate plummeted to 39%. By the end of the war requests for nurses stabilized somewhat but were still filled only about 50–60% of the time.[97]

As the NPR experienced more and more difficulty filling requests for nurses, a vicious cycle began to play out. Unable to depend on the private duty field for an adequate supply of nurses, hospitals resorted to other means of supplementing short staffs. Hospitals discovered they could easily hire nurses on either a temporary or permanent basis without registry help and started bypassing the registry, choosing to deal directly with nurses when they needed to fill either general or private duty jobs. As nurses found that they could find work through hospitals, they often neglected to place themselves on call with the registry. This further reduced the number of nurses available to the NPR and made it even harder to fill requests. Some nurses most likely left the field of private duty altogether, taking positions as staff nurses instead.[98] As the registry experienced more and more problems filling requests, it came to be viewed as an unreliable source of nurses.

Post–World War II nurses tended to accept hospital employment.[99] New graduates did not consider the private duty field the best venue in which to practice. Other measures instituted by hospitals further endangered the private duty market. Hospitals found that using a differentiated nursing staff composed of several different types of nurse workers met the need for staff and decreased the need for private practitioners.[100] This success allowed them to employ more lesser-trained, cheaper workers and fewer more expensive registered nurses. The cumulative effect of the changes occurring during the 1940s was to marginalize private duty nursing as a viable occupational field.[101] With fewer nurses entering the market, fewer nurses hired for private duty, and hospitals initiating strategies to reduce the need for private nurses and turning away from the private duty market as a source of nurses, the private duty field passed into decline.

A speaker at the 1948 ANA convention summed up the changes in the field and asked poignantly:

> How secure is the future of private duty nursing? . . . The age group of the present membership would indicate that the younger nurse is not interested. Why? Is the answer a question of income, a seven-day week, lack of self-confidence? Does the nurse assume it is her responsibility to remain for staff duty with the hospital from which she is a graduate? Are the rules for accepting calls unsatisfactory? Is the yearly fee unattractive? Are we overlooking opportunities to advance private duty nursing by not promoting good personnel practices? Salary increases in other fields of nursing must be equally balanced by the private duty nurse if we expect to replace the older nurse resigning from our registries.[102]

Despite this nurse's uncertainties over private duty's future, she remained hopeful that the field would continue, concluding, "Collectively, we may establish a satisfactory attractive private duty program that will continue to meet the expected demands of each community for special nursing." Given the contemporary circumstances in the nurse labor market, this nurse's optimism that private duty nursing would survive seemed misplaced.

For the NPR, the downturn in private duty did not result in immediate closure. The registry remained open for another 30 years, but as a greatly reduced business. It did attempt to improve its rate of filling requests for nurses. It also expanded services in the 1950s, when it opened a registry placing private duty practical nurses. But it would never regain its earlier status as the center of nurse distribution for the Chicago area. In 1980, the Chicago Nurses Association, citing financial concerns, closed the 69-year-old NPR.

CONCLUSION

Providing private nursing services on a one-to-one basis made a great deal of sense to early practitioners of nursing. Late nineteenth- and early twentieth-century hospitals were not yet interested in hiring the nursing staff necessary to deliver the technical care required by advances in modern medicine. The private duty market bridged the gap in nursing services by supplying professional graduate nurses to hospitals and to those patients fortunate enough to afford private care. Private duty registries functioned as an important source of jobs for the increasing numbers of nurses graduating from schools nationwide.

Analyses of private duty tend to emphasize the system's weaknesses. Private duty was an inefficient, expensive, and unreliable method through which to distribute nurses. Nevertheless, despite its problems, the field operated with a fair degree of success. The private duty market was the largest and most structured job market for nurses in the early years of the profession. The professional registry system offered nurses a unique opportunity to control, organize, and systematize their work. The registries that connected nurses with patients provided not just employment for nurses but also a significant barometer of labor market functioning in supplying enough work for nurses and meeting demands for nurse services. Moreover, when times were bad, such as during the Great Depression, professional private duty registries offered a support system to help nurses survive.

Hospitals used the private duty system to their full benefit. During the first half of the twentieth century, they remained committed to student-centered care, relying on the private duty market to obtain a graduate nursing staff for patients willing and able to pay for private care without the expense and bother of employing nurses. During the 1930s, hospitals became savvy consumers of the registry system, using registries as a source of temporary general duty nurses. This arrangement permitted hospitals to continue avoiding employing permanent staff.

However, it was an arrangement with significant liabilities for both nurses and hospitals. Hiring temporary nurses allowed hospitals to ignore provision of proper working conditions and created considerable dissatisfaction among nurses. Little incentive existed for nurses to remain loyal to hospitals. Speculations only are in order as to the influence of hospital behavior on nurses' decisions to enter, remain in, or leave the labor market. It is unlikely that the treatment hospitals afforded nurses encouraged them to work.

Relying on temporary nurses for delivery of nursing care, whether at a private or institutional level, was a fundamentally flawed system. An increased demand for nurses beginning around World War II demonstrated the precarious nature of their employment situation. As more nurses were required and fewer were available, a crisis atmosphere caused hospitals to take actions that resulted in the marginalization of the private duty market as an employment field. Distributing nurses to patients, one nurse at a time, became an anachronism.

Placing the decline of the private duty market in the context of a nurse shortage has meaning beyond just situating an event in a specific time and place. Analyses of periodic nurse shortages over the century predominantly focus on causative factors and solutions. But shortages create consequences that are important to both recognize and explain. Meeting demand for nurses was a tenacious problem throughout the twentieth century. In mid-century, unmet demand resulted in the slow death of the private duty market and the adoption of alternative employment arrangements for nurses.

This serves as a cautionary tale as the profession approaches supply-and-demand issues today. Critical nurse shortages have long-standing effects beyond the very serious and immediate outcomes at the patient's bedside. For better or worse, they may also carry the potential to change the very structure of nurses' employment and frustrate nurses' attempts to manage their own practice.

ACKNOWLEDGMENTS

This research was made possible by a National Research Service Award (#NR07270 1997–99) and grants from Sigma Theta Tau Xi Chapter, Sigma Theta Tau International, the American Nurses Foundation Eleanor Lambertson RN Scholar Award, and a Rockefeller Archive Center Grant. Versions of this chapter were presented at the national meeting of the American Association for the History of Nursing, Milwaukee, Wisconsin, September 19, 2003, and at the 37th Biennial Convention of Sigma Theta Tau International, Toronto, Ontario, November 3, 2003. The author gratefully acknowledges the guidance and support of Karen Buhler-Wilkerson, Joan Lynaugh, and Walter Licht in carrying out the original research for this project, to Patricia D'Antonio for her suggestions, to Robin Cheung for her thoughts and comments, and to the reviewers at the *Nursing History Review* for their useful critiques.

NOTES

1. The name of the association changed several times. Originally known as the Graduate Nurses' Association of the State of Illinois, it became the Illinois State Association of Graduate Nurses in 1902 and the Illinois State Nurses Association in 1929. It acquired its present name, the Illinois Nurses Association, in 1956. See Mary Dunwiddie, *A History of the Illinois State Nurses Association, 1910–1935* (Chicago: Illinois State Nurses Association, 1937), and Karen J. Egenes and Wendy K. Burgess, *Faithfully Yours: A History of Nursing in Illinois* (Chicago: Illinois Nurses Association, 2001). I use the contemporary name Illinois State Nurses Association (ISNA) throughout this chapter.

2. Terms used to categorize private duty registries for nurses changed over time. "Central registry" was used at the turn of the twentieth century for registries in a central location in a city or town. In 1924, as professional nurse groups enlarged their interest in the operations of central registries, private duty nurses at the American Nurses Association (ANA) annual convention recommended adopting the term "official registry" as more fitting. See "Central Registries for Nurses," *Trained Nurse and Hospital Review* 73 (July 1924): 57. The term "professional registry" came into use during the 1930s to identify a registry approved by a local district nurse association. See "Meetings of the Board of Directors," *American Journal of Nursing* 38 (March 1938): 329 (hereafter *AJN*). This chapter uses the term "central registry" either in its historic sense to refer to a registry operating in the initial decades of the twentieth century or to a specific registry named a central registry. It uses the term "professional registry" as a generic term for registries operated by and for nurses.

3. Lucy Van Frank, "The Problems of a Registrar," paper presented at the Annual Meeting of the Illinois State Nurses Association, Peoria, October 10–12, 1923, Illinois Nurses Association Papers, Illinois State Historical Library, Springfield, box 2, folder 1 (hereafter INAP).

4. See, for example, "Official Registries and Professional Progress," *AJN* 26 (February 1926): 91–94; Elizabeth Burgess, "The Future of the Central Registry," *AJN* 15 (August 1915): 1033–35; Editor, "Registries," *AJN* 26 (March 1926): 206–7.

5. Several excellent studies on the change of employment status for nurses from private duty to staff nursing exist. See, for example, Marilyn Flood, "The Troubling Expedient: General Staff Nursing in United States Hospitals in the 1930's: A Means to Institutional, Educational, and Personal Ends" (PhD dissertation, University of California at Berkeley, 1981) and Susan M. Reverby, *Ordered to Care: The Dilemma of American Nursing, 1850–1945* (Cambridge: Cambridge University Press, 1987).

6. For the number of schools of nursing, see Department of Health and Human Services, Public Health Service, Human Resources Administration, *Source Book—Nursing Personnel,* DHHS publication (HRA) 81–21 (Hyattsville, MD: U.S. Department of Health and Human Services, Public Health Service, Human Resources Administration, 1981), 83.

7. For a contemporary description of early twentieth-century private duty nursing see Katherine De Witt, *Private Duty Nursing,* 2nd ed. (Philadelphia: Lippincott, 1917; reprint New York: Garland, 1984). For the best historical analyses of early private duty nursing and nurses, see Susan M. Reverby, "'Neither for the Drawing Room Nor for the Kitchen': Private Duty Nursing in Boston, 1873–1920," in *Women and Health in America: Historical Readings,* ed. Judith Walzer Leavitt (Madison: University of Wisconsin Press, 1984), 454–66; Reverby, *Ordered to Care.*

8. For the ways patients and physicians secured nurses at the turn of the century, see Sister M. Ignatius Feeny, "Central Directories," *AJN* 4 (July 1904): 796–99; Elizabeth Scovil, "Openings for Nurses," *AJN* 1 (March 1901): 439.

9. Many discussions on the best types and ways to organize hospital-based registries took place in the late 1890s at conventions held by the American Society of Superintendents of Training Schools for Nurses. See, for example, Louise Darche, "Training School Registries," in American Society of Superintendents of Training Schools for Nurses, *Annual Conventions 1893–1899* (New York: Garland, 1985), 22–31. For a concise contemporary history of the evolution of hospital-based registries, see Ella Best, "Nursing Supply—How To Balance Supply and Demand," *Modern Hospital* 39 (August 1932): 97–102.

10. The exact number of hospital-based registries is indeterminate. At the Third Annual Convention of the American Society of Superintendents of Training Schools for Nurses, held in 1896, Sophia Palmer reported 40 alumnae associations in existence in the United States and Canada. How many of them operated private duty registries was not mentioned. See Sophia Palmer, "Discussion," in *Annual Conventions 1893–1899,* 63.

11. For the evolution of central registries see Best, "Nursing Supply"; Lavinia L. Dock, "Nursing in the United States," in *Transactions of the Third International Congress of Nurses in Buffalo, September 18–21, 1901,* ed. the Committee on Publication, Isabel Hampton Robb, Lavinia L. Dock, and Maud Banfield (Cleveland: J. B. Savage, 1901), 481–82.

12. For the number of commercial employment agencies in Chicago, see Van Frank, "The Problems of a Registrar." Using commercial employment agencies either to obtain work or to hire employees was a common practice for both workers and employers at the turn of the century. For a history of private employment agencies, see Tomás Martinez, *The Human Marketplace: An Examination of Private Employment Agencies* (New Brunswick, NJ: Transaction Books, 1976).

13. For negative reports of commercial registries, see Minnie Aherns, "Discussion, 18th Annual Convention, ANA," *AJN* 15 (August 1915): 1036; Editor, "The Commercial Registry," *AJN* 14 (February 1914): 329–30; Martha Russell, "Club Houses, Hostelries, and Directories for Nurses," *AJN* 5 (August 1905): 803. Nurses were particularly critical of agencies that placed them with other domestic workers, such as chambermaids and scrubwomen. See, for example, Editor, "Commercial Directories," *AJN* 9 (July 1909): 723–24; Mary Thornton to Editor, *AJN* 3 (December 1903): 243–44. For Lavinia Dock's comments, see Dock, "Nursing in the United States," 481–82.

14. For a discussion of the Boston Medical Library Directory for Nurses, see Reverby, "Neither for the Drawing Room Nor for the Kitchen"; Reverby, *Ordered to Care.*

15. For a history of the Philadelphia Directory, see Frederick Fraley, "History of the Directory for Nurses of the College of Physicians," *Transactions and Studies of the College of Physicians of Philadelphia* 4, 1 (1936): xi–xvi.

16. Dock, "Nursing in the United States," 482.

17. See, for example, Helen MacMillan, "Central Registration," *AJN* 4 (July 1904): 791–94; Mary Thornton, "The Organization and Management of Clubs and Homes for Graduate Nurses," *AJN* 1 (February 1901): 378–80.

18. Lavinia L. Dock, "Directories for Nurses," in *Annual Conventions 1893–1899,* 57–60; Isabel Hampton Robb, "Discussion," in *Annual Conventions 1893–1899,* 63.

19. See Elizabeth Burgess, "The Future of the Central Registry," *AJN* 15 (August 1915): 1033–35; Editor, "Central Registries and the Idle Nurse," *AJN* 9 (December 1909): 145–47; Marion Mead, "Registry from the Point of View of the Registrar," *AJN* 14 (July 1914): 827–29. Early twentieth-century nurse-run central registries were also often associated with dub houses or living quarters for nurses and provided a spectrum of services, including meals, recreation, and educational opportunities. See MacMillan, "Central Registration"; Feeny, "Central Directories." Some believed a nurse registry should offer a variety of services to patients, in effect serving as a one-stop nursing

shopping center for the community. Paying individuals could use the registry not just for nursing services when ill but also for purchasing special diets and sickroom supplies. See, for example, Sophia Rutley, "Private Duty Nurses and Their Relationship to the Directory," *AJN* 15 (August 1915): 939–43.

20. Editor, "Central Registries and the Idle Nurse."

21. The establishment of central registries often paralleled the organization of state and local nurse associations. State nurse associations began forming in the early years of the twentieth century, many with the specific purpose of passing nurse practice acts. Although variation existed in the ways in which each state association organized, eventually state associations included smaller, locally based units called district associations. District associations were considered to be the best sponsor of a central registry. For discussions regarding the organization and ownership of central registries, see Katherine De Witt, "The County Association and Its Relationship to the State," *AJN* 9 (August 1909): 809–15; Janette Peterson, "Central Directories—The Nurse's Obligation to Support Them," *Nurses' Journal of the Pacific Coast* 7 (October 1911): 441–49. In 1911, the conglomeration of state, district, and alumnae associations became the American Nurses Association. For the organization of the ANA and its constituent state associations, see Lyndia Flanagan, *One Strong Voice: The Story of the American Nurses Association* (Kansas City: ANA, 1976).

22. Nurse association–run central registries were reported in Boston, Denver, Washington, D.C., Minneapolis, Philadelphia, Oklahoma City, and Kansas City. See Editor, "Central Registries," *AJN* 12 (January 1912): 281–82; Reba Thelin Foster, "The Organization of Nurses Clubs and Directories Under State Association," *AJN* 9 (January 1909): 247–52; Grace Holmes, "An Ideal Central Directory," *AJN* 6 (June 1906): 606–8; Susan Bard Johnson, "The Boston Nurses Club," *AJN* 9 (April 1909): 662–63; Lily Kanely, "A Successful Central Registry," *AJN* 9 (April 190?): 496–98; Sarah F. Martin, "Central Directories," *AJN* 10 (December 1910): 162–67; Marion Mead, "Registry System of the Hennepin County Graduate Nurses Association, Minneapolis, Minn.," *AJN* 10 (August 1910): 819–24.

23. Exact estimates of how many professional central registries existed prior to the mid-1930s are difficult to obtain. In 1915, the Special Registry Committee of the ANA located more than 40 central registries; see "Report of the Special Registry Committee," *AJN* 15 (September 1915): 1121–22. A 1924 ANA survey reported on 75 professional registries; see "Official Registries and Professional Progress," *AJN* 26 (February 1926): 92. In the mid-1930s the ANA began compiling statistics on professional registries, providing a more accurate estimate of the number of such agencies. Prior to World War II, the ANA recorded as many as 145 professional registries in business. The number fluctuated during the 1940s but began rising steadily after the war until 1956, when 176 registries were in operation. After 1956, the number of professional registries fell, but as late as 1965 there were 153 professional registries listed with the ANA. For numbers of professional registries, see the ANA annual publication *Facts About Nursing: A Statistical Summary* (New York: ANA, 1935–): 1939, 43; 1953, 80; 1957, 109; 1966, 116.

24. For the organization of nursing in Illinois, see Dunwiddie, *A History of the Illinois State Nurses' Association;* Egenes and Burgess, *Faithfully Yours.*

25. In the first decades of the twentieth century, Chicago was the second largest city in the nation in population, with 2,701,705 inhabitants in 1920. See U.S. Department of Commerce, *Fifteenth Census of the United States: 1930,* vol. 1, *Population* (Washington, DC: U.S. Government Printing Office, 1930), 18.

26. For a history of the Chicago medical world, see Thomas Neville Bonner, *Medicine in Chicago, 1850–1950,* 2nd ed. (Urbana: University of Illinois Press, 1991).

27. Egenes and Burgess, *Faithfully Yours,* 23.

28. The registry took on many names during its years of operation. For the first 30 years, Central Directory, Registry, or Official Registry were names commonly used. Sometime in the 1940s the name was changed permanently to Nurses Professional Registry (NPR), the name I use throughout this article.

29. For rules and regulations, see "Regulations," undated, most likely 1935, Chicago Nurses Registry Collection, Midwest Nursing History Center, College of Nursing, University of Illinois, Chicago, box 1 (hereafter CNRC).

30. Dunwiddie, A History of the Illinois State Nurses Association, 94; Minnie Aherns, "Discussion, 18th Annual Convention," 1035–36.

31. "Nurses Professional Registry, Average Number of Registrants and Average Monthly Number of Private Duty Assignments, 1917–1946," July 26, 1947, CNRC, box 1.

32. For the amounts of contributions made by area alumnae associations, see Dunwiddie, A History of the Illinois State Nurses Association, 163–65.

33. The twelve alumnae associations were those of the Illinois Training School, Presbyterian, Augustana, Chicago Memorial, Merry, Mt. Sinai, St. Elizabeth's, St. Joseph's, St. Luke's, Washington Boulevard, Wesley Memorial, and West Suburban Schools of Nursing. See Dunwiddie, A History of the Illinois State Nurses Association, 94; "Annual Report Club and Registry, 1926," First District Bulletin 24 (February 1927): 10–11, INAP, box 3, folder 10.

34. Exact statistics are not available on the number of patients NPR nurses cared for in the home versus in the hospital. In 1929, Van Frank reported that the majority of cases were in the hospital and that nurses clearly preferred hospital to home care. See Lucy Van Frank, "The Private Duty Nurse," paper presented at the Annual Meeting of the Illinois State Nurses Association, Moline, October 10, 1929, INAP, box 4, folder 12. The Committee on the Grading of Nursing Schools (CGNS), which carried out a study of private duty nursing in 1928, estimated that about 79% of private duty cases were in the hospital. See May Ayres Burgess, ed., Nurses, Patients, and Pocketbooks: A Study of the Economics of Nursing (New York: Committee on the Grading of Nursing Schools, 1928; reprint New York: Garland, 1984), 74.

35. "Nurses Professional Registry, Average Number of Registrants and Average Monthly Number of Private Duty Assignments, 1917–1946."

36. For the number of graduate nurses in Illinois and Chicago, see U.S. Department of Commerce, Fifteenth Census of the United States: 1930, vol. 4, Occupations, 428.

37. For the number of beds in Chicago hospitals, see "Hospital Service in the United States," Journal of the American Medical Association 94 (29 March 1930): 941–43 (hereafter JAMA).

38. "Nurses Fees, 1913–1980," April 7, 1976, CNRC, box 1; "Annual Report, Private Duty Section, Illinois State Nurses Association, 1926–1927," INAP, box 3, folder 10.

39. "Income over Expenses," undated, most likely 1947, CNRC, box 1. As a nonprofit agency the NPR did not make profits in a commercial sense. I use the term profit to indicate income over expenses.

40. "Annual Report, First District, 1924," INAP, box 2, folder 2; "Annual Report Club and Registry Committee, 1926," 11.

41. "Report of the Registry Committee," June 7, 1930, INAP, box 4, folder 13.

42. Hourly nursing services were private nursing services paid for by the hour, as opposed to the patient hiring a nurse for a designated shift. For a description of the NPR's hourly nursing program, see Jean C. Whelan, "Smaller and Cheaper: The Chicago Hourly Nursing Service 1926–1950," Nursing History Review 10 (2002): 83–108. Institutional placement services offered registered nurses a means to obtain permanent or temporary positions in hospitals and other health care agencies. The NPR's attempts to expand the institutional placement service were never very successful. For a contemporary discussion of institutional placement services in the Chicago area and

the efforts of the Chicago Nurses Association to enter this market, see "The Registry as Placement Bureau," *First District Bulletin* 24 (August 1927): 4, INAP, box 3.

43. "Registry," *First District Bulletin* 23 (March 1926): 3, INAP, box 3, folder 8.

44. Ethel Johns, "A Study of the Present Status of the Negro Woman in Nursing, 1925," unpublished report, Exhibit B-2, folder 1507, box 122, series 200 United States, Record Group 1.1 Projects, Rockefeller Foundation Archives, Rockefeller Archives Center, North Tarrytown, NY. Darlene Clark Hine recorded the difficulties African American nurses experienced because of exclusionary, segregated policies; see Darlene Clark Hine, *Black Women in White: Racial Conflict and Cooperation in the Nursing Profession, 1890–1950* (Bloomington: Indiana University Press, 1989).

45. 1 have used Mary Roberts's estimate of the number of schools for the 1920s; see Mary Roberts, *American Nursing: History and Interpretation* (New York: Macmillan, 1954), 110. According to Roberts, the number of schools of nursing peaked in 1927 at 2,286 and by 1930 had declined to 1,844. See Department of Health and Human Services, *Source Book—Nursing Personnel,* 83; for the number of nurses, see p. 26.

46. Estimating the number of nurses working as private duty nurses is problematic. The best contemporary estimate is from the CGNS; see Burgess, *Nurses, Patients, and Pocketbooks,* 249. The Committee surveyed 24,389 nurses from ten states selected by the CGNS on a nonrandom basis; the results indicated that 54% of the nurses worked as private duty nurses. This statistic has been generally accepted as reflecting the size of the private duty market in the late 1930s. It is also the statistic frequently compared to figures cited by the 1923 Rockefeller study on nursing (which estimated that 80% of all nurses were in the private duty field) as indicative of a movement of nurses out of private duty. For the Rockefeller study, see Josephine Goldmark, *Nursing and Nursing Education in the United* States (New York: Macmillan, 1923; reprint New York: Garland, 1984). Caution needs to be exercised when using these percentages. First, the nonrandom nature of the sample used by the CGNS might or might not reflect an accurate measure of the population. Second, percentages can be indicative of different phenomena. For example, a declining percentage might reflect a decrease in the total number of private duty nurses or a stable or even increasing number of private duty nurses in an increasing population.

47. For a discussion of the cost of private duty nursing, see Elizabeth Gordon Fox, "The Economics of Nursing," *AJN* 29 (September 1929): 1037–44. Fox estimated that only about 1.5–2.0% of the population could afford private duty nurses. The CGNS also addressed the cost of private duty, concluding that many patients needed nursing care but failed to receive it because of high cost. See Committee on the Grading of Nursing Schools, *Nursing Schools Today and Tomorrow* (New York: Author, 1934), 237–38.

48. See Burgess, *Nurses, Patients, and Pocketbooks,* 83–85, 304–9. Another study on private duty nursing, completed in 1926 in New York state, found results similar to chose of the CGNS; see Janet Geister, "Hearsay and Facts in Private Duty," *AJN* 26 (July 1926): 515–28.

49. Burgess, *Nurses, Patients, and Pocketbooks,* 311.

50. See, for example, Geister, "Hearsay and Facts in Private Duty"; Janet Geister, "The Economics of Nursing," *Bulletin of the American College of Surgeons* 13 (December 1929): 14–17.

51. Burgess, *Nurses, Patients, and Pocketbooks,* 500–551; CGNS, *Nursing Schools Today and Tomorrow,* 233–49.

52. Burgess, *Nurses, Patients, and Pocketbooks,* 311. The study found private duty nurses were hesitant about whether to stay in or leave the field.

53. Ibid., 318.

54. Ibid., 320.

55. Van Frank, "The Private Duty Nurse."

56. For an analysis of the Great Depression, see William Leuchtenberg, *Franklin D. Roosevelt and the New Deal, 1932–1940* (New York: Harper & Row, 1963). Leuchtenberg estimated that the number of unemployed was as high as fifteen million.

57. "Report to the State Private Duty Section, Annual Business Session," ISNA, October 16 1930, INAP, box 4, folder 13.

58. "Report of the State Private Duty Section, Regular Meeting, Board of Directors," ISNA, October 13, 1931, INAP, box 4, folder 14.

59. "Registry," *ISNA Bulletin* 30 (April 1933): 6, INAP, box 5, folder 16.

60. "Nurses Professional Registry, Average Number of Registrants and Average Monthly Number of Private Duty Assignments, 1917–1946."

61. "Income over Expenses."

62. "Unemployment and Relief," *ISNA Bulletin* 30 (April 1933): 7–8, INAP, box 5, folder 16.

63. "Annual Report, Private Duty Section, First District, 1933," INAP, box 5, folder 20.

64. "Registry," *ISNA Bulletin* 30 (April 1933): 6.

65. "Objectives of the Private Duty Section for the Coming Year," *ISNA Bulletin* 29 (March 1932): 7–8, INAP, box 5, folder 16.

66. "Minutes, Annual Meeting, Private Duty Section, ISNA, 13 October 1933," INAP, box 5, folder 20.

67. "Education and Distribution of Nursing Services," *ISNA Bulletin* 29 (December 1932): 6, INAP, box 5, folder 16.

68. "Annual Report, Private Duty Section, First District, ISNA, 1933."

69. "Education and Distribution of Nursing Service," 6; "Report of Illinois Committee on the Distribution of Nursing Service Organization, Questionnaire No. II, 1933," INAP, box 5, folder 20; "Report of Committee on Distribution of Nursing Service, ISNA, 11 October, 1933," INAP, box 5, folder 20.

70. "Annual Report, Private Duty Section, First District, ISNA, 1933." See also Egenes and Burgess, *Faithfully Yours,* 77.

71. For the best discussions of this period, see Flood, "The Troubling Expedient"; Susan M. Reverby, "'Something Besides Waiting': The Politics of Private Duty Reform in the Depression," in *Nursing History: New Perspectives, New Possibilities,* ed. Ellen Conlife Lagerman (New York: Teachers College Press, 1983), 133–56. The various terms used to identify nurses employed by hospitals for bedside patient care included *general duty nurse, floor duty nurse, institutional nurse,* and *staff nurse.* This chapter uses the term *general duty nurse.*

72. Estimates of how many general duty or staff nurses existed during this time period are difficult to make. Contemporaries generally cited statistics generated from CGNS studies in the late 1920s as a base from which to measure the growth of staff nursing during this period. See, for example, Roberts, *American Nursing,* 286; "Did You Ever See a Nurse Nursing?" *AJN* 38 (April 1938): 30(s). The CGNS found approximately 4,000 nurses employed as floor duty nurses (general duty or staff nurses) in a survey of 1,397 hospitals affiliated with schools of nursing in 1929. See CGNS, *Results of the First Grading Study of Nursing Schools, Section III—Who Controls the Schools* (New York: Author, 1930), 24. At the time of this survey, there were 6,665 hospitals in the country, leaving a significant number of hospitals unaccounted for in the estimate. For numbers of hospitals, see "Hospital Service in the United States," 921. It is possible to track the growth of staff nursing in hospitals associated with schools of nursing. In 1937 the National League for Nursing surveyed 1,259 schools of nursing, finding that in hospitals associated with schools, 27,000 general staff nurses were employed. This represented a sevenfold increase in the number of staff nurses from 1929 levels, at least in hospitals associated with a school of nursing. See "More General Staff Nurses," *AJN* 38 (February 1938): 186.

Whatever the exact figures, it was accepted at the time that the growth in the number of general duty nurses was remarkable.

73. For an analysis of the factors leading to the employment of staff nurses, see Flood, "The Troubling Expedient"; Reverby, *Ordered to Care,* 180–98. Contemporaries attributed the rise of staff nursing to a decrease in the number of student nurses, a growing awareness that a graduate nursing staff was essential, an increase in the number and occupancy rates of hospital beds, and the growth of hospital insurance plans that contributed to increased hospital usage. See "Did You Ever See a Nurse Nursing?" 17(s)–34(s).

74. This statement is based on a number of indicators. Professional nurse registries nationwide began reporting an increase in the number of calls received for private duty nurses to fill temporary staff nurse positions. Between 1937 and 1940, professional nurse registries recorded an increase of 10,000 calls received for temporary staff positions. See "What Registries Did in 1937," *AJN* 38 (October 1938): 1115–23; "What Registries Did in 1938," *AJN* 39 (September 1939): 998–1006; "What Registries Are Doing," *AJN* 41 (August 1941): 902–8. The 1936 ANA study of working conditions of nurses highlighted the widespread practice of using private duty nurses as temporary staff nurses. See American Nurses Association, *Study of Incomes, Salaries and Employment Conditions Affecting Nurses* (New York: ANA, 1938). See also "The American Nurses Association and the Eight-Hour Schedule for Nurses," *AJN* 36 (October 1936): 979–83; Barbara Hunter, "An All Graduate Staff and the Eight-Hour Day," *AJN* 37 (May 1937): 473; Margaret Tracy, "The Eight-Hour Day for Special Nurses: At the University of California Hospital," *AJN* 35 (January 1935): 29–32.

75. See, for example, reports from professional nurse registries as published in the *AJN*: "What Registries Did in 1937," "What Registries Did in 1938," and "What Registries Are Doing."

76. See "Nurses Professional Registry, Average Number of Registrants and Average Monthly Number of Private Duty Assignments, 1917–1946." This is not to suggest that the private duty market had completely recovered from the economic effects of the Great Depression. Despite the improved overall conditions, other indices reveal a less positive picture. Although the number of requests for nurses rose, the NPR continued to record large numbers of nurses as on call and without patient assignments. See "Annual Report, Executive Committee, Board of Directors, ISNA, 1936," INAP, box 6, folder 26. In 1938, bad economic conditions caused the NPR to limit its membership to graduates of hospitals affiliated with the registry. See "Annual Report, First District, ISNA, 1938," INAP, box 7, folder 28.

77. For the use of private duty nurses as temporary general duty nurses, see "The American Nurses Association and the Eight-Hour Schedule for Nurses"; Hunter, "An All Graduate Staff and the Eight-Hour Day"; Tracy, "The Eight-Hour Day for Special Nurses."

78. For the problems private duty nurses experienced with temporary general duty, see "The American Nurses Association and the Eight-Hour Schedule for Nurses."

79. Fees paid by patients for private duty nurses dropped during the Great Depression and did not return to pre-Depression levels for several years. By 1936, the fee charged by NPR nurses for an 8-hour shift was $5. Nurses working 12-hour shifts received $6. See Retta Gasteyer, Secretary, First District, ISNA, to Directors of Nursing, January 23, 1936, CNRC, box 1.

80. ANA, *Study of Incomes, Salaries and Employment Conditions,* 509.

81. Complete statistics on how many calls for temporary general duty were received and filled by the NPR are lacking. In 1936, the NPR filled 448 calls for temporary general duty; see "Annual Report, First District, ISNA, 1936," INAP, box 6, folder 26. Reports for later years mention filling calls for general duty nurses but do not estimate

the numbers of calls fitting this category; see, for example, "Annual Report, First District, ISNA, 1940," INAP, box 7, folder 33. By the early 1940s, filling calls for general duty nurses seems to have increased, as noted in discussions on the matter; see "Annual Report, Private Duty Section, ISNA, 1942," INAP, box 8, folder labeled "Minutes, Board of Directors and Annual Meeting, 1942"; "Annual Report, First District, ISNA, 1942," INAP, box 8, folder 37.

82. "Report of the Private Duty Round Table, 1940," INAP, box 246, folder 1.

83. "Annual Report, Private Duty Section, ISNA, 1942."

84. "Proceedings, Round Table for General Staff Nurses, American Nurses Association, June 23, 1936," American Nurses Association Papers, Mugar Library, Special Collections, Boston University, Boston, box 87 (hereafter ANAP).

85. See, for example, "Board of Directors Meeting, American Nurses Association," January 28–31, 1936; June 20–26, 1936, ANAP, box 18; "Board of Directors Meeting, American Nurses Association," January 25–29, 1937, ANAP, box 19.

86. See ANA, *Study of Incomes, Salaries and Employment Conditions*.

87. "Board of Directors Meeting, American Nurses Association," January 25–29, 1937, ANAP, box 19.

88. ANA, *Study of Incomes, Salaries and Employment Conditions*, 499–512.

89. "Board of Directors Meeting, American Nurses Association," January 24–28, 1938, ANAP, box 20.

90. Alma Scott, "Status of Graduate Nurse Service as Indicated by Recent Studies Conducted Through the American Nurses Association Headquarters," *Transactions of the American Hospital Association* 60 (1938): 410–17.

91. This era, from the late 1930s to the early 1940s, a time when nurses became more vocal regarding their working conditions and the ANA began to take very tentative steps in addressing the needs of working nurses, is worthy of further investigation by historians.

92. "Annual Report, First District, ISNA, 1940."

93. "Income over Expenses."

94. Roberts, *American Nursing*, 343.

95. This estimate of the percentage of nurses serving in the military is based on dividing the 70,000 nurses in the armed services as reported by Roberts by the total number of nurses as enumerated by the 1940 U.S. Census. For the number of nurses in 1940, see *Source Book—Nursing Personnel*, 26.

96. Numerous contemporary articles appeared in professional journals describing and analyzing the increased demand for nurses. See, for example, "Why America Needs More Nurses," *AJN* 43 (February 1943): 132–33; "Wartime Nursing Is Different," *AJN* 43 (September 1943): 835–38; Joseph Mountin, "Nursing—A Critical Analysis," *AJN* 43 (January 1943): 29–34.

97. "Annual Report, Private Duty Section, ISNA, 1942"; "Annual Report, First District, 1944," INAP, box 9, folder labeled "Minutes, Board of Directors and Annual Meeting; "Annual Report, First District, 1945," INAP, box 9, folder labeled "Proceedings House of Delegates 20 October, 1945." Nationally as well, professional registries experienced low rates of filling calls. Between 1946 and 1950, professional registries reporting to the ANA recorded unfilled calls ranging from 29% to 46%. See *Facts About Nursing: A Statistical Summary* (New York: ANA, 1963), 126.

98. For the difficulties the NPR experienced in filling calls, see "Annual Report, First District, 1942"; "Summary of Activities, First District, 1942," INAP, box 313; "Annual Report, First District, 1945," INAP, box 9.

99. The number of nurses employed in hospitals increased considerably in the 1940s. The 1941 National Inventory of Registered Nurses listed 81,708 nurses as employed in hospitals, 47% of the active employed registered nurses surveyed. See Pearl McIver,

"Registered Nurses in the United States," *AJN* 42 (July 1942): 769–73. No indication is given in what positions these nurses were employed, so it cannot be determined how many were general duty or staff nurses. The 1944 annual survey of hospital data carried out by the Council on Medical Education and Hospitals of the American Medical Association listed 64,741 nurses employed as general duty nurses (56,766 full-time and 7,975 part-time); see "Hospital Service in the United States," *JAMA* 127 (March 31, 1945): 780. Four years later, in 1948, this figure had almost doubled to 121,318 general duty nurses (104,041 full-time and 17,277 part-time); see "Hospital Service in the United States," *JAMA* 140 (May 7, 1949): 34. It is also likely that in different parts of the country, staff nursing became the norm at different points in time. For example, Flood notes that hospitals in California may have instituted staff nursing earlier than did other parts of the country. See Flood, "The Troubling Expedient."

100. As with registered nurses, obtaining accurate counts of nursing assistive personnel is problematic. In many cases, different names and categories were used when estimating the number of assistive personnel, making an exact count difficult. The 1943 American Medical Association annual survey of hospital data listed 175,677 individuals in the categories of practical nurse, nurse's aide, attendant, and orderly. In 1949 there were 225,001 persons listed in similar categories. See "Hospital Service in the United States," *JAMA* 124 (March 25, 1944): 848; "Hospital Service in the United States," *JAMA* 140 (May 7, 1949): 34.

101. For a discussion of the post–World War II health care environment and the many problems facing nursing during this time period see Joan E. Lynaugh and Barbara L. Brush, *American Nursing From Hospitals to Health Systems* (Malden, MA: Blackwell, 1996), 1–15.

102. "ANA, Proceedings, Private Duty Section," May 31–June 4, 1948, ANAP, box 89.

CHAPTER 8

The Cost of Caring: The Metropolitan Life Insurance Company's Visiting Nurse Service, 1909–1953

Diane Hamilton

In the spring of 1909, a firm handshake sealed a contract between Haley Fiske, vice-president of the Metropolitan Life Insurance Company (MLI) and Lillian Wald, director of the Henry Street Settlement House (HSS). The agreement stated that, for a period of three months, trained nurses from HSS would provide health teaching and home care to MLI policy-holders within a section of New York City. In return, Metropolitan agreed to pay the nurses 50 cents for each visit.[1]

On June 9, 1909, Ada Beazley, a Henry Street nurse, reported to the Metropolitan office on Broadway to collect a list of industrial insurance policyholders who had requested nursing care. After discussing the social background of her patients with the Metropolitan superintendent, she walked through the alleys and over the rooftops of New York City's Richmond district to locate Ellen Daly, the first Metropolitan visiting nurse service client. Daly, an Irish immigrant suffering from varicose leg

This chapter was originally published in the *Bulletin of the History of Medicine*, 1989; 63:414–434. Copyright Johns Hopkins University Press. Reprinted with permission.

ulcers and isolation, blessed both Nurse Beazley and the Metropolitan Life Insurance Company for attending to her affliction and discomfort. Daley and thousands of immigrants like her had accepted the insurance agents' sales offer promising that for just pennies a week the immigrants could avoid a pauper's grave while receiving skilled nursing care to alleviate the physical and psychological pain of tenement life.

Metropolitan policyholders embraced the security the firm's sales agents described to them, and Nurse Beazley and her colleagues anticipated that their work with MLI would give them an opportunity to realize their humanitarian ideals, rescue poor patients from death and disease, and earn income and recognition as visiting nurses.[2]

When the initial experiment proved advantageous for both Metropolitan and the Henry Street House, Metropolitan extended an invitation for contracts to other visiting nurse associations (VNAs) across the United States and Canada, creating the Metropolitan Visiting Nurse Service. From the nursing service's inception in 1909 through its termination in 1953, approximately twenty million policyholders received home nursing care as a benefit of their insurance policy.[3]

VNAs had experienced phenomenal growth in the United States between 1877 and 1909. By 1909, over 566 associations offered nursing home visits and health teaching to the sick poor.[4] As Karen Buhler-Wilkerson has noted, VNAs in the United States were an extension of the English system of district nursing, where the nurse taught the poor the value of exercise, proper diet, sunshine, and cleanliness.[5] As the United States experienced urban growth, industrialization, and immigration, women philanthropists supported the development of American VNAs, viewing the trained nurse as a messenger of care, cleanliness, and character for the hordes of poor, sick immigrants who disrupted the order of American cities. The "care of strangers" lay within the boundaries of the sphere of women. Women's duty to care was joined with ideas of reform, and a new opportunity for nurses was created.

This growth of visiting nursing (later called public health nursing) has been documented by historians,[6] but the corporate sponsorship of public health nursing has not been analyzed. While many reform organizations (the New York City Mission and Tract Society, 1877; the Society for Ethical Culture, 1879; United Hebrew Charities, 1885), settlement houses, churches, hospitals, and businesses (Suit, Skirt, Dress, and Waist Industry, 1903; Joint Board of Sanitary Control, 1904) organized VNAs, Metropolitan Life was the first insurance company to establish its own visiting nurse service.[7]

Throughout the Metropolitan Visiting Nurse Service's history, businessmen and nurses held different views. Although Metropolitan executives admired the selfless art of nursing, they perceived nurses as company employees whose skills and knowledge offered a pragmatic solution to the business problems of finances and company image. And the Metropolitan men believed that nurses, as company employees, needed their guidance. From Metropolitan's perspective, nursing was a business. Nursing leaders understood the financial advantages of business sponsorship, but they viewed visiting nursing not as a business but as an emerging profession whose primary goals were to raise the profession's status and provide high-quality care for patients. These differences in perspective affected the course of the Metropolitan Visiting Nurse Service until finally, in 1950, amidst business and social changes, Metropolitan executives decided that the liaison with nursing no longer constituted a wise business investment.

ORIGINS OF THE METROPOLITAN VISITING NURSE SERVICE

Beginning at the end of the Civil War, "life assurance" was sold by lawyers to middle-class men concerned about the welfare of their families. This type of life insurance, called ordinary insurance, was advertised not only as a method of financial investment, but as a way for men to demonstrate the fulfillment of their duty in protecting their families against poverty. By the end of the nineteenth century, life insurance companies had multiplied, and competition among them was fierce. While most companies competed in a headlong chase for larger, more expensive policies, a small New York company, Metropolitan Life Insurance, sought to be distinctive by selling small ($500) life insurance policies costing 35 cents a week. Company executives marketed their idea as "insurance for the masses," selling the majority of policies to laborers who belonged to the Hildese Bund, a mutual assistance organization for German immigrants. Bund officers collected premiums, and thus Metropolitan saved money on commissions, sales promotions, and salaries, making the company's strategy profitable as well as unique.[8]

When membership in the Hildese Bund declined, lapses in Metropolitan insurance policies escalated. Seeking a new market and sales methods that would provide low-income families with affordable life insurance, the Metropolitan executives were attracted to a new type of insurance called "industrial insurance," which had been developed by the Prudential of London. In contrast to ordinary insurance, industrial insurance was sold door to door by an insurance agent who also collected the 3- to 10-cents weekly premium in the homes of poor urban industrial workers. Unlike ordinary insurance, industrial insurance was sold to women and children as well as to men, with the rationale that loss of income due to the death of any family wage earner would threaten the family's survival. Moreover, the sales agent had the power to issue industrial insurance policies without the usual medical examination. Thus, housewives often purchased policies for every family member without their knowledge. From the Metropolitan executives' perspective, the purpose and methods of industrial life insurance were congruent with the company's philosophy of life insurance. Hoping to saturate the working-class market, Metropolitan began selling industrial life insurance in 1879.[9]

In just two decades (1879–1900) Metropolitan rose from a national ranking of eighteenth to the fourth-largest insurance company in the United States, with industrial insurance sales averaging 2,000 new policies a day. Only the top three ordinary insurance companies (New York Life, Mutual Life, and Equitable of New York) outranked Metropolitan in sales and assets.

The success of industrial insurance was no surprise to Haley Fiske. Evangelistic, perspicacious, and obsessively religious, Fiske had an unshakable conviction that he had been chosen to serve God's children using industrial insurance as his instrument of service.[10] Yet Fiske was a man of contrasts. Although he righteously advocated life insurance as a means of teaching immigrants American values, Fiske, a pragmatic lawyer, also believed that selling insurance was a method of obtaining power, profits, and success. Thus, for Fiske, humanitarian concern and profit were interdependent ideas. Good intentions reaped profit, profits increased power, and power allowed one to help the disadvantaged.

Fiske's beliefs were shaken in 1904 when the journalist Thomas Lawson's muckraking exposé *Frenzied Finance* was published. Lawson described corrupt practices within the life insurance industry and condemned the "Big Three" insurance companies (Equitable, New York Life, and Mutual Life) as scoundrels of the first order. He accused the companies of speculation and misuse of policyholders' money, of issuing dishonest contracts, and of fraudulent alliances with large companies such as Standard Oil. Moreover, Lawson reported that the insurance commissioners knew of and reported on the deceitful practices but that their reports were ignored by state officials. When newspapers across the country published the story and aroused the public, New York legislators demanded an investigation.[11]

In July 1905, the New York Assembly and Senate resolved to examine the affairs of life insurance companies authorized to do business in the state of New York. The resolution directed a committee of eight, chaired by State Senator William Armstrong, to examine the investments of companies, the relationship between companies and subsidiary organizations and their policyholders, and any other phases of life insurance business deemed to merit examination. Charles Evans Hughes, the examining attorney, convened the Armstrong Committee hearing on September 6, 1905, in the city hall in New York. It remained in session

until December 30. The 7,000 pages of information collected during the
Armstrong investigation supported Lawson's earlier charges and revealed
dishonest practices of nepotism, blackmail, and mismanagement of funds
in the Big Three companies. The investigators' belief that the Big Three
were responsible for forcing smaller companies to compete dishonestly
meant that the smaller companies, including Metropolitan, were treated
relatively easily by the committee.[12]

Although the Armstrong Committee sought only to investigate the
practices of life insurance companies, there is little doubt that newspapers across the country had placed the companies on trial. News
accounts, editorials, and cartoons portrayed insurance companies as corrupt, depraved, and unethical. Moreover, the press assumed that the
charges it published were true and demanded that prosecution follow the
investigation to protect the future of democracy.[13]

While the public digested the startling revelations of the news
reports, the Armstrong Committee's Report, dated February 2, 1906,
described in detail the serious problems with the insurance industry and
called for immediate action to correct the deficiencies. Once the
Armstrong Report appeared, the presidents of the Big Three companies
resigned and several officers of the Mutual Life and New York Insurance
companies were charged with grand larceny and forgery.[14] Clearly, the
insurance industry had been disgraced.

Discouraged by the outcome of the Armstrong hearings, Haley Fiske
formulated strategies to defend his company and improve its image.
Considering the hearings a threat to private insurance companies and to
his personal cause, Fiske initiated a series of public forums in which he
emphasized Metropolitan's commitment to social responsibility. Publicly,
Fiske promised to liberalize contracts, increase benefits, lower premiums,
and maintain honest business practices.[15]

In December 1908, Fiske was invited to a forum at the Charities
Building in New York City to discuss industrial life insurance. After the
meeting, Lee Frankel, director of United Hebrew Charities, approached
Fiske to continue the dialogue. Frankel had just returned from Germany,
where he and the social activist Miles Dawson had been sent by Robert
DeForest, head of the Russell Sage Foundation, to study workingman's
insurance. Frankel favored state-sponsored life insurance for the working
class and believed private insurance companies in the United States were
profit mongers not interested in helping the workingman. Frankel, a
chemist by training who received his doctorate from the University of
Pennsylvania in 1891, spent the major part of his career as a social
worker with Jewish immigrants. In an autobiographical sketch, Frankel
stated that he had accepted the position with United Hebrew Charities in
order to serve his people with "the Hebrew ideals of love, justice, and

mercy." Shocked by the egregious conditions in which Jewish immigrants lived, Frankel noted that he eventually learned that the goals of social work were more effective when money, legislation, and organization supported one's high ideals.[16]

In response to Fiske's evangelical speech defending life insurance, Frankel suggested that Metropolitan implement its rhetoric by organizing a division to provide directly for the health care of policyholders. When convinced that such a plan might lower mortality rates, enhance the image of the company, and increase sales and profits, Fiske challenged Frankel in return by agreeing to the idea on the condition that Frankel join Metropolitan. Thus, in January 1909, Lee Frankel accepted the position of manager of Metropolitan's new Welfare Division. According to Frankel, Metropolitan had moved into "a new era which joined in the battle against disease and in which it hoped to lead the world in preserving lives."[17]

Frankel had a clear vision of what he hoped to accomplish. To launch the Welfare Division, he decided to target one disease at a time. Yet the question remained: Which disease? Because Metropolitan statistics suggested that tuberculosis was responsible for 20% of the death claims made to the company, Frankel decided to wage war against the "white plague." Although he consulted with Lawrence Veiller, director of the National Tuberculosis Association, Frankel clearly wanted to lead a distinctive national health movement. Frankel and Fiske believed that neither the established organizations nor the medical profession had the vision to fight tuberculosis effectively. In addition, Frankel wished to maintain control of the funds and manpower required to implement his plan. With his goals clear, he decided to write a health pamphlet on tuberculosis; to convert his insurance agents (who would distribute the pamphlet to policyholders) into messengers of health education; to build a tuberculosis hospital for Metropolitan employees, demonstrating that tuberculosis could be cured; and to advertise health services and life insurance through magazines and speeches.[18]

Proud of his strategies for health reform, Frankel spoke to many organizations about his plan. After one such speech, in February 1909, Lillian Wald, director of the Henry Street Settlement House, approached Frankel and suggested that although his plan had merit, trained nurses would be more effective than insurance agents in teaching good health practices to policyholders.[19]

Wald needed no introduction to Lee Frankel. With funds provided by the philanthropists Mrs. Solomon Loeb and Jacob H. Schiff (Mrs. Loeb's son-in-law), Wald and her associate Mary Brewster had begun the Henry Street Settlement House (originally the Nurse's Settlement House) in 1893. Like nurses in other settlement houses, Henry Street nurses lived among the poor and attempted to create a household for the benefit of immigrants. According to Wald, her nurses accomplished this by providing home care "in a manner which upheld the dignity and independence of the patient." By 1909, Lillian Wald was directing eleven Henry Street subresidences and four county rest homes in the New York City area.[20]

Adept at establishing contacts and at using the art of persuasion, Wald performed her work with the financial support of various social organizations: During Frankel's tenure with United Hebrew Charities, its medical bureau had employed physicians, midwives, and nurses to care for Jewish immigrants. When the supervision of staff proved difficult, Frankel arranged for patients to see physicians in various dispensaries and in 1902 had contracted with Wald's Henry Street nurses to visit patients in their homes.[21]

Wald's suggestion for the utilization of nurses by Metropolitan extended the Wald-Frankel working relationship. Despite Frankel's familiarity with Wald's work, he knew he must convince the Metropolitan board of directors of the value of her idea. At the invitation of Frankel, Wald spoke to the board, explaining to the men that Henry Street nurses made visits in eleven Manhattan districts to give home care and teach elements of health such as cleanliness and nutrition. The directors were only mildly interested until Wald presented her Henry Street statistics, which suggested that mortality rates declined due to nursing visits. Immediately, the men saw an opportunity to decrease mortality rates, increase profits, and enhance the image of the company.[22]

The Metropolitan Visiting Nurse Service began in June 1909 as a three-month-long experiment on the west side of New York City. The visiting nurses, advertised by Metropolitan as friends of the poor, were quickly appreciated by policyholders. Thousands of letters scratched on scraps of paper poured into Metropolitan offices from these grateful policyholders. The *humanitarian* Frankel delighted in the policyholders' response, but the statistics teased the *businessman* Frankel. Louis Dublin, the chief MLI statistician, suggested that in neighborhoods where nurses visited, insurance sales increased and mortality rates declined. The positive data prompted Haley Fiske to announce publicly "that nurses demonstrated in a practical, visible way the responsibility which Mother Met feels towards her children."

Before the experiment ended, the board of directors decided to extend the nursing service throughout Manhattan and then in swift succession to Washington, D.C., Baltimore, Boston, St. Louis, and Cleveland.[23] Generally in these ventures in other states Metropolitan followed the precedent established by its liaison with Henry Street and cooperated with existing VNAs. Anxious to receive additional income and to make nursing more visible to the public, VNAs welcomed an alliance with the company.[24] Yet, in their initial enthusiasm, they failed to recognize the impact that corporate sponsorship might have on their organizations.

DISCORD AND ITS AFTERMATH

Initially it appeared that nursing and business had similar beliefs and goals. Both stated an interest in the welfare of policyholders and a desire to increase income and decrease mortality rates. Beneath the superficial agreement, however, lay an unspoken assumption that would prove discordant. Metropolitan businessmen assumed that nurses were employees under the jurisdiction of the company, while nursing leaders believed that staff nurses were accountable to the patient, to professional ethics, and to nursing leaders.

As businessmen, Fiske and Frankel believed that the Metropolitan Visiting Nurse Service was a marketable entity that should be administered as a business. Metropolitan statistics indicated that the company provided between 20% and 50% of the service's annual incomes. Using this datum as justification, Frankel and Fiske concluded that they had a duty and a right to supervise, and demand efficiency from, visiting nurses. At Metropolitan, efficiency meant systematic recordkeeping, time management, and accurate cost accounting for each visit. Visiting nurses believed that they already functioned efficiently, but Frankel had his own efficiency standards for nurses. He calculated that a nurse should work ten hours each day, average twelve visits a day, and accumulate 250 visits every month. From Frankel's viewpoint, a performance below this standard could not justify the nurse's monthly salary of $74.[25]

In 1914 Frankel decided to document nurses' efficiency by conducting a study of twelve large urban VNAs. The data revealed a wide variance in the number of daily visits made by nurses. In New York City the average number of visits made by a nurse per day was 12 (more than one per hour, given the ten-hour day), while in Baltimore nurses averaged six visits per day (less than one per hour). Discovering that an average Metropolitan patient was a female (67%) under the age of forty (73%), Frankel initially suspected that Baltimore nurses (and their sisters in other cities who did not achieve the twelve-visit standard) lingered in the homes to chat with patients. But upon further thought, Frankel realized that the data reflected a range of *actual* nursing care. For instance, in New York City, the average number of visits per case was 8.5, while visits per case in Baltimore averaged 5. The number of days a patient remained on the VNA's rolls before discharge ranged from 12 (New York City) to 36 (Baltimore). Frankel concluded that the philosophy of care in New York was to work as intensively as possible with patients, whereas Baltimore nurses advocated a philosophy of health supervision and teaching over a longer period. Moreover, in studying the condition of patients upon discharge, Frankel found that the New York City VNA recorded 56.8% of patients as "improved," while that of Boston, for example, recorded only 13%. Although the demographics of all patients were similar, the rates of recovery differed radically. Frankel concluded that neither the philosophy of care nor the criteria of what determined improvement were standardized among the various associations.[26]

As manager of Metropolitan's Welfare Division and an advocate of the theories of Frederick W. Taylor, the father of "scientific management," Frankel believed he should determine what constituted standardized nursing care and terminology. But he would learn that viewing nursing as a business was foreign to nurses. As Barbara Melosh and Susan Reverby have pointed out, the "traditionalist" or "worker nurse" in the field at the time had been trained in a culture of nursing which emphasized character, duty, and spirituality.[27] Visiting nurses were intent in acting out their mission of caring. While the Progressive era's ideas of efficiency were not unknown to visiting nurses, nurses remained dedicated to their duty as efficient mothers of the world, not efficient workers of business.

Worker nurses, dedicated to patients, passively resisted Frankel's expectations, but nursing leaders frankly rejected the notion that nursing was a business. Fighting to convince the public of the value of the trained nurse, Wald and other national nursing leaders had a clear vision of the definition, role, and potential of the visiting nurse. Convinced that the nurse should be an independent practitioner, nursing leaders could not view the nurse as an employee of Metropolitan and would not allow business to define or control nursing practice.[28]

Publicly, Frankel stated his support of public health nursing's development, but privately he doubted that nurses or the "lady managers" supporting the VNAs possessed the business acumen needed to manage the associations effectively.

In his endeavor to dissuade nursing from what he labeled its "charity attitude," Frankel criticized the VNAs' management practices, arguing that the associations' costs were too high, nursing visits too few, and paying patients too scarce. As Buhler-Wilkerson has noted, the women managing the VNAs could hardly disagree with his facts, but they reacted negatively to his attempts to control nursing.[29]

Generally, the "lady managers" of the associations were philanthropic women from the "gentle [upper] class." Although middle-class nurses were perceived as hardworking and pragmatic, they lacked access to the persons of influence who associated with upper-class women. Nurses were not "ladies," and therefore the so-called *lady* managers were uniquely qualified to appropriate the money, the time, and the power that was needed to manage a VNA and its nurses. Despite the absence of social or professional equality, the nurses and the lady managers shared an enthusiasm for the elements of reform. They agreed that cleanliness, empathy, order, and morality must be provided for the multitude of patients they served.

The VNAs valued reform principles. Frankel's worldview was rooted in business concepts and efficiency. The differences between the business perspective and the nursing perspective led to discord. For example, as part of an attempt to collect health statistics, Frankel demanded that detailed records be kept on patients. Lillian Wald perceived this demand as an attempt to use nurses as data collectors and argued that patient care could not be sacrificed for the sake of Metropolitan paperwork. As the nurses' employer, Frankel disagreed. When Chicago visiting nurses did not comply with his wishes and continued to obtain lengthy social histories rather than health statistics, Frankel ordered the practice to cease. In another incident, Frankel suggested that as a cost-containment measure, practical nurses be assigned to chronically ill patients. Edna Foley, superintendent of the Chicago VNA, exploded in anger, insisting that patients could not be placed at the "mercy of . . . half-trained and counterfeit workers."[30]

In each of these episodes Frankel stood firm, arguing that philanthropic attitudes and ineffective management practices damaged the company's image and threatened its financial stability. And in each case, Frankel used his cost argument to shape nursing practice: Nurses began to collect detailed health statistics, the practice of obtaining lengthy social histories stopped, and chronically ill patients were limited to six nursing visits. Frankel believed that finances should shape nursing-care policy, whereas nursing leaders maintained that the nurses' assessment of patient care should govern policy. In an effort to define nursing and control their own practice, nurses clung to issues of quality of care and resisted business values. Frankel interpreted this resistance as incompetence in business skills; thus, he took control of financial issues and used cost arguments as his entitlement for power. Nursing became engulfed in a power struggle. A few years later Mary Beard stated, "Frankel frightened the nurses and because of this they were unable to communicate their professional standards to him or hear his business needs."[31]

Arguments between nursing leaders and Frankel continued for a decade. Each year the VNAs increased their charges to Metropolitan for the cost of a nursing visit. And each year Metropolitan required factual justification from the associations for the increases. The continuous debate effectively polarized cost against quality of care. Finally, in 1922, public health nursing leaders agreed with Frankel that a scientific determination of nursing visit costs might resolve the problem, and a committee was set up to investigate. With the John Hancock Mutual and Aetna Insurance companies planning to open visiting nurse services, nursing leaders believed the cost issue had to be settled.[32]

The cost study, which was financed by Metropolitan and published in 1924, concluded that the variability of patient needs made the calculation of nursing visit costs impossible. Frankel, who had always maintained that the cost of a nursing visit could be determined through scientific inquiry, was chagrined by the results. Yet he gained some satisfaction from the fact that the independent committee agreed with him that the cost of a nursing visit was a critical issue.[33]

Despite his impatience with nursing leaders, Frankel remained dedicated to the idea and cause of visiting nursing. Believing that "reality comes slowly to nurses," Frankel abandoned his polemical relationship with national nursing leaders, hired his own superintendent of nursing, and set out to prove that the Metropolitan Visiting Nurse Service could function as an efficient business with high productivity and low cost.[34] The new nursing superintendent, Helen LaMalle, was a trusted ally of Frankel's. When she suggested that increased supervision and education would increase nursing efficiency, Frankel hired twelve area nursing supervisors and 23 clerks to handle records, revised the nursing manual, opened practice centers for in-service education, implemented a correspondence course to teach nurses public health principles, increased nurses' salaries, designed a safe driving course for nurses, and wrote two nursing textbooks. In 1929, LaMalle and Frankel decided the programs should be evaluated. At the completion of an evaluation study, Frankel announced that research had determined that the Metropolitan Visiting Nurse Service was functioning with high efficiency and low cost. According to company statistics, nurses made four million visits annually and saved the company millions of dollars a year in death claims. Moreover, nurses completed records accurately, gave quality patient care, and visited ten patients each day.[35] Frankel had reached his goals. The nursing service functioned as an efficient business according to Frankel's standards. But the efficient humanitarian reveled in his success for just over a year. In the spring of 1931, Lee Frankel died. His death foreshadowed changing times: Fiske had died two years earlier; the old guard of nursing leaders had faded; and idealism and reform within Metropolitan was waning.

THE UNRAVELING OF THE NURSING SERVICE

The Fiske-Frankel era was over and with it the expansive humanitarian worldview that had characterized Metropolitan's activities. Although the Welfare Division remained concerned with conservation of life, by 1935 changes in disease patterns in American society, medical treatment, public health, and lifestyle of policyholders undermined the original justification for Metropolitan's emphasis on health reform programs. Metropolitan policyholders were now one or two generations removed from immigrant status and were accustomed to employment, education, and upward mobility. While communicable disease and other acute illness and child-birth had once formed the basis of the nursing cases, the later, more sophisticated, policyholders had been immunized against communicable disease and were choosing hospitalization for childbirth. As Charles Rosenberg has shown, medicine's advancing diagnostic and treatment capacities convinced patients and physicians that the hospital, not the home, was the center for legitimate care of any person with an acute illness. The growing acceptance of the physician's "cultural authority" in curative treatment effectively relegated public health and its preventive focus to secondary status.[36]

Metropolitan executives were aware that sick policyholders at this time had more health care options available to them than had the immigrant policyholders of earlier years. According to company statisticians, policyholders were more capable of treating themselves at home, were more accustomed to physicians and hospitals, and had higher salaries with which to pay for health care. In addition, it was clear to company executives that with the passage of the Sheppard-Towner Act (1921), the federal government had entered the area of health care on a large scale. By 1935, Franklin Roosevelt's New Deal offered funding for hospital construction, medical and public health programs, and support to children, the blind, the disabled, and the aged through the Social Security Act.[37]

In this changing pattern of provision of health care, the men who replaced Fiske and Frankel did not feel a need to claim responsibility for the health of the American public. Metropolitan's new president, Fred Ecker, believed that in the future the responsibility for disease treatment and prevention would be shared between government agencies and the individual. As a pragmatic businessman, Ecker viewed the life insurance industry as a corporate giant, not a social cause. Labeling Metropolitan "the largest Company in the world," Ecker emphasized real estate sales, investments, and profits and delegated social concerns to social scientists.

Donald Budd Armstrong, a physician with a master's degree in public health, replaced Frankel as vice-president in the Welfare Division.

He agreed with Ecker that Frankel's social work approach was outdated, and he believed that the Welfare Division needed to embrace a more modern public health outlook, one that identified health issues and transferred the work to local, state, and federal health authorities. Armstrong, as a physician, did not wish to duplicate the work of or compete with his medical colleagues. Physicians had gained power through the years, and as Paul Starr had noted, they objected to any middleman—whether company, agency, individual—coming between them and their practice.[38] Anxious to maintain and widen their power, physicians wanted neither persons in auxiliary roles nor the realm of public health to challenge their authority or economic position. Ecker and Armstrong believed that Metropolitan could continue to enhance the company image through its Welfare Division work without antagonizing physicians or duplicating the health care efforts of other agencies.

Armstrong stated that the Welfare Division would support health programs, but he emphasized that physicians held the primary obligation for direct patient care. In Armstrong's view, nurses were trained auxiliary personnel who could detect health problems and obtain business for physicians, but who could not practice independently due to their lack of judgment. The new director of Metropolitan's nursing service, Alma Haupt, heartily disagreed and hoped to change Armstrong's attitude. A graduate of the Johns Hopkins Nursing School in 1929, Haupt had held the position of acting director of the National Organization of Public Health Nursing prior to her employment at Metropolitan. Although aware of the rapid growth of hospital nursing during her career, Haupt remained convinced that the visiting nurse was a distinctive kind of nurse and one who had a bright future. In light of the rising costs of medical care, Haupt believed that the expansion of public health, education, and environmental programs would secure public health nursing's future.[39]

Haupt also believed that quality of patient care, facilitated through nursing education and supervision, would provide public health nurses with leverage to control their own practice. Backed by a powerful company like Metropolitan, she planned to improve the standards of nursing care and convince executives of the value of the nurse. With these goals in mind, Haupt insulated herself with a nurse executive staff and then implemented an industrial model for the nursing service, adding layers and layers of educators, peer reviewers, and supervisors. Between 1935 and 1940, Haupt and her nurse executives strengthened the educational focus of the nursing service, transformed practice centers into teaching centers, and initiated a quality assurance program, an in-service education program, and a peer review program.[40]

Armstrong offered no objections to Haupt's new programs until she decided to define the functions of the Metropolitan visiting nurse.

Believing that physicians should determine nursing practice, Armstrong objected to the idea that nurses should take blood pressures, complete urinalyses, and administer intramuscular injections. Even though nurses had successfully performed these tasks during the years of Frankel's leadership, Armstrong now argued that these procedures called for a physician's judgment. But Haupt contended that these treatments were a function of the professional nurse. Incensed with Haupt's rebellion, Armstrong asked the Metropolitan Law Division for a decision. When the lawyers ruled in favor of the nurses, Haupt believed she had outmaneuvered Armstrong and instructed her nurse executives to begin a multitude of projects aimed at defining and evaluating nursing practice.[41]

The nurse executives naively thought they had won their point. They did not seem to understand that their educational and credentialing programs would prove inadequate against social trends, the growing authority of physicians, and the business needs of Metropolitan. Nor did the nurses comprehend that the extensive educational programs increased the operating costs of the nursing service and that, as in the days of Frankel, Metropolitan was a business in which finances influenced policy. Nurses could argue for autonomous functions and plan educational programs, but the issue of finances belonged to Metropolitan executives. The precedent had been set by Frankel and would not be reversed. Cost issues would again serve as a powerful argument for policy formation.

In 1939, Jerome Apfel, head of the Metropolitan Accounting Division, reported that, over seven years, nursing visits had declined at a rate of 200,000 per year. Apfel added that the large supervisory and educational programs had resulted in lower productivity of nurses. With fewer visits, increased overhead expenses, and a sharp decline in industrial insurance sales, Apfel warned Metropolitan executives that the cost of a nursing visit was out of proportion to the industrial insurance premiums collected. Although the inverse relationship between cost and volume alerted executives to the financial problems of the nursing service, it was the Temporary National Economic Committee (TNEC) that motivated the company seriously to reassess nursing's benefits.[42]

The TNEC, a federally sponsored committee, began in 1938 as a result of a business recession the year before. A group of economists convinced President Franklin Roosevelt that the United States economy had reached maturity, that private enterprise could not offer sufficient investment opportunities for the American public, and that only the government was capable of running the economy. Big business in this view was to blame for economic problems in the United States, and big government was the solution. As Arthur Krock wrote in his syndicated column, "insurance companies are too large; they now rival the federal government in the amount of money they invest and tax the public."[43] Insurance premiums were viewed as being equivalent to a tax, insurance companies were competitors of the federal government, and Metropolitan was the largest company. With assets of $5 billion, Metropolitan came to be a prime target for questions regarding the methods it used to obtain wealth.

During the two-year proceedings of the TNEC, lawyer Gerhard Gesell accused Metropolitan of using the nursing service as a sales gimmick to obtain insurance business. He charged that this method of sales amounted to unfair competition, resulting in the excessive size of Metropolitan. Furthermore, Gesell questioned the legality of Metropolitan spending policyholders' money on nursing services. He charged that the practice was a misuse of funds. Although Metropolitan's president, Leroy Lincoln, defended the tradition of the nursing service, the tone of the questioning convinced him that the committee's ultimate goal was to highlight defects within the insurance industry and demand federal regulation of the industry. The final report of the TNEC confirmed Lincoln's suspicions. It stated: "A fundamental change in the conduct of industrial insurance should occur, otherwise its elimination will be necessary."[44]

In addition to making this terse recommendation, the final report pointed to failures of state supervision and suggested that state insurance boards strengthen their insurance commissions, supervise agency practices, standardize policy forms, and limit insurance companies' expenditures on policyholders. In response to the recommendations, the New York State legislature proposed legislation limiting insurance companies' expenditures on policyholders to 1.5% of income from industrial insurance. The proposed legislation led to a $1 million decrease in the nursing service budget. As an attorney himself, Lincoln knew that the law offered no elasticity, and he feared that expenditures on the nursing service increased the company's vulnerability to federal regulation.[45]

Threats of war forestalled decisions regarding the future of the nursing service. Metropolitan executives concentrated on inserting war clauses into policies and approving military leaves, while Welfare Division personnel worked to create programs for blood donation, venereal disease eradication, and industrial safety.[46]

By 1946 the Metropolitan Visiting Nurse Service was in a vulnerable position. The overhead expenses of both the contracting VNAs and Metropolitan's visiting nurse centers continued to rise.[47] Escalating costs of automobiles, gasoline, rent, supplies, and staff contributed to the cost of a nursing visit rising from $1 in 1935 to $3 in 1946. At this point Metropolitan executives decided to conduct a study to determine the reasons for continued declining utilization of the service. Results of 3,000 interviews suggested that policyholders no longer wanted nursing services. Although the nation's birthrate had increased after the war, with 10%

of policyholders adding a baby to the family, 72% of the affected families had not requested a nurse. Of policyholders who reported a serious medical illness within the family, only 24% used nursing services, while 96% reported using physician services. When families were asked if there was any occasion when the family would have liked to have had a nurse, only 12% responded affirmatively. The results of the study forced Louis Dublin, a longtime supporter of visiting nursing, to speculate that despite the hopes of public health leaders, health care had moved to hospitals.[48]

In the face of the grim findings of the study, Metropolitan nurses conducted business as usual. Despite the declining volume of cases, nurses still hoped for a brighter future. While penicillin, sulfonamides, insecticides, and vaccines had all but conquered dysentery, communicable diseases, and pneumonia, the number of patients suffering from chronic diseases such as cancer and heart disease increased. Metropolitan nurses thought that as the number of chronic patients increased, Metropolitan would lead a national movement to include nursing in health care insurance plans. Blinded by their commitment to public health, nurses remained convinced that their role would change from acute care expert to caretaker of chronic patients. They failed to comprehend that Metropolitan had little to gain from financial sponsorship of nursing care for chronic patients. As Melosh has noted, larger social and cultural expectations of medicine militated against a broader commitment to chronic patients.[49] Public health programs, once the champion of preventive and acute care, had been overshadowed by mainstream medicine and its aggressive curative interventions.

TERMINATION OF THE NURSING SERVICE

Although nurses remained optimistic, it was clear to Metropolitan executives that the Metropolitan Visiting Nurse Service had outlived its usefulness. The final decision to terminate the nursing service was made at the board of directors' meeting on June 27, 1950, three days before President Leroy Lincoln announced publicly, "Metropolitan Life Insurance Company has reached the conclusion that its visiting nurse service is no longer needed to meet the important health needs for which it was organized."[50]

After one hour of discussion, the board of directors decided to put an end to the company's 41-year tradition of providing nursing services. Louis Dublin, chief company statistician since 1911, presented data that described the changing state of health in America. He argued that since 1911 the life expectancy of industrial insurance policyholders had increased 17.2 years (from 46.6 years to 63.8 years). Changing patterns of disease, improved diet, water, and milk, and new medical therapies had led to the replacement of the high mortality rate from acute diseases by escalating morbidity rates for chronic diseases. Dublin paraphrased the opinions of other experts on health care by stating that the responsibility for the care of chronic patients rested with various hospitals, nursing homes, and federal health agencies, not with the private sector or with corporations such as Metropolitan. Moreover, Dublin predicted that as voluntary sickness insurance programs grew in popularity and workers' earnings escalated, policyholders would accept financial responsibility for their own health care. The original purpose of the visiting nurse service had been to care for patients with acute diseases in the home, but times had changed. The care of patients suffering from acute illness had moved to hospitals, and Metropolitan was not interested in absorbing the moral or the financial responsibility for the home care of chronically ill patients.[51]

Donald Armstrong added that agents, the public, and even lay members of VNAs had lost interest in public health nursing. Moreover, Armstrong speculated that as the caseload of chronic cases increased, nurses would need to make longer home visits, driving the volume of visits even lower and the cost higher. From Armstrong's perspective, the cost of the nursing service was prohibitive to the company.[52]

Dublin had presented arguments against continuing the nursing service from a social perspective, while Armstrong had presented arguments reflecting the company's perspective. No arguments surfaced in favor of retaining the nursing service, although George Wheatley, vice-president of the Health and Welfare Division, suggested that the nursing service be discontinued over a period of two years. The decline in Metropolitan cases had reduced the amount of income for VNAs, but the company still provided many VNAs with 10% to 20% of their annual income. Wheatley argued that it was only fair to give associations and policyholders time to adjust to the loss of the nursing service. The board voted to close the Metropolitan Visiting Nurse Service on January 1, 1953.

After the board meeting, Armstrong informed Haupt and the nurse executives of the decision. Nurses had been neither informed of, nor invited to attend, the meeting. Caught unaware, the nurses reacted with shock and anger, calling the decision unfair. For years nurses had dedicated themselves to the efficient care of patients and the management of the visiting nurse service. They were stunned at the company's lack of appreciation. Although nurses knew about the inverse relationship between cost and volume, they anticipated that the trend would reverse when the public and the business world realized the importance of the nurse to the health of Americans. When Haupt made an attempt to convince

Armstrong of public health nursing's bright future, he flatly stated that the board's decision was irreversible. This cold dismissal starkly accentuated the nurses' awareness of their powerlessness, and they humbly prepared to dismantle the nursing service.[53]

The Metropolitan Visiting Nurse Service closed quietly. Although a few policyholders wrote to the company protesting the decision, the vast majority did not view the visiting nurse as an important component of their health care and accepted the company's decision in silence. Haupt stopped the nursing advertisement and closed the 300 Metropolitan Visiting Nurse agencies one by one. Many of the VNAs that were dependent on company monies were absorbed by communities, merged with public health agencies, or simply closed. Metropolitan nurses either retired with a separation allowance or found employment elsewhere. Nurses completed the tasks of termination efficiently, quietly, and sadly. Despite their feelings of hurt and rejection, their faith in public health nursing remained strong. Nurses proudly compiled an eight-volume scrapbook of their nursing service. They believed that the Metropolitan Visiting Nurse Service had contributed to the health of Americans. Haupt was convinced that the scrapbook would leave a written legacy of nurses' accomplishments and would provide guidance for the leaders of the next golden era of public health nursing.[54]

CONCLUSIONS

The Metropolitan Visiting Nurse Service closed on January 1, 1953. Ironically, the nursing service ended as it began. In 1909, the effects of a national inquiry into insurance companies intersected with grim social conditions to stimulate Wald, Frankel, and Fiske to form the Metropolitan Visiting Nurse Service. For years, company statistics supported the notion that the nursing service was a wise business venture. According to Dublin's interpretation of the data, nurses lowered mortality rates and raised the company's image, sales, and profits. For years, Metropolitan staff nurses cared for the ill in their homes and taught the principles of health to millions of industrial insurance policyholders. While staff nurses labored at the bedside, nursing leaders fought to define public health nursing and increase its status, power, and autonomy. They hoped that their association with a large corporation like Metropolitan would provide a means to their goal of independent nursing practice. But Metropolitan nurses were inextricably linked to business and medicine and caught in a dependent web without economic, social, or contractual power. Their attempts to gain self-definition and autonomy by increasing performance and educational standards did not provide visiting nurses with sufficient power to function separately from medicine and business. And as the focus of health care moved from prevention within the home environment to curative treatment in hospitals, visiting nursing had less appeal to physicians, businesses, and policyholders.

In the 1940s, social conditions, health trends, and policyholders' health needs intersected with a second national insurance investigation. In contrast to those of 1909, statistics in 1947 portrayed visiting nurses as a liability to the company and provided pragmatic Metropolitan executives with objective evidence for terminating the nursing service. In a sense, nursing had reached its goal. The nurses of the 1950s were better educated, more skilled, and more sophisticated than their counterparts of 1909. Nursing had demonstrated growth and strength. Yet nursing possessed no power. The liaison with Metropolitan had given visiting nurses visibility and income, but it failed to provide nurses with the prestige, autonomy, or conception of themselves that the early leaders had envisioned for the profession. Nursing seemed to have little control over its destiny. In the end, business judged nursing as unnecessary for the health needs of policyholders and, thus, expendable.

ACKNOWLEDGMENTS

This chapter is an expansion of a paper presented at the 60th annual meeting of the American Association for the History of Medicine, Philadelphia, Pennsylvania, May 1, 1987.

NOTES

1. Lillian Wald and Mary Gardner determined the cost of a nursing visit by dividing their total expenditures by the number of patients. See Lillian Wald to Mrs. Jacob Schiff, April 17, c. 1905, box 40, reel 37, Lillian D. Wald Papers, Manuscript Section, New York Public Library; Lee Frankel, "The Visiting Nurse Service;" speech to International Congress on Hygiene and Demography, 1912, Health and Safety Files, Metropolitan Life Insurance Company Archives, New York (hereafter MLIC Archives); Mary Gardner, "Dr. Frankel's plan," *Quarterly Bulletin* 1 (July 1937): 1-2; Lillian Wald to Alma Haupt, February 1937, Health and Safety Files, MLIC Archives.

2. Nursing legend states that Metropolitan's nursing service began on the Lower East Side of Manhattan. Although Henry Street was also located on the lower east side, District 12, where Ellen Daly lived, was on the west side of Manhattan. See report of Beazley's activities in Ruth King to Alma Haupt, March 31, 1939, Health and Safety Files, MLIC Archives.

3. Metropolitan statistics suggest that at the peak of the nursing service, in 1931, 35 out of every 1,000 policyholders received nursing care. The company's statistics record a

total of 102.5 million visits from 1909 through 1953. On the average, each patient received five visits during an illness. Thus, the chief Metropolitan statistician estimated that approximately 20.5 trillion policyholders received nursing care during the tenure of the nursing service. See Louis Dublin, *A Family of Thirty Million: The Story of the Metropolitan Life Insurance Company* (New York Metropolitan Life Insurance Company, 1943), 11–86. See also Marquis James, *The Metropolitan Life: A Study in Business Growth* (New York Viking Press, 1947), 111–12; Maurice Taylor, *The Social Cast of Life Insurance* (New York: Alfred A Knopf, 1933).

4. Annie Brainard, *The Evolution of Public Health Nursing* (Philadelphia: W. B. Saunders, 1922); Yssabella Waters, *Visiting Nursing in the United States* (New York: New York Charities Publication Committee, 1909), 516–26; William Rathbone, *Sketch of the History and Progress of District Nursing from Its Commencement in the Year 1859 . . .* (London: Macmillan, 1890); Yssabella Waters, "The Rise, Progress, and Extent of Visiting Nurses in the United States," *Charities and Commons* 16 (1906): 16–19.

5. See Karen Buhler-Wilkerson, "False Dawn: The Rise and Decline of Public Health Nursing, 1900–1950" (PhD diss., University of Pennsylvania, 1984); idem., "Left Carrying the Bag: Experiments in Visiting Nursing, 1877–1909," *Annual Review of Nursing Research* 36 (1987): 42–47.

6. Gloria Caliandro, "The Visiting Nurse Movement in the Borough of Manhattan" (EdD diss., Columbia University, 1970), 71–105; Barbara Mclosh, *The Physician's Hand: Work Culture and Conflict in American Nursing* (Philadelphia: Temple University Press, 1982); Susan Reverby, *Ordered to Care: The Dilemma of American Nursing, 1850–1945* (Cambridge: Cambridge University Press, 1987); Charles E. Rosenberg, *The Care of Strangers: The Rise of America's Hospital System* (New York Basic Books, 1987); Buhler-Wilkerson, "False Dawn."

7. Following Metropolitan's lead, other insurance companies formed visiting nurse services. John Hanoodt's nursing service began in 1925 and Aetna's in 1929. Caliandro, "Visiting Nurse Movement," 103; Taylor, *Social Cast*, 127; Lillian Wald to Alma Haupt, December 5, 1938, Health Education Files, MLIC Archives.

8. Ordinary or class insurance had been available in the United States since 1762, but only after the Civil War did it gain popularity. This shift was due in part to the conceptual shift in the meaning of death. Death was no longer a predestined punishment from God, it was a force over which men could exercise control by insuring their families against poverty—despite the inevitability of death. J. Owen Stalson, *Marketing Life Insurance: Its History in America*, 2d ed. (Cambridge, Mass.: Harvard University Press, 1984); Malvin Davis, *Industrial Life Insurance* (New York: McGraw-Hill, 1964); James, *Metropolitan Life*, 43.

9. Directors' Minutes, October 28, 1879, Vertical Files, MLIC Archives; Taylor, *Social Cast*, 47–60; R. Carlyle Buley, *The American Life Convention, 1906–1952: A Study of the History of Life Insurance*, 2 vols. (New York: Appleton-Century-Crofts, 1953), 1: 268–80.

10. According to Fiske's daughter Helen, shortly after his marriage to a devout Catholic, Fiske had a vision in which St. Thérèse of Lisieux appeared. The saint instructed him to live a life for others. His colleagues attributed his vigor, confidence, and devotion to God and life insurance directly to the vision. Fiske was a stubborn, principled man who, according to his associate Lee Frankel, "would not budge one-tenth of an inch if right were on his side." Darwin Kingly of the New York Life Insurance Company eulogized Fiske as "the Jupiter of Life Insurance Heaven." Fiske described himself as a pragmatist who "feared God, paid cash, and kept his bowels open." Despite the

theatrical descriptions, the historical record suggests that Fiske was the patriarch of Metropolitan Life who ruled the "Met family" with a mixture of discipline, caring, arrogance, wit, and shrewdness. See Helen Fiske, *The Garden of Little Flowers* (Baltimore: Southland Press, 1907).

11. Thomas Lawson's book *Frenzied Finance* (New York: Ridgway-Thayer Co., 1905; Books for Business, 2004) was written in the genre of Lincoln Steffens's *The Shame of the Cities,* Ida M. Tarbell's *History of Standard Oil,* and Ray Baker's *The Backroads on Trial.* Lawson hoped to be a member of the Steffen, Tarbell, Baker, Upton Sinclair, group of forceful young writers, but his book is less factual and more hysterical than those of the classic Muckrakers. "Frenzied Finance" was first published in *Everybody's Magazine* in 1904, then in book form.

12. Armstrong Committee, Record, Testimony, Exhibits, and Reports, New York State Legislature, 7 vols., 1906, vol. 1: 130–80.

13. Accounts can be found in most daily newspapers across the nation: *New York World, New York Evening Post, Chicago Tribune, Philadelphia Inquirer, Richmond Dispatch, Detroit Journal,* to name a few.

14. Armsttong Committee, Report, February 2, 1906, vol. 7: 336. A copy can be found in MLIC Archives.

15. "The Search for a Remedy," *Outlook,* November 4, 1905, 12; Haley Fiske, *Triennial Addresses 1–3* (New York: Metropolitan Life, 1900–1928).

16. Lee Frankel, *In The Early Days of Charity* (New York: National Conference of Jewish Social Services, 1930), 1; "Tribute to Lee Frankel," transcript, December 9, 1927, MLIC Archives.

17. Lee Frankel, memorandum (date-stamped 1909), Fiske File, MLIC Archives.

18. Lee Frankel to Haley Fiske, February 9, 1909, MLIC Archives; Harold Howk, "Modern Life Insurance Company's T.B. sanatorium," *Modern Hospital* 7 (October 1916): 278–87.

19. Lillian Wald, *The House on Henry Street* (New York: Henry Holt 1915), 29–32; idem., *Windows on Henry Street* (Boston: Little, Brown, 1934); George Rosen, *A History of Public Health* (New York: MD Publications, 1958); Lillian Wald to Alma Haupt, February 26, 1937, Health and Safety Files, MLIC Archives.

20. Originally, Wald's Settlement House was located on Jefferson Street in Manhattan. In 1895 Jacob Schiff purchased the home at 265 Henry Street on the Lower East Side. See also Clack Chambers, *Seedtime of Reform: American Social Service and Social Action, 1918–1933* (Ann Arbor: University of Michigan Press, 1967); Louis Dublin, *After Eighty Years: The Impact of Life Insurance on the Public Heath* (Gainesville: University of Florida Press, 1966); Allen Davis, *Spearhead for Reform: The Social Settlements and the Progressive Movement, 1890–1914* (New York: Oxford University Press, 1967). The quotation and descriptions of the Henry Street expansion are in Wald to Haupt, February 26, 1937, Health and Safety Files, MLIC Archives.

21. Caliandro, "Visiting Nurse movement," 71–105; Dorothy Jansen, "The Henry Street Settlement: A Response to the Needs of the Sick Poor" (EdD diss., Columbia University, 1979), 78; Robert Duffers, *Lillian Wald: Neighbor and Crusader* (New York: Macmillan, 1938).

22. Lillian Wald collected statistics on the nursing visits from the founding of the Henry Street settlement. By 1909, Wald employed a full-time statistician, Mabel Curan. For her presentation, see Haley Fiske, "Meet Metropolitan Life Insurance Company," July 1909, Fiske File, MLIC Archives. Lavinia Dock, "The Nurses [sic] settlement," 1900, Visiting Nurses Association of New York Archives (the collection

is uncatalogued); Lillian Wald, "The Henry Street Settlement," *Charities and Commons* 16 (1906): 35.

23. By 1931, there were 843 agencies contracting with Metropolitan and 346 Metropolitan stations. Some of the visiting nurse stations sponsored by MLI employed one or two nurses. Nurses cared for policyholders in more than 7,000 cities in the United States and Canada. See "Summary of Welfare Division," 1930 (uncatalogued), Health and Safety Files, MLIC Archives.

24. A few national nursing leaders such as Lillian Wald and Edna Foley were suspicious of Metropolitan's economic motives in joining with nursing. Wald remarked to Mrs. Jacob Schiff, "We must take care not to enhance a great marketing scheme, but to carry on our nursing work." Lillian Wald to Mrs. Jacob Schiff; April 1911, Health and Safety Files, MLIC Archives; Edna Foley to Lillian Wald, April 1910 (uncatalogued), Chicago VNA Archives; Lillian Wald to Eugene Liaes, October 1910, Lillian D. Wald Papers, Manuscript Division, New York Public Library.

25. Metropolitan's financial support of visiting nurse associations ranged from 20% to 50% of expenses. For instance, MLI paid for 32% of cases carried by Philadelphia VNA nurses in 1911, 20% of Providence, RI, VNA cases in 1913, and 25% of Henry Street cases in 1916. Francis Curtis, "Relative functions of health agencies: IV. Relation between official and non-official health agencies," *American Journal of Public Health* 10 (1920): 956–60; Buhler-Wilkerson, "False Dawn," 69; Caliandro, "Visiting Nurse Movement," 182; Louis Dublin, "Statistics," 1910–20, Health and Safety Files, MLIC Archives.

26. Lee Frankel, "Standards of VNA Work," 1915, Welfare Division Files, MLIC Archives; idem., "Visiting Nursing from a Business Viewpoint," 1913, Welfare Division Files, MLIC Archives.

27. Melosh, *Physician's Hand*, 124; Reverby, *Ordered to Care*, 145; Buhler-Wilkerson, "False Dawn," 69.

28. Lillian Wald to Lee Frankel, May 21, 1913, Health and Safety Files, MLIC Archives. For nursing leaders' attitudes on the issue, see Maybelle Welch, "Standardizing Qualifications for Public Health Nursing Positions," *Public Health Nursing* 17 (1923): 297–99.

29. Buhler-Wilkerson, "False Dawn," 70–112. Lee Frankel to Mrs. Joseph Cudahy, December 20, 1916, Chicago VNA Archives.

30. Lillian Wald to Lee Frankel, April 7, 1919, Health and Safety Files, MLIC Archives; Frankel to Louis Dublin, July 1919, Health and Safety Files, MLIC Archives; Edna L. Foley, "Concerning the Employing of Practical Nurses by Visiting Nurse Associations," *American Journal of Nursing* 12 (1912): 328–30 (quotation is on 328).

31. Mary Beard, President's Address, *Proceedings of the Twenty-Third Annual Convention* (New Orleans: National League for Nursing Education, 1917), 6.

32. *Report of the Committee to Study Visiting Nursing* (New York: MLIC, 1924), 11–13; Lillian Wald to Louis Dublin, August 12, 1922, Health and Safety Files, MLIC Archives; "John Hancock Nursing Service Overview," 1925, Health and Safety Files, MLIC Archives.

33. Lee Frankel, "Report of Round Table on the Visiting Nurse Study," June 20, 1924, Health and Safety Files, MLIC Archives.

34. Lee Frankel to Louis Dublin, c. 1924, Health and Safety Files, MLIC Archives.

35. According to Metropolitan, nurses had always saved the company money. According to Dublin's calculations, from 1909 to 1918, the nurses saved Metropolitan $18 million in death claims. These claims cannot be substantiated by the historical record. Lee Frankel, "Stabilization of MVNS," 1930, Welfare Division Files, MLIC Archives; Louis Dublin, Nursing Data, 1909–19, Health and Safety Files, MLIC Archives.

36. Rosenberg, *Care of Stranger,* 262–85. See also Paul Starr, *The Social Transformation of American Medicine* (New York: Basic Books, 1982).

37. Donald Armstrong, "Time and Methods of Transferring Health Work to Public Authority," June 20, 1928, Armstrong File, MLIC Archives; "About Fred Ecker" (c. 1950), typescript, Health and Safety Files, MLIC Archives; Louis Dublin and Alfred J. Lotka, *Twenty-Five Years of Health Progress: A Study of the Mortality & Experience among the Industrial Policyholders of the Metropolitan Life Insurance Company, 1911 to 1935* (New York: MLIC, 1937).

38. "The largest Company in the world," was a favorite description of Ecker's and was imprinted on MLI stationery. James, *Metropolitan Life,* 292–93; Donald Armstrong, "The physicians and the VNA," *Public Health Nursing* 27 (1934): 279, Armstrong Files, MLIC Archives; Donald Armstrong to Fred Ecker, November 1931, Health and Safety Files, MLIC Archives; Starr, *Social Transformation,* 217.

39. Lloyd Taylor, *The Medical Profession and Social Reform, 1885–1945* (New York: St Martin's Press, 1974), 121–27; *Committee on the Cost of Medical Care for the American People* (Chicago: University of Chicago Press, 1924), 42; Alma Haupt, "The Metropolitan Nursing Story," *Quarterly Bulletin* 15 (1951): 19; idem., "Some new emphasis on public health nursing," *Public Health Nursing* 27 (1935): 626; Alma Haupt to Margaret Reed, August 18, 1939, Health and Safety Files, MLIC Archives. For Armstrong and Haupt's positions, see Alma Haupt Supervisory Minutes, July 20 and 27, 1939, Health and Safety Files, MLIC Archives.

40. Alma Haupt, "Supervisory Nurses," 1937, Health and Safety Files, MLIC Archives; Alma Haupt "Progress Report," 1937, Health and Safety Files, MLIC Archives; "Official Statement of Functions of Public Health Nursing," 1936, microfilm 19, National Organization of Public Nursing Archives, New York.

41. See Donald Armstrong to Law Department, June 1936, Health and Safety Files, MLIC Archives.

42. Jerome Apfel to Donald Armstrong, December 1939, Health and Safety Files, MLIC Archives; Buley, *American Life Convention,* 2: 800–60; Temporary National Economic Committee, *Final Report and Recommendations* (Washington, D.C.: U.S. Government Printing Office, 1941), 40–43; idem., Hearings, 1940, pt. 28, 15671–731, Health and Safety Files, MLIC Archives.

43. TNEC, *Final Report,* 559–609; Henry Stodard, "The great monopoly mystery," *Saturday Evening Post,* March 30, 1940, 212; Arthur Krock, "The prompters: stage managers of TNEC hearings," *New York Times,* June 7, 1939.

44. TNEC, *Final Report,* 500.

45. Leroy Lincoln, "Effects of TNEC," Report to Welfare Division, 1941, Health and Safety Files, MLIC Archives; "Leroy Lincoln: 1880–1957," Lincoln Files, MLIC Archives.

46. "War Work," 1940–42, Welfare Division Files, MLIC Archives.

47. In 1946 there were 845 "affiliated services" (VNAs) and 327 "salaried centers" (MLI-sponsored agencies) covering 7,737 towns in the United States and Canada. *Survey of Metropolitan's Nursing Service* (New York: MLI Press, 1947), 27–35; "Nursing Service: 1935–1950," Health and Safety Files, MLIC Archives.

48. "MVNS Annual Report," 1946, Health and Safety Files, MLIC Archives; Marion Randall, "Home nursing service in the health insurance plan of Greater New York," *American Journal of Public Health* 39 (1949): 167; Alma Haupt to Marie Johnson, August 1946, Health and Safety Files, MLIC Archives; Survey of Metropolitan's Nursing Service.

49. Melosh, *Physician's Hand,* 112–18.

50. Leroy Lincoln, "An Announcement concerning the Health Conservation Program of MLIC," June 30, 1950, Lincoln File, MLIC Archives; "An Analysis of Volume of

Service in Relation to Its Costs," 1949, Health and Safety Files, MLIC Archives; Donald Armstrong, "Conference with NOPHN," June 30, 1950, 3–15, Lincoln File, MLIC Archives; George Wheatley, interview June 1984, Lincoln File, MLIC Archives; James Fillmore, Termination" (c. 1953), typescript, MLIC Archives.
51. Lincoln, "Announcement concerning the Health Conservation Program;" "Analysis of Volume of Service;" Armstrong, "Conference with NOPHN": Wheatley, interview.
52. Armstrong, "Conference with NOPHN."
53. "Transition," 1951, typescript, Health and Safety Files, MLIC Archives; Alma Haupt to Helen LaMalle, September 16, 1922, Haupt File, MLIC Archives; "A Report of the Study of the Effect of the Termination of Metropolitan Contracts," 1951, Health Welfare File, MLIC Archives; Jerome Apfel, "Nursing Cost Guide," 1950, Health and Safety Files, MLIC Archives.
54. Nursing Bureau Scrapbook, 1950, MLIC Archives.

SECTION 3

Doing Nurses' Work

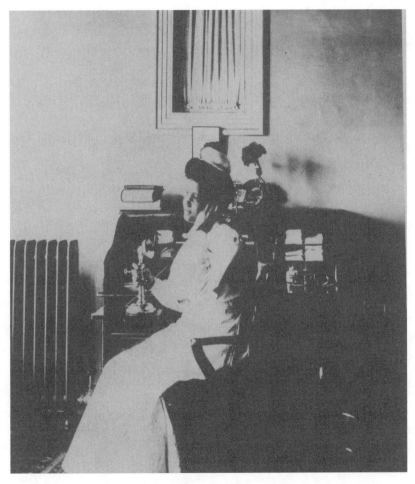

A nurse at Douglas Hospital, Philadelphia, circa 1898. Reprinted with the permission of the Barbara Bates Center for the Study of the History of Nursing.

Introduction

Sylvia D. Rinker

There is in this work (nursing), room for exercise of talents of the highest and virtues of the rarest order . . . it is a field of usefulness such as is nowhere else afforded, and a woman with the requisite qualifications, who desires to be really of service to her fellow creatures, and to adopt an employment of absorbing interest, can not do better than to train herself for a nurse.[1]

Writing one of the earliest textbooks in nursing, Clara Weeks-Shaw introduced the practice of nursing as both an inspiring and challenging occupation. The primacy of practice is the overarching concept in nursing that unites the diversity of nursing's educational programs, research agendas, knowledge paradigms, and various practice initiatives. The complexities faced by nurses as they engaged in their work—the practice of nursing—is the focus of this section. A recent recognition of the need to understand how the practice of nursing has evolved over time declares that "to be blind to the skill and competence of ordinary nurses in the past is to risk denying the skill and competence of nurses in the present."[2] It is vital to explore what nurses have done and what they have known because the historical antecedents of nursing practice shaped the ambiguities, challenges, and, yes, successes that define current nurses' clinical practice.

The personnel who performed nurses' work, their compensations, and the rapidly changing expectations for nursing practice are all made visible in the articles selected for this section, which deal specifically with nurses' responses to the needs of society through an ever-evolving nursing practice. The environments in which the early practice of nursing occurred both shaped and were shaped by the initiatives of nurses who cared for patients within various contexts. The chapters in this section provide glimpses into a variety of places where nursing was practiced, offering insight into the influence of environment on practice.

ENVIRONMENT OF CARE

Most readers will be familiar with hospital-based training schools and the early use of student nurses as laborers within burgeoning hospital institutions at the beginning of the twentieth century. The first chapter in this section explores nurses' work in a slightly different place, that of the early twentieth-century tuberculosis (TB) preventoriums.[3] As in hospitals, nurses' efforts made the institutions possible. Their persuasive demeanors, careful documentation of every aspect of care, and attention to the teaching needs of their patients and families led to the gradual recognition of TB preventoriums as health care facilities. Preventorium nurses oversaw children's daily needs, instructing parents on the importance of cleanliness, hygiene, rest, and good nutrition. Recognizing the importance of care beyond the institutions' walls and the diversity of their patient population, TB nurses made home visits and developed written teaching pamphlets that were translated into immigrants' native languages. Their efforts were well-received and effective. By 1910, TB nurses represented the vanguard of public health.[4] The shift from treatment to prevention required an expanded role for nurses that fit the needs of early twentieth-century American society and meshed well with other public health initiatives of the time. Cynthia Connolly clearly presents the dilemmas faced by TB nurses that sound all too familiar today.[5] Encouraged to be authoritative with patients, nurses were reminded that they were to look always to physicians and medical science for direction. According to Mary Gardner, author of an early public health text, society wanted TB nurses to be visible and "pile up brilliant results" but did not understand the structural impediments that made their work difficult, such as inadequate resources, too few numbers, physician resistance to their efforts, and, in many instances, weak authority to structure their own practices."[6] The story of the TB preventorium, while a relatively short lived type of nursing, highlights ongoing opportunities as well as frustrations experienced as nursing practice grew.

ORGANIZATION OF CARE

In the second chapter in this section, Lynne Dunphy details the intensive care required by the use of the iron lung to combat the effects of the polio epidemic, 1929–1955.[7] The introduction of the frightening but lifesaving iron lung complicated the already difficult care of polio patients and required extensive teamwork from the nurses involved. For example, since patients weakened by the disease were unable to sustain their own respirations, basic hygiene procedures required that two to four nurses work rapidly together to complete the care in as short a time as possible.[8] Nursing care during polio epidemics provides an early example of patient triage and grouping of very ill patients together to render more effective care—foreshadowing later intensive-care-unit environments and illuminating the commitment and power of nurses who knew their patients' very lives depended on their efficient nursing actions.

Traveling from epidemic to epidemic, "polio nurses" used their ingenuity, effectively gaining expertise that provides an early example of specialization in nursing. Growing expertise led to pushing the boundaries of nursing practice: "Although it was clearly designated to be the domain of medicine to 'set' the particular pressure gauges on the machines, the nurses monitored the settings, adjusting and individualizing them to each patient and situation, and troubleshooting when problems arose."[9]

The work was arduous. Nurses wrote of the long hours without days off and the relentless "mental stress" of having to deal with constant power outages, when the cumbersome iron lungs had to be operated manually to preserve the patient's life.[10] Iron lung patients called for nurses to care concurrently for both patient and machine, and much can be learned from nurses' responses to and use of this early technology.[11] Because nurses worked closely with their patients, they could see firsthand the effects of their practice. The practical constraints of too few nurses caring for extremely ill patients shaped nursing practice in the early twentieth century in ways that today's nurses can surely recognize.

TECHNOLOGY

Enduring issues of power and authority surround the evolution and use of technology in nursing practice. Nurses have shown themselves very willing to adopt and use new technology as it has become available. In fact, nursing practice has always been as "advanced" as the science and technology of the era in which it was practiced.[12] Julie Fairman has noted, "By the way nurses organized their work, their consent to go beyond boundaries of nursing practice of the time or simply their decision to use their clinical judgment when the rationality of physicians' orders was in question, nurses made choices about technology that deeply influenced patient care."[13]

The third chapter in this section is a fascinating exploration of the impact of technology on nursing practice as revealed in nurses' roles related to the technology surrounding blood transfusion.[14] Part of the attraction that technology has posed for nursing practice has been its usefulness to distance nurses from their domestic roots.[15] Cynthia Toman's article raises thoughtful questions about what is gained and what is lost as professional nurses take on and let go of technological roles in changing practice environments.[16] "Blood Team" nurses gained proficiency in their practice, just as the TB preventorium nurses, polio nurses, and later coronary care unit nurses gained expertise in their particular areas of practice. Toman notes that interns at the Ottawa Civic Hospital rotated through a month's experience with the Blood Team, is an example of doctors learning from nurses, a complete reversal of the tradition that posited the physician as unquestioned authority and the nurse as subordinate learner.[17] Nurses' constant presence with patients, incorporating technology as it becomes available, provides the environment in which nursing practice grows and changes. It was the accumulated "tricks of the trade" that provide the practical solutions to problems that nurses encountered in assisting, maintaining, and monitoring patients in iron lungs, as well as in caring for patients receiving blood transfusions. Nursing evolves as the result of the accumulated, embodied wisdom acquired in practice.

The wisdom that nurses have acquired over time has "elasticized" the sphere of the nurse.[18] In describing the inception and proliferation of coronary care units in the United States in the 1960s, for example, Arlene Keeling notes in Chapter 12 that in the interest of saving lives, nurses were given special training to recognize deadly cardiac arrhythmias, and they accepted the responsibility of taking the actions needed to correct them.[19] The artificial disciplinary boundaries between medicine and nursing were blurred when nurses assumed the technological skills of cardiac monitoring and defibrillation in early coronary care units. As coronary care units developed, what was new to nursing practice was that nurses had to move from simply collecting data and reporting their findings to physicians to acting on their own assessment of data when necessary, prior to reporting it to a physician: "That nurses could interpret EKGs and defibrillate patients represented a radical change for all concerned."[20] Keeling concludes that nurses who had been "ordered to care" now stepped over the nursing practice domain into the realm of scientific medicine and "cured" patients' arrhythmias in lifesaving moments. In so doing, these pioneers set the stage for continued expansion of nursing's scope of practice.

According to Margarete Sandelowski, nurses have always sought to understand and make the best of the things that have increasingly and paradoxically defined and blurred the definition of their practice.[21]

CONCLUSION

The chapters in this section inform us, and yet, our understanding remains incomplete.[22] The spaces where nurses and patient meet become the arenas where practice develops. The ways nurses organize their responsibilities within the constraints and benefits of environments infused with technology create patients' expectations and shape patients' experience of nursing care; the possibilities are endless. Patricia Benner et al. remind us that nursing praxis is broader than the science guiding it and includes the working out of knowledge, inquiry, and relationships in practice.[23] The challenge is to create organizational and unit cultures that can accommodate both the science and the human goods associated with confronting the human realities of risk, suffering, loss, and death, and offering whatever comfort measures possible.[24] Accepting and striving toward such a goal does indeed require nurses with "talents of the highest and virtues of the rarest order."[25]

NOTES

1. Clara Weeks-Shaw, *A Text-Book of Nursing*, 3rd ed. (New York: D. Appleton and Co., 1912), 2–3.
2. Sioban Nelson and Suzanne Gordon, "The Rhetoric of Rupture: Nursing as a Practice with a History?" *Nursing Outlook* 52 (September/October 2004): 260.
3. Cynthia Connolly, "Nurses: The Early Twentieth Century Tuberculosis Preventorium's 'Connecting Link,'" *Nursing History Review* 10 (2002): 127–57.
4. Ibid., 134.
5. Ibid.
6. Mary S. Gardner, Letter to the Editor, *Public Health Nursing* 21 (February 1929): 66–67. Quoted in Connolly, "Nurses," 140.
7. Lynne Dunphy, "'The Steel Coccoon': Tales of the Nurses and Patients of the Iron Lung, 1929–1955," *Nursing History Review* 9 (2001): 3–33.
8. Ibid., 17.
9. Ibid., 24.
10. Ibid.
11. Ibid., 4.
12. Nelson and Gordan, *Rhetoric of Rupture*, 258.
13. Julie Fairman, "Alternative Visions: The Nurse-Technology Relationship in the Context of the History of Technology," *Nursing History Review* 6 (1998): 142.
14. Cynthia Toman, "Blood Work: Canadian Nursing and Blood Transfusions, 1942–1990," *Nursing History Review* 9 (2001): 51–78.
15. Ibid., 51.

16. Ibid. 52.
17. Ibid., 160.
18. Margarete Sandelowski, "The Physician's Eyes: American Nursing and the Diagnostic Revolution in Medicine," *Nursing History Review* 8 (2000): 8.
19. Arlene Keeling, "Blurring the Boundaries Between Medicine and Nursing: Coronary Care Nursing, circa the 1960s," *Nursing History Review* 12 (2004): 139–64.
20. Ibid., 156.
21. Margrete Sandelowski, "'Making the Best of Things:' Technology in American Nursing, 1870–1940," *Nursing History Review* 5 (1997): 4.
22. Toman, "Blood Work," 71.
23. Patricia Benner, Patricia Hooper-Kyriakidis, and Daphne Stannard, *Clinical Wisdom and Interventions in Critical Care* (Philadelphia: W. B. Saunders, 1999), 19.
24. Ibid., 291.
25. Weeks-Shaw, *A Text-Book of Nursing*, 2.

CHAPTER 9

Nurses: The Early Twentieth-Century Tuberculosis Preventorium's "Connecting Link"

Cynthia A. Connolly

INTRODUCTION

Speaking to her colleagues at the nineteenth annual National Tuberculosis Association (NTA) meeting in 1923, Colorado public health nurse Ida Spaeth stressed the nurse's importance to a newly founded institution, the tuberculosis preventorium, for indigent children presumed "pretubercular":

> The service the public health nurse can render the preventorium and the tuberculous child is invaluable. She is the connecting link between the home and the institution; between the child and his physician; between the public and the tuberculous child in need of preventorium care. Whether she works out from the institution or in the community as the public health nurse, her responsibility and opportunity toward the tuberculous child and the preventorium are alike.[1]

The preventorium strove to prevent children infected with the tubercule bacillus from developing active tuberculosis (TB), and there is ample

This chapter was first published in the *Nursing History Review*, 2002; 10:127–157. Copyright Springer Publishing Company. Reprinted with permission.

evidence to support Spaeth's claim that nurses were integral to the institutions. In New York City, for example, nurses practicing in dispensaries,
schools, and community-based settings such as the Henry Street
Settlement identified pretubercular children and referred them to the
Charity Organization Society's association of TB clinics, the primary
referral base for that city's biggest preventorium, located at Lakewood
(later Farmingdale), New Jersey.[2] Nurses staffing the preventorium oversaw children's daily health needs, managed its programs, and worked
alongside teachers, a matron, and other employees.[3]

Still other nurses from New York City's Department of Health conducted mandatory home visits throughout a child's preventorium stay.
Nurses in all the aforementioned capacities instructed parents on the
importance of cleanliness and hygiene. When feasible, nurses facilitated
sanatorium admission for the tubercular parent. Nurses visited the home
for years after children left the preventorium; if their assessment revealed
deteriorating home conditions or former patients' weight loss, they usually recommended readmission to the preventorium.[4]

In this chapter I examine the role of nurses in the preventorium
movement. To understand nurses' thoughts and actions related to these
institutions, it is necessary first to describe the preventorium and outline
the relevant medical, social, and cultural frameworks in which it evolved.
Second, I trace nurses' efforts with regard to the preventorium movement
within the context of early twentieth-century public health nurses' antituberculosis work. Finally, I argue that nurses' efforts made the institutions possible, and describe the ways in which preventoria relied on
nurses at every juncture.

CHANGING IDEOLOGIES OF TB CAUSATION

The youngsters sent to preventoria often remained there for months or
years and generally came from poor, often immigrant, families in which
at least one parent suffered from tuberculosis. The first preventorium
opened in 1909 at Lakewood, New Jersey, and the nation's last, San
Diego's Rest Haven, closed in 1951. During the preventorium's heyday,
from the 1920s through the early 1930s, at least 26 institutions in
15 states cared for children labeled at-risk for TB. California, home of at
least eight preventoria, dominated the landscape of the preventorium
movement, while the rest of the institutions were scattered throughout
the United States, with concentrations in rural areas surrounding the
large urban centers of the Midwest and Northeast.[5]

The preventorium idea originated during frustrating times in the
early twentieth-century antituberculosis movement. As the nation's most

visible infectious disease, TB was a national preoccupation during most of the late nineteenth and early twentieth centuries. Although many people died from the disease, many more experienced long periods of tuberculosis-related debilitation. Minimizing TB's toll on society became the focus of numerous public and private endeavors.[6]

Throughout the first three quarters of the nineteenth century, tuberculosis, like most diseases, was postulated to be hereditary and noncontagious. The concept of disease as a discrete entity did not exist in its contemporary form. Physicians as well as the lay public believed that constitutional endowments, hereditarily transmitted, promoted or resisted illness.[7] Notions of TB were radically changed in the 1880s by new frameworks through which disease and illness came to be understood.[8] While Robert Koch's 1882 isolation of the tubercule bacillus facilitated the emergence of the germ theory, many scientists did not immediately discard sanitarian and hereditarian philosophies. Instead, as Nancy Tomes has argued, these older ideas were accommodated, and in many instances incorporated, in newer infectious-disease explanatory models.[9] Thus, most health care providers continued to interpret racial, ethnic, and socioeconomic variations in TB's incidence as evidence that certain groups needed moral, not just material, uplift.

The first years of the twentieth century, the period of time during which the germ theory's acceptance evolved, were tumultuous ones for the United States. As the pace of industrialization accelerated, many North Americans moved to urban areas seeking greater opportunities. In addition, waves of immigrants, many of them indigent, poured into U.S. cities. People crowded into tenements, were often unable to speak English, and frequently engaged in cultural practices foreign to earlier arrivals and the native-born. Poverty, inadequate sanitation, crime, and infectious diseases, especially tuberculosis, became rampant in the poorer districts."[10] Widespread fears of contamination from immigrants and the poor spurred health care professionals to practice what Alan Kraut has labeled "medicalized nativism."[11] Indeed, most nurses, physicians, and others active in the fight to eradicate TB considered race, ethnicity, and social class critical variables in their estimation of patients' TB risk. They cited research published in prestigious professional journals to justify their positions.[12]

Moreover, although the germ theory enriched scientists' and society's understanding of TB and spurred the creation of newly formed antituberculosis organizations, it added no effective tools to the curative arsenal. Treatment in the early twentieth century, whether in the home or the sanatorium, remained much the same as in the nineteenth century. Adjusting patients' environment, nutrition, and exercise-to-rest ratio remained therapeutic mainstays, along with providing health advice and encouraging the modification of deleterious behaviors.[13] As a

result, the era bookended by Koch's findings and the widespread availability of an antibiotic cure in the 1940s was a time not just of enormous hope, but also of frustration for antituberculosis activists in the
United States. Furthermore, the intricate interplay between bacteria,
host, and environment proved difficult to unravel. Epidemiological
investigations revealed that host factors such as individual behaviors,
heredity, and environment all played a role in disease progression,
though researchers often disagreed with one another on the extent of
their influence.[14]

Fears of contagion did lead to legislative approaches to control of
TB's spread. These laws, mandating registration and segregation of the
tubercular, were enacted in many cities during the early twentieth century.
Many of these regulations generated controversy and fear among the
poor.[15] Reformers seeking to arrest TB's spread sought less contentious
solutions, and found one in the idea of two prominent New Yorkers.

PROGRESSIVISM, CHILD-SAVING, AND THE EVOLUTION OF THE PREVENTORIUM CONCEPT

Nathan Straus, member of the wealthy New York retailing family, was a
well-known benefactor and activist. Alfred F. Hess was a respected pediatrician. These men became the chief protagonists in the development of
the first preventorium. Together, they galvanized support among the rest
of New York's social and medical elite. Their outlook, that the tuberculosis movement needed to be less treatment oriented and more prevention focused, reflected a growing philosophy among public health
leaders.[16]

While poverty-related conditions such as an inadequate living environment, excessive crowding, overwork, and insufficient nutrition clearly
enhanced one's risk for developing TB, these social problems were, by
themselves, too nonspecific to categorize as predisposing criteria unique
to TB. Clemens von Pirquet's 1908 discovery that a by-product of tubercule bacilli culture, known as tuberculin, could be used to identify those
individuals who were infected with TB before they developed actual
symptoms further energized public health experts.[17] Before tuberculin,
physicians classified children into two groups with regard to TB, the sick
and the well. After 1908, a third disease category was created, compris-
ing those infected with the organism but without active disease. Referred
to as "pretubercular," these children became the target population for the
preventorium. New York City's activist public health officer Herman
Biggs estimated that approximately 40,000 such children resided in the
city's tenement districts.[18]

The tuberculin test's discovery illuminated individuals' infection status, but it raised new questions as well. For example, almost all people over the age of 14 reacted positively to tuberculin, indicating widespread exposure to TB.[19] Only some infected youngsters actually developed TB symptoms, however. Many concluded that these data implied the influence of an intervening variable, perhaps resistance to infection. Low resistance, termed "physiological poverty" by New York physician Sigard Adolphus Knopf, condemned a child to a life of indigence and ill health.[20]

Seizing upon the tuberculin test's objectivity, Hess, Straus, and their colleagues sought to use it as an efficient tool to identify the pretubercular child. Once recognized, children at risk could be admitted to the preventorium and have their health preserved or restored. Preventorium supporters believed this outcome would be achieved not just by removing the child from the source of the infection, but also by re-creating within the institution the social conditions and moral climate of the wealthier classes. With the preventorium's founding, both men hoped to combine the best elements of a home, school, and sanitorium into one pediatric institution.[21]

Its founders designed the preventorium to articulate with the New York City Charity Organization Society (COS) and its programs by emphasizing the importance of choosing COS trustees to serve as preventorium medical board directors. For the first several years of the preventorium's operation, at least four individuals served jointly: physicians Herman M. Biggs, Abraham Jacobi, and James Alexander Miller, and social worker Lawrence Veiller.[22] Because of this close affiliation, the preventorium was influenced by many of the same principles that guided the COS. Many COSs in the United States conflated the medical and social problems faced by their clientele. This resulted in interventions that reflected a desire to improve patients' morality and reshape what they saw as inappropriate behaviors and patterns of thought, in addition to providing health care services and material assistance.[23]

The campaign to institutionalize pretubercular children was strengthened by the national reform-oriented ethos of the time known as Progressivism, and a media barrage in the professional literature as well as the lay press helped popularize the movement. Subsequent institutions patterned their therapeutics and daily operations after the New Jersey preventorium, but, unlike that institution, many newer facilities restricted admission by sex, ethnicity, race, or religion. Some operated as private, voluntary institutions similar to Farmingdale, while others were founded with private capital but grew to be managed by public agencies such as health departments or school districts. Still others functioned in association with public or private sanatoria.[24]

The numbers of preventoria grew after World War I, partly due to the fact that the massive preparedness efforts revealed that more than 80,000 young recruits were unfit to serve in the military because of active or suspected TB.[25] Most institutions drew patients from within a several-hour train or automobile ride. Several new preventoria opened in the early 1930s, but by that decade's end, falling numbers of new cases of TB and its champions' inability to quantify the institution's efficacy eroded its mission. In addition, a growing number of 1930s child welfare interventions, such as those implemented by the 1935 Social Security Act, prioritized family preservation, making the preventorium out of step with the times. The advent of antibiotics represented the single most damaging factor to the preventorium's existence, however. The discovery of streptomycin in 1943 followed by isoniazid in 1952 reframed TB as a disease treatable with outpatient therapy. The incidence of TB in the United States declined rapidly, and the era of the preventorium was over.

The preventorium never became a fixture in every community in the way its loyalists had hoped. Preventoria remained few in number and were usually located adjacent to cities with large numbers of TB sufferers or regions with many TB migrants. However, the institutions received a great deal of attention in the lay and professional TB literature as well as from local, state, and national antituberculosis organizations. One reason for the preventorium concept's popularity may have been its emphasis on children in a time period rich with child-saving rhetoric. Moreover, in an era in which no TB vaccine or cure existed but many people were exposed to the tubercule bacillus, interventions with potential to prevent morbidity and mortality appeared to many people to offer the best hope of eradicating the epidemic. That they were expensive to operate and required a relatively sophisticated public health infrastructure for maintenance probably limited their number, but not the idea's popularity.

Throughout the duration of the preventorium movement, the presence of trained nurses emphasized founders' vision of the preventorium as a health care facility. To date, however, there has been little research into nurses' duties with regard to individual preventoria, and no one has described what role, if any, nurses played within the broader effort to institutionalize pretubercular children. Many of the nurses who interfaced with the preventorium, its child clientele, and their families carried out one of public health nursing's most visible and prominent campaigns, tuberculosis eradication.[26] In the next section, I explore preventoriurn nursing in the context of public health nursing as well as antituberculosis public health efforts.

NURSES AND THE ANTITUBERCULOSIS MOVEMENT

Public Health Nursing in the United States

While fewer in number than their colleagues in private-duty and hospital work, public health nurses exerted a profound impact on early twentieth-century health care.[27] Despite the emergence of a professionally driven health care delivery infrastructure over the course of the early twentieth century and a growing number of institutions devoted to the sick, many ill people could afford no services whatsoever. Poverty and crowding overwhelmed city governments' outdated mechanisms for monitoring water quality and eliminating sewage and other waste. Infectious diseases spread rapidly among those crowded into tenement slums. Public health officials recognized that these illnesses could easily spread to the general population because the indigent sick often prepared food, cleaned houses, or sewed clothes worn by those who could afford to purchase such services.[28]

Reform-oriented men and women struggled to respond to the social and public health problems caused by the rapid pace of immigration, industrialization, and urbanization. Drawing upon the British concept of district nursing, they formed charitable organizations such as visiting nurse societies. By sending trained nurses out into the community to care for, educate, and monitor the sick poor, they hoped to ameliorate disease and improve living conditions.[29] Some Progressive activists even moved into residences, known as settlement houses, in the most destitute neighborhoods, with the goal of studying, and hopefully remediating, the social conditions surrounding poverty, crime, and disease.[30]

Nurse Lillian Wald developed the philosophical framework for public health nursing in the United States. In 1893, she and a colleague merged the concepts underlying district nursing and settlement houses by creating the nurse-managed Henry Street Settlement. Wald believed that bringing subsidized nursing care to the poor in their homes, as with the care that the middle and upper classes could afford for themselves, both heightened the chances for its success and made treatment more humane.[31]

Public health nurses' work differed from that of their peers in several substantive respects. Though they worked long hours in dangerous neighborhoods, unlike their colleagues in private-duty or institutional settings, nurses in public health negotiated more autonomy and less physician control for themselves. Furthermore, since the class relationship between patient and nurse was usually reversed from that of private-duty nursing and the care was subsidized by a third party, public health nurses held more authority than did other nurses.[32]

Public health nurses often worked 6–6 1/2 days a week. They usually visited between 8 and 12 patients over the course of an 8–10-hour day. These nurses maintained responsibility for the nursing care of both pediatric and adult patients suffering from a variety of acute and chronic illnesses. Some patients were so sick that the nurse visited them once in the morning and again in the evening before she went home. Because many patients were immigrants, their cultural background and ethnic origins often differed from that of the nurse.[33]

Public health nursing quickly evolved to become the province of a certain type of nurse, the graduate of a premier nursing school or a woman with the means to seek postgraduate training at one of the programs designed to supplement the narrow hospital nurse training with subject material related to economics, sociology, psychology, and public health.[34] In addition to having a broader knowledge base, nursing leaders believed that public health nurses needed more sophisticated skills than those of their colleagues in hospitals and private duty, along with better critical thinking and more initiative. They also had to be highly flexible and well versed in the social service and health care resources available within their communities. Since patient education constituted an important part of their role, they also needed to be articulate.[35]

Wald and her fellow public nurses successfully created an expanded nursing role that fit the needs of early twentieth-century American society. They made health care more accessible and less threatening to the poor by providing it within the social and economic context of New York's vulnerable populations. Since eradicating a "house disease" such as TB required the trust and cooperation of the poor in their homes, public health nurses' success made them indispensable to early twentieth-century public health efforts.[36]

The deftness with which public health nurses worked in the interstices of traditional health care ensured them a unique niche within the antituberculosis movement.[37] The shift in emphasis from treatment to prevention in the antituberculosis crusade mandated an intensive campaign based in homes, schools, and community settings, focused on people before they developed TB symptoms. Though nurses continued to care for ill and dying tubercular patients at home as well as in sanatoria, clinics, and dispensaries, those who specialized in TB prevention represented the vanguard of public health nursing by 1910.[38] Public health nurses recognized that their work differed from that of the general nurse. Both because they faced issues that other nurses did not and in an effort to establish themselves as an elite corps within nursing, public health nurses founded their own organization in 1912, the National Organization for Public Health Nurses (NOPHN).[39]

The Beginnings of Tuberculosis Nursing

Tuberculosis public health nursing evolved out of experiments in both Baltimore and New York City. In 1903, amid growing concerns about New York's TB problem, the city's COS and the health department made provision for a nurse to visit TB patients in their homes. Public health officials quickly deemed the nurses' efforts a success, and 13 more nurses were hired over the next two years.[40]

Although Baltimore's Johns Hopkins Hospital had developed a program a few years before New York did, it did not initially involve nurses. Beginning in 1899, the hospital's physician-in-chief William Osler assigned female medical students to monitor TB dispensary patients at home. Osler believed that the work required supervising patients' household cleanliness as well as personal hygiene, and saw these functions as women's roles. In 1904, Mary Adelaide Nutting, American nursing pioneer and superintendent of nurses and principal of the Nurse Training School at Hopkins, convinced Osler that nurses could do the work more effectively.[41] Soon after, Baltimore's Instructive Visiting Nurses Association (IVNA) added nurses devoted exclusively to tuberculosis public health nursing.[42]

Many TB nurses had themselves battled TB. While a few had contracted the disease while caring for tuberculous patients, many were recruited into sanatorium nursing schools from among the healthier female patients. Since TB's stigma, even for those considered cured, was potent, nurse training often represented the best option for many women who needed to work. Like public health nurses everywhere throughout the United States, tuberculosis nurses visited patients in their homes. In many instances, they combined dispensary work with patient visits. For example, in both Baltimore and New York, nurses made home visits for part of the day and staffed the dispensary with the time left.[43]

While tuberculosis nurses needed to possess all of the characteristics of other public health nurses, they especially needed a persuasive demeanor so that patients could be induced to follow directions. Tuberculosis public health nurses filled the bulk of their time with patient education because unless they were near death, patients could usually care for themselves. Nurses kept careful records of their work, monitored patients' progress or deterioration with each visit, and searched for new TB cases in the community as they made their rounds.[44] They instructed patients about every aspect of daily living, including matters related to personal hygiene and habits, food preparation and diet, childrearing, and the importance of home ventilation and cleanliness. Nurses also developed written teaching points and distributed them in pamphlet form in immigrants' native languages.[45]

Much of the information nurses taught patients could, if followed assiduously, protect the health of the tuberculous and those with whom they lived. For example, tuberculous parents who collected their sputum in a cup and discarded it appropriately reduced the chances that children in the household would come in contact with infectious materials. But differences in social class, culture, and ethnicity between nurses and their patients often made it difficult for them to understand one another. In 1915, for example, tuberculosis public health nurse Sarah Stevens shared with her colleagues the way in which cultural differences sometimes made TB care more difficult and confusing for all involved. She described her frustration with a Jewish woman who refused to let her child be sent away for "fresh air" after his father had died of TB because the mother believed that Judaism dictated that children must pray daily in a synagogue for a deceased parent.[46]

Stevens recounted another instance in which an Italian immigrant woman who had lost her husband and oldest child to TB brought her two remaining children to a dispensary. When the nurse began to prepare one child's arm for the von Pirquet tuberculin test, the mother screamed, swept up both children, and ran from the clinic. Stevens later learned that the mother told neighbors that nursing personnel wanted to burn a hole in the child's arm.[47] Though some nurses acknowledged the importance of learning about different cultures and customs alien to them, most did so only to be better able to sway patients from their beliefs and practices, not to incorporate them together in a way that met the demands for public health safety but also preserved patients' cultural practices.[48]

Stevens, for example, did caution nurses to respect patients' "racial and religious preferences," noting: "The mere fact that a certain dish does not appeal to our American palate is not proof positive that it is unfit to eat. . . . It is not unlikely that some of our own table delicacies seem quite as impossible to our friends from across the water." She asserted that such "unlimited forbearance toward the ignorant and superstitious" paid off because the nurse gained the trust of the family more quickly, which made it easier to persuade them to make changes the nurse suggested.[49] Delores Gladys Spicer informed her colleagues that "the cultural level of many a tenement house mother is not far removed from that of her primitive ancestors," reminding nurses that tact will encourage a prospective mother to try "'American ways' because she wants her child to be a real American, and because she trusts the nurse and wants to do all she can to please her."[50]

Physicians and philanthropists who funded public health initiatives usually came from the upper classes and viewed public health nurses as a conduit between themselves and the indigent people they perceived to be in need of moral uplift, education, and other direct assistance. By design, therefore, nurses in the antituberculosis movement laced their interventions with educative functions reflecting white, middle-class cultural practices.[51]

As a result, some of the information that nurses dispensed to sick TB sufferers had less to do with minimizing contagion but was instead more oriented toward inculcating bourgeois behaviors into patients' personal habits and daily activities. For example, Sara Shaw, the supervising nurse at New York's Bellevue TB program, emphasized the importance of a plain (nonethnic) diet and wrote condescendingly of patients' tendencies toward "delicatessen knickknacks." She also stressed to her patients the importance of properly served meals, cleaning house, arranging furniture, behaving patriotically, and using childrearing techniques aimed at making "enthusiastic little [American] homemakers" of the girls and "strong, manly men" with "fine ethical codes . . ., champions of a clean city."[52]

Furthermore, nurses did not always recognize the economic barriers that prevented full compliance for many tuberculosis sufferers. For example, in 1904 Jane Delano, superintendent at Bellevue Hospital's nurse training school, published the hospital's 41-point educational protocol, which all nurses followed when they visited TB patients in their homes. Delano made no mention, however, that certain of the recommendations were not feasible for the very poorest patients. Although many TB sufferers themselves agreed that it made sense for the tuberculous not to work or become overtired, and to have their own beds and bedrooms, those living in poverty had little control over these factors. Thus, patients' ability to adhere to many of the instructions dictated to them by nurses was hampered by the fact that, in many instances, compliance was economically untenable.[53]

Nurses often felt angry and frustrated when patients disregarded their directions, and often attributed noncompliance to a lack of intelligence, self-discipline, or callousness toward the health of others.[54] For example, Winifred M. Allen and Elizabeth McConnell, nurses at New York City's tuberculosis clinic at Gouverneur Hospital, signaled their attitude toward the dispensary's patients, 94% of whom were immigrants, by stratifying them by race and ethnicity into the following categories: "(A) fairly intelligent, (B) stupid, (C) inexpressibly stupid or defective."[55]

Such attitudes were not limited to nurses in the northeastern United States. California's Elsie M. Courrier, an Oakland tuberculosis nurse, presented a paper at the 1909 convention of the Nurses' Associated Alumnae in which she complained about the difficulty of inculcating better health practices into immigrants and the poor. Seemingly oblivious to the formidable cultural and economic obstacles that made such changes difficult, Courrier vented her frustrations: "What is to reach the army of ignorant, vicious, depraved, and often non-English-speaking people whom poverty, overcrowding, and our pernicious system of foreign immigration have placed among us? Can they be taught a sufficient knowledge of the subject to be anything but an ever-present menace in our midst?"[56]

In yet another instance, Rose MacGowan of Los Angeles alphabetized the nationalities of the patients with whom she interacted in her role as a school nurse. Based on her experiences, she described her interactions with children and their parents, attributing their behaviors and responses to her interventions to racial or ethnic characteristics. MacGowan's two-page summary of 16 different minority characteristics reflected prevailing early twentieth-century stereotypes. For example, MacGowan believed Mexicans to be shiftless and dirty and assumed that Jewish children shrewdly accepted her interventions primarily because they knew she could get them free services if they cooperated with her.[57]

In addition to case-finding new TB patients, educating patients about health-related issues, and monitoring their progress, an important nursing role also consisted of policing indigent communities for compliance with public health measures. Patients who did not follow nurses' instructions could lose part or all of their charitable assistance. Nurses could also recommend forcible removal of noncompliant patients, or their at-risk children, to sanatoria or other institutions.[58]

Nurses' authority to withhold much-needed assistance, as well as attitudes such as those expressed by Stevens, Shaw, Delano, Allen, McConnell, MacGowan, and Courrier, caused at least some patients to perceive TB nurses' efforts as coercive and threatening. Tuberculosis nurses themselves generally viewed their work as rewarding and contributory to society, however. Most considered their role a pivotal one, possessed of what Lillian Wald termed "civic intelligence."[59]

The Maturation of Tuberculosis Nursing

While the efforts of nurses at prestigious hospitals such as Johns Hopkins, as well as those in large cities such as New York, garnered the most attention, public health nurses throughout the nation joined the antituberculosis movement. National, state, and local nursing organizations convened committees and task forces to fight the TB epidemic. Articles, letters to the editor, and editorials on TB-related issues proliferated in nursing journals such as the *American Journal of Nursing, Trained Nurse and Hospital Review, Public Health Nurse,* and the *Pacific Coast Journal of Nursing.* Almost every issue of the aforementioned nursing journals between 1903 and the late 1920s emphasized some aspect of TB nursing work or highlighted issues and controversies related to its practice.

In addition to their activities within the profession, many TB nurses played influential roles within the wider antituberculosis community. The media paid attention to their accomplishments and rewarded them for their activism as well as their ability to link health care's public sphere of dispensaries and sanatoria to private spheres such as patients' neighborhoods and homes.[60] Many tuberculosis nurses participated in local, state, and national antituberculosis organizations as well. The National Tuberculosis Association (NTA) valued its nurse members' opinions. As a result, TB nurses as a group did not experience the invisibility faced by many private-duty and hospital-based nurses.[61]

The NTA highlighted nurses' contributions at its annual meetings, and especially emphasized their work at the widely publicized 1908 International Congress on Tuberculosis in Washington, D.C. The organization sought their opinions on major issues, organized a nursing section within its membership, and regularly included features by nurses and about tuberculosis nursing issues in publications such as the *Journal of the Outdoor Life, Transactions of the National Tuberculosis Association,* and the *Bulletin of the National Tuberculosis Association.*

Several TB nurses became famous as a result of their activism, and one, Ellen La Motte, emerged as an early leader and spokeswoman for tuberculosis nurses.[62] La Motte's thoughts, and those of her colleague Mary Lent, published in articles and books over the next few years, emerged as TB nurses' manifesto.[63] The influence of both women, particularly La Motte, was so substantial that many of their philosophies and ideas were propagated almost without revision in texts of both public health and tuberculosis nursing from 1915 until streptomycin came into use as a treatment for TB in the 1940s.[64]

La Motte and Lent had long championed nurses' role as patient educator. In 1908, both women, discouraged by the unwillingness or inability of many patients to comply with that which they had been taught, began to advocate for more patient incarceration. No longer did they see the nurse's primary role as a teacher—they now fervently deemed it her duty to enlighten the public about the virtues of institutionalization for the tuberculous and to encourage sufferers to "submit to the state's demands" in all matters, including segregation and even institutionalization.[65]

Not everyone agreed with La Motte and Lent, however. Their colleague 100 miles to the north in Philadelphia, Mabel Jacques, thought their stance too harsh. She argued that La Motte and Lent could not expect appreciable changes in TB mortality based on their interventions in just a few years, especially given the fact that Baltimore had hired only a few nurses to serve a large population of indigent TB sufferers. While Jacques agreed that some patients did need to be institutionalized, she scolded La Motte and Lent for being too quick to break apart families and for what she saw as their insensitivity.[66]

In addition to conflict surrounding the better place for treatment—home or institution—another issue divided tuberculosis nurses. Disagreement centered around whether the same nurse should provide preventive as well as curative care. Most health systems lacked a unified framework that allowed the nurses to provide both direct and preventive care. Care of the sick at home, considered therapeutic rather than preventive, fell increasingly under the purview of voluntary organizations such as visiting nurse societies, who called their staff "visiting nurses." By 1910, more and more health departments hired public health nurses and classified their efforts as purely preventive, partly to avoid strife with private physicians who saw these nurses as a threat to their economic livelihood.[67]

Lillian Wald opposed the idea of one nurse delivering bedside care while another provided education, but Ellen La Motte thought it made good sense.[68] Like many of her physician colleagues, La Motte saw this trend toward greater specialization as positive. She and her supporters hoped that specialization might afford nurses greater recognition as well as opportunities for leadership, both within professional nursing and in the public health world.[69]

But nurses received mixed messages from physicians about their place in the antituberculosis movement. Allowed to be authoritative with patients, they were not permitted to forget their place in the professional hierarchy. For example, the Johns Hopkins physician who wrote the introduction to La Motte's book on TB nursing admitted as much when he emphasized that nurses must look to medical science for direction, a good nurse being one whose "attitude always conform[ed] to [that of] medicine."[70] Physicians, while recognizing nurses' contribution to the antituberculosis movement, may also have attempted to moderate TB nurses' power to stifle competition and protect their own status. Even though he praised nurses' value to the antituberculosis movement, Dr. Theodore B. Sachs reminded them that "the physician designates the method of treatment and the nurse puts it into action."[71] In order to preserve her role as the nurse "most equal to physicians," in the words of one physician, TB nurses maintained this status only by being "as wise as a serpent and as harmless as a dove," as another doctor admonished.[72]

Tuberculosis nurses received other confusing and frustrating messages as well. As nurse Mary Sewall Gardner, author of a prominent text on public health nursing, noted, society wanted TB nurses to be visible and "pile up brilliant results" but did not understand the structural impediments that made their work difficult, such as inadequate resources, too few numbers, physician resistance to their efforts, and, in many instances, weak authority to structure their own practices.[73] Gardner wrote in reference to a report published in *Public Health Nurse* the month before by Linsley R. Williams, M.D., and Alice M. Hill of the National Tuberculosis Association, wherein the authors concluded that TB nurses were not doing all they should to address the disease, even when taking into account forces over which nurses had no control.[74]

Nurses even received conflicting signals from one another. For example, although one 1908 *American Journal of Nursing* editorial encouraged nurses to "make practical application of the plans established by the medical men and the lay public," it did not encourage them to lead or innovate.[75] The outspoken La Motte, however, did not believe that nurses needed to subjugate themselves to doctors; in her 1915 treatise on TB nursing, she charged her colleagues with the task of subverting unqualified medical practitioners at every juncture.[76]

Tuberculosis nurses themselves counted leadership, intelligence, their thorough knowledge base regarding the disease, relevant legislation, and the latest therapeutics among their most important attributes; however, they also encouraged one another to be cooperative, cheerful, tactful, and patient, and to adapt their roles to accommodate other professionals and community agencies.[77] Margaret G. Weir, for example, a TB nurse from Massachusetts, encouraged nurses to keep their work health-oriented, and not to provide "material relief." Weir recognized, however, that when "no such agencies exist in her community [and] if relief agencies are not doing their job," nurses were obligated to take on this responsibility in addition to their other duties.[78] Grace L. Anderson, director of the East Harlem Nursing and Health Demonstration in New York City, asserted that the successful TB nurse was one who synthesized those health services already present in the community into her role formulation.[79] Thus, nurses needed to design their interventions not just based on what they saw as patients' most pressing nursing care needs, but also in such a way as to fill gaps left by others in the community.

In spite of the controversies between TB nurses and others, and the many issues related to the nurses' role, however, the numbers of TB nurses grew. In 1912, Lillian Wald estimated the number of TB public health nurses to be approximately 3,000. National Tuberculosis Association records indicated that, of these nearly 3,000 TB nurses in practice in 1912, most (2,809) worked for charity organizations, churches, state and local health and education departments, dispensaries, the Metropolitan Life Insurance Company, hospitals, clinics, factories, and shops. Not counted in these numbers were private-duty nurses hired to care for ill tubercular patients in their homes.[80]

NURSES AND THE PREVENTORIUM

Nurses' Support for the Preventorium Idea

Nurses found the concept of institutionalizing pretubercular children attractive for several reasons. First, in the preantibiotic era the preventorium seemed to many nurses to offer the most potential for reducing TB morbidity and mortality. Second, many of the factors believed to cause pretuberculosis, such as poverty, poor hygiene, inadequate nutrition, and ignorance, were also implicated in other diseases that afflicted large numbers of children, such as infant diarrhea. As a result, those nurses who became interested in the preventorium movement often found that their antituberculosis work put them at the leading edge of not just one popular reform movement but two: child-saving and tuberculosis prevention. Third, the preventorium underscored a fundamental Nightingalean precept, that of health promotion, and did so definitively because of its focus on not-yet-ill children.

The concepts underpinning the preventorium were not new to nurses. In fact, years before the advent of the first preventorium, some nurses suggested that circumstances sometimes warranted separating children from tubercular parents. In 1903, for example, nursing leader Lavinia Dock advocated removing not just ill tubercular children (and adults) from their homes, but also children "strongly predisposed to consumption."[81] Influenced by the growing eugenics movement, some public health nurses, like their physician colleagues, believed that a mixture of genetics and environment caused TB predisposition.[82]

Such assumptions not only gave nurses an imperative to assert control over minute aspects of patients' lives, but cloaked their biases, as well as those of the physicians and philanthropists with whom they worked, with a veneer of objectivity. Many antituberculosis activists did not even believe that their actions breached the family unit. La Motte, for example, asserted that *TB*, not the actions of the nurse who removed the ill parent or at-risk child, disrupted the home.[83] According to her thinking, nonremoval of the child constituted abuse and the state's abrogation of its responsibilities, to the child as well as to society. She argued that since the law prevented parents from abusing or neglecting their children, authorities must intervene to protect children from parents with tuberculosis. Otherwise, La Motte noted: "A father may not beat his child or brutally misuse it, [but] he is quite within his rights in giving it whatever disease he pleases."[84]

Jacques took a more muted stance on the issue of removing children from tuberculous parents, perhaps a reflection of her ambivalence. In Jacques's prizewinning educational leaflet from the 1908 International

Congress on TB, she wrote that with proper hygienic practices and family education, children of tubercular parents were at low risk for contracting the disease.[85] In another article published the same year in the *Trained Nurse and Hospital Review,* however, she seemed to support segregating such children and parents from one another.[86]

Public health nurses were on the front lines in the search for pretubercular children. In fact, they could make the difference between a success" preventorium and an unsuccessful one. For example, in her aforementioned presentation at the 1923 NTA meeting, Ida Spaeth described the use patterns of that city's two preventoria, arguing that their difference in occupancy rates demonstrated the need for more public health nurses. She noted that the preventorium affiliated with public health nurses and a referring clinic enjoyed a long waiting list, while the second preventorium with neither of these features always posted patient vacancies.[87]

As the preventorium movement gathered momentum just after World War I, nurses proclaimed their support for the idea.[88] Elizabeth Stringer, supervising nurse for the Metropolitan Life Insurance Company, summarized the beliefs of many nurses when she wrote: "Where the father or mother of a family has been tuberculous, the children should be watched for symptoms. Even before they develop, if the child does not seem to have the necessary resistance, it should be sent to one of the many institutions provided for such cases."[89]

In 1925, the NTA asked its nursing subcommittee for a recommendation on the preventorium's value to the antituberculosis campaign. Oklahoma nurse Mary Van Zile, the chair of the subgroup, reported to the NTA that her membership supported the preventorium idea with conviction. In its recommendation the nursing subgroup urged the NTA to strengthen the affiliations between children's hospitals and preventoria, both to reduce the institutions' chronic financial straits and to standardize nursing and medical care.[90] There is no evidence that the NTA acted on any of these recommendations, although during the 1930s, as fewer children sought preventorium care, individual institutions did respond to nurses' suggestions to broaden admissions policies and seek out different types of children.[91]

PREVENTORIUM NURSING

Though preventoria everywhere in the United States depended on nurses to locate prospective patients, manage the institutions, care for their pediatric clientele, and monitor children's status postdischarge, in at least one state, California, nurses created them.[92] Sidney Maguire, the first public health nurse in Los Angeles and later the secretary of the city's TB association, founded California's first preventorium in 1917.[93]

Maguire, struck by the number of pretubercular children she encountered and the paucity of public and private resources for their care, took action. With very few resources and only one helper, she gathered 20 of the sickliest children she could find and kept them for an entire summer at Long Beach, California, where they lived outdoors in tents and ate nutritious food. As a result of her efforts, this health camp grew into a year-round preventorium in the San Gabriel Mountains, wherein public health nurses oversaw the typical preventorium routine of fresh air, exercise, good food, sunshine, play, and hygienic education.[94] In 1921 Maguire, proud of her efforts and anxious to promote the preventorium concept, addressed her colleagues at the annual convention of the California State Nurses Association and touted her preventorium's contribution to the child welfare and antituberculosis campaigns.[95]

While they were not listed among the founders of the first preventorium in New Jersey, prominent nurses such as Lillian Wald maintained an active interest in the institution's affairs and supported its efforts. Wald's Henry Street Settlement referred prospective admittees for admission, and Wald herself attended the dedication of a new preventorium building in 1912.[96] Alfred F. Hess, the physician who oversaw the New Jersey preventorium, recognized nurses' critical importance to the institution's success from its inception. In a letter written in August of 1909 to Marcus Marks, a wealthy New York philanthropist and president of the preventorium, Hess expressed his concern for an unnamed nurse whom he deemed "not quite suitable." He went on to note the need to replace her "if she cannot get the affection of the children."[97]

In his first formal summary of preventorium activities to the institution's board of trustees, delivered in November 1909, Hess noted trained nurse Ella Wheelwright's responsibility for children's care and physical welfare "from the day she fetches them from the railroad station until she returns them to their families 2–3 months later."[98] Anne Thompson, listed as a former "nurse" for the Grover Cleveland family, is also acknowledged, but her role is elusive. Hess did not mention whether or not Thompson had formal nurse training, and her duties appear to have been subordinate to those of Wheelwright. She may have served as matron.

Subsequent to Wheelwright, J. Palmer Quimby, a trained as well as registered nurse, became the preventorium's supervisor.[99] Both Wheelwright and Quimby lived at Farmingdale, as did many of their counterparts at similar institutions. Since the preventorium strove to be a health care facility, nurses needed to be available 24 hours a day in the event that a child became ill or suffered an accident. Hess charged the preventorium nurse with monitoring children's welfare, observing for illness, educating about hygiene, and supervising all aspects of life at the institution.[100]

Most preventoria strove to have a nurse available at all times, although it is not clear how many institutions actually achieved this goal. At San Diego's Rest Haven Preventorium, for example, it was not until 10 years after its opening, in 1931, that children had 24-hour access to a graduate nurse. This meant that while children received the requisite nursing care during the day, at night no health care providers were on site should their services be needed.[101]

Since overseeing the daily operations of the institution consumed nurses' days, they must have been exhausted when a sick child kept them on duty into the night. At Farmingdale, the nurse's time was almost as regimented as that of her patients, with little time to catch up on rest. Upon the arrival of each patient, she performed an initial health assessment and weighed the child. New admissions spent their first few weeks isolated from the other children in an effort to minimize widespread outbreaks of infectious disease. During this time, nurses got to know the patient and made general estimations of his or her health and symptomatology, the results of which she reported to Hess.[102] Although isolating children may have prevented communicable disease outbreaks within the preventorium population, such a practice must also have been psychologically traumatic for the child just wrenched from the familiar surroundings of home and family.

The preventorium's therapeutics deviated little from day to day. The central nursing role included the creation and maintenance of an environment superior to that of the child's home. To this end, the nurse managed the institution, making sure that food and supplies got ordered, laundry was washed, and the physical plant remained in working order. She addressed issues related to the preventorium's operations as they arose and determined which crises needed to be forwarded to the board of directors.[103]

The nurse also needed to address children's emotional needs and development. If they acted out, she dealt with the problem. She comforted them when they were homesick or upset. Like her physician colleagues, however, Quimby minimized the family disruption and potential for emotional turmoil resulting from family separation. She stressed children's improving health and believed the patients to be happy at the preventorium.[104] Quimby was also a link between parents and children. She responded to inquiries from parents worried about their children. Finally, she designed and implemented educational programs on TB-related issues for both parents and children.

In addition to the Farmingdale nurse's role as chief operating officer, educator, disciplinarian, counselor, and substitute mother, she also needed to attend carefully to children's health, monitoring their nutritional intake, weight, temperature, and other barometers of physical well-being. Since the nurse oversaw every aspect of the children's strict schedule, it became her timetable as well. As a result, her days were full, as this 1912 Farmingdale schedule of children's daily activities reveals:

7 a.m.	Rising bell
8 a.m.	Breakfast: cereal, milk or cocoa, stewed fruit, bread and butter
9 a.m.	Clear tables and make beds
9:30 a.m	School
10:45 a.m.	Luncheon of crackers and milk
10:45 a.m.–12 noon	Recess and play in the fields or in the laurel grove
12:30 p.m.	Dinner: Meat, fish, or eggs; potatoes, green vegetables, pudding, milk, and bread
1:30–2:30 p.m.	Rest in bed (no talking)
2:30–3:30 p.m.	Play
3:30–4:30 p.m.	School
4:30–5:30 p.m.	Play
5:30 p.m.	Supper: One egg, stewed fruit, bread and butter, cocoa made with milk
6:30 p.m.	Sleep (winter)
7:30 p.m.	Sleep (summer)[105]

Quimby worked at the New Jersey preventorium for more than 20 years. The National Tuberculosis Association's *Directory of Sanatoria, Hospitals, Day Camps, and Preventoria for the Treatment of Tuberculosis in the United States* lists her as the nursing superintendent in its 1916 through 1938 editions.[106] She evidenced her strong commitment to the preventorium's mission in a 1917 article published in the journal *Modern Hospital,* wherein she described the institution, offering many of the same justifications for its existence as did Hess.

Quimby also unwittingly pointed out a fundamental flaw in preventorium supporters' thinking when she noted that, even when a tuberculous mother was willing to go to a sanatorium rather than have her child sent to a preventorium, she could not be spared if there were other children in the home. In such instances, Quimby argued, the preventorium protected the "delicate" child while preventing the disruption of the entire family.[107] However, since Quimby presumably knew the germ theory's basic precepts, the rationale behind leaving an infectious mother at home to care for children not yet labeled "pretubercular" or "delicate" is difficult to understand, since this practice potentially doomed siblings to the same fate as that of their sickly brother or sister.

Rules governing parental visitation varied from preventorium to preventorium, but the practice was generally discouraged or at least limited in order to minimize contact with the tubercular parent. Quimby did not mention it in her descriptions of the preventorium's practices. Perhaps she was ambivalent about parental/child contact, or maybe she did not consider it noteworthy because it was not a medical or nursing intervention.[108] Hess, in a description of his effort to broaden the preventorium to provide care for at-risk infants, noted that he believed the institutions should be at least "far enough away from the city [Hess suggested 2 hours] for the items of expenditure of time and money to act as a deterrent to frequent visits on the part of mothers."[109]

Before a child's discharge, either a preventorium nurse or a public health nurse visited the home to make sure it met specified requirements, which included recovery or death of the afflicted parent or at least a cleaner, more hygienic, better ventilated environment. Nurses followed former patients indefinitely. As one Farmingdale report emphasized: "No child is returned from the Preventorium until the nurse reports home conditions safe. The children are followed up [by nurses] for years. . . . Our purpose is to permanently save every child that comes to us."[110]

CONCLUSION: THE DECLINE
OF PREVENTORIUM NURSING

Through their publications, we know that Quimby and Maguire ardently believed in the preventorium cause.[111] But what of other preventorium nurses? We know little of their thoughts. In fact, the nursing perspective on preventoria is framed largely by the public health nurses who referred patients to the institutions and followed them once they were discharged back into their communities, and not by those nurses employed by the preventoria.

Even basic demographic information is missing about most preventorium nurses. What, for example, were their ages? Marital status? Tuberculosis status? Where did they train? Furthermore, we don't know how they came to be working in such a role. Did they feel their work conferred greater status than that experienced by other nurses, or was it the only job they could get?

We also know little about preventorium nurses' professional activities. Were they leaders in the nursing profession? Maguire, for example, served as executive secretary of the Los Angeles TB Association in 1921, but was she similarly active in the California State Nurses' Association?[112] While nurses who belonged to the NTA supported the preventorium idea, was there broad support for the preventorium movement within the National Organization for Public Health Nursing? How many nurses practiced in preventoria throughout North America? What was the nurse's work environment really like?

No conclusive answers to these questions exist. Moreover, since preventoria themselves varied widely, so did the roles of the nurses who worked there. Quimby and Maguire seem to have had at least as much power and autonomy as public health nurses. This was not true for all preventorium nurses, however, since those at Rest Haven appear to have had no more authority than did their peers in a hospital or private-duty setting.

Ida Spaeth summarized the public health nurse's role succinctly when she referred to her as the "connecting link" among all aspects of the campaign to institutionalize pretubercular children.[113] The nurses who worked within the preventorium performed a similar function, though in a more circumscribed environment. They linked the community within the preventorium to the outside world of parents, schools, physicians, public health nurses, and other resources.

While nurses' contributions to preventoria made them invaluable assets to the movement, there was a downside to serving as the glue that held the system together. In most communities, tuberculosis prevention and treatment were linked together through a complex web of public and private initiatives. It was the nurse's job to fit people and resources together appropriately, as both Margaret G. Weir and Grace L. Anderson noted.[114] As a result, however, public health nurses often found themselves caught between different parties with competing agendas.

Part of nurses' success depended on their ability to buffer tensions between groups and make a particular community's programs articulate with one another in a meaningful fashion. Although some nurses, such as Lillian Wald, Mabel Jacques, Ellen La Motte, and Sidney Maguire, for example, did press their own antituberculosis agendas, other nurses may have been inhibited from doing so. While nurses were usually well positioned to make determinations regarding community needs, forging their own initiatives may have subverted their ability to mesh together what was already in place. Using Spaeth's words to examine the potential negative outcomes inherent in her "connecting link" metaphor, it is difficult to be in a position both to create a chain's links and to weave them together. In other words, it is not easy to be ubiquitous as well as unique.

Though preventorium and TB public health nurses both focused their energies on the same disease, their roles did differ. At least some preventorium nurses lived at the institutions, which perhaps rendered their work more similar to that of nurses who worked in sanatoria or hospitals than of those in the public health arena who visited patients at home.[115] Preventorium nurses also appear to have remained employed by their institutions, unlike many other public health nurses, whose affiliation shifted from voluntary agencies such as TB associations to city and state health departments between 1900 and 1920.[116] In at least one respect, preventorium nurses and TB public health nurses' roles bore a striking similarity. Both appeared to accept their Americanization mission with vigor, believing, like their employers, that children could be used as "little missionaries that can be sent back into the home."[117]

The paucity of surviving evidence makes it difficult to make sweeping comparisons between preventorium nurses' work and that of their peers in private duty or other institutions, but a few similarities and differences stand out. Since a certain fluidity of roles existed between the nurse and the institution's social worker or teacher, preventorium nursing may have been more interesting than private-duty nursing work. Just as with other nursing specialties, however, the boundaries between physicians and nurses remained impermeable in most instances. Moreover, some preventorium nurses may have felt their professional actions and judgment constrained, not just by their relationship to physicians but also by the institution's board of directors, an experience shared by many public health nurses.[118] Finally, both preventorium and TB public health nurses shared the almost universal feature of early twentieth-century nursing practice in that they struggled with too few resources to fully achieve their own ambitious goals as well as those set for them by others.

In the late 1920s, the economic, social, and medical trends that had made the need for TB and other public health nurses seem so compelling a few years earlier began to erode, the result of a growing trend toward fee-for-service hospital care, the falling incidence of infectious diseases in the United States, and reduced immigration.[119] By the end of the 1940s, preventorium nursing had virtually disappeared as the institutions closed or became converted for other uses. Although nurses remained heavily invested in children's health, after World War II they did so in a very different environment, one increasingly bureaucratized, hospital-based, and technologically driven.

NOTES

1. Ida Spaeth, "The Public Health Nurse, the Tuberculosis Problem, and the Child in the Sanatorium," *Transactions of the National Tuberculosis Association* 19 (1923): 438–39.
2. "Organization Report of the Tuberculosis Preventorium." Nathan Straus papers, Box 8, New York Public Library, New York City (hereafter cited as NYPL).
3. First Medical Report of the Preventorium, July-November 1909. Straus papers, Box 8, NYPL. Annual Report of the Tuberculosis Clinic for Bellevue Hospital, New York, for the Year 1909; Alfred F. Hess, "The Tuberculosis Preventorium," *Survey* (August

1913): 666–68. Nurses in other regions performed functions similar to those of their New York counterparts. For example, one Pennsylvania public health nurse detailed her efforts with a tuberculous mother to protect her children from infection. This article described in depth the nurse's assessment of the home and family situation, the way in which she coordinated social welfare services for the family, and her efforts to work through family resistance to get a child to the preventorium. See Anonymous, "The State Nurse Goes 'A-Visiting,'" *Listening Post* (January 1923): 18–22. For a Pennsylvania nurse's description of a preventorium case, see a letter from Elizabeth M. Dennie in *Listening Post* (May 1924): 21–22.

4. Annual Report for the year 1912, The Tuberculosis Preventorium for Children. Straus papers, Box 8, NYPL. These same functions were carried out by nurses in other cities with preventoria. For examples, see John B. Hawes of Boston's Prendergast preventorium, 336–42, and Henry Farnum Stoll, "The School Child and Tuberculosis: A Plea for Preventoria," 122–31, in *Transactions of the National Tuberculosis Association* 6 (1910).

5. National Tuberculosis Association, *A Directory of Sanatoria, Hospitals, Day Camps, and Preventoria for the Treatment of Tuberculosis in the United States* (New York: National Tuberculosis Association, 1926).

6. Mark Caldwell, *The Last Crusade: The War on Consumption, 1862–1954* (New York: Atheneum, 1988), 9; Sheila M. Rothman, *Living in the Shadow of Death: Tuberculosis and the Social Experience of Illness in American History* (Baltimore: Johns Hopkins University Press, 1990), 179–84.

7. Rene and Jean Dubos, *The White Plague: Tuberculosis, Man, and Society* (New Brunswick, NJ: Rutgers University Press, 1952), 3–11.

8. Charles E. Rosenberg, "The Bitter Fruit: Heredity, Disease, and Social Thought in Nineteenth Century America," in *From Consumption to Tuberculosis: A Documentary History,* ed. Barbara G. Rosenkrantz (New York: Garland, 1994), 154–94.

9. Nancy J. Tomes, "American Attitudes Toward the Germ Theory of Disease: Phyllis Allen Richmond Revisited," *Journal of the History of Medicine and Allied Sciences* 52 (January 1997): 17–50.

10. Rothman, *Living in the Shadow,* 179–84.

11. Alan M. Kraut, *Silent Travelers: Germs, Genes, and the "Immigrant Menace"* (Baltimore: Johns Hopkins University Press, 1994), 2–4, 31–78.

12. For examples, see Sigard Adolphus Knopf, "What Shall We Do with the Consumptive Poor?" *Proceedings of the National Conference of Charities and Corrections at the 29th Annual Session* (Boston: Lea and Febiger, 1902): 219–31, and Arnold C. Klebs, *Tuberculosis: A Treatise by American Authors on Its Etiology, Pathology, Semeiology, Diagnosis, Prevention, and Treatment* (New York: Appleton and Company, 1909), 120–30.

13. Barbara Bates, *Bargaining for Life: A Social History of Tuberculosis, 1876–1938* (Philadelphia: University of Pennsylvania Press, 1992), 25–41.

14. Klebs, *Tuberculosis,* 120–130.

15. Hermann M. Biggs, "The Administrative Control of Tuberculosis;" *Medical News* 84 (20 February 1908): 338–45.

16. Preventing TB in New York City. *Ninth Report of the Committee on the Prevention of TB of the Charity Organization Society of New York, 1911, 1912, 1913* (New York: M. B. Brown).

17. Clemens von Pirquet, "Frequency of Tuberculosis in Childhood," *Journal of the American Medical Association* (February 1909): 675–79 (hereafter cited as *JAMA*).

18. Biggs is quoted in Linsley L. Williams, "Tuberculosis in Children," *Journal of the Outdoor Life* 9 (August 1907): 241–44.

19. von Pirquet, "Frequency of Tuberculosis," 675–79.

20. Sigard Adolphus Knopf, "Overcoming the Predisposition to Tuberculosis and the Danger From Infection During Childhood," in *Sixth International Congress on Tuberculosis*, vol. II (Philadelphia: William F. Fell, 1908), 635–47.

21. Hess, "Tuberculosis Preventorium," 666–68.

22. "Tentative Scheme for the Operation of the Proposed Preventatorium [the word was later shortened to preventorium] for Children." Straus papers, Box 8, NYPL.

23. For more on the New York COS, see Emily K. Abel, "Medicine and Morality: The Health Care Program of the New York Charity Organization Society," *Social Service Review* 71 (December 1997): 634–49. For more on the COS movement in the United States in general, see Michael B. Katz, *In the Shadow of the Poorhouse: A Social History of Welfare in the United States* (New York: Basic Books, 1986), 66–80.

24. National Tuberculosis Association, *Directory*, 1911, 1916, 1923, 1926, 1928, 1931, 1934, 1938, 1942, and 1948.

25. Merritte W. Ireland, "Physical Defects Discovered in Selective Draft Men During the World War," *JAMA* 79 (November 1922): 1579–81.

26. Karen Buhler-Wilkerson, "Left Carrying the Bag: Experiments in Visiting Nursing, 1877–1909," *Nursing Research* (January/February 1987): 42–47.

27. Susan Reverby, *Ordered to Care: The Dilemma of American Nursing, 1850–1945* (New York: Cambridge University Press, 1987), 109–110; Barbara Melosh, *"The Physician's Hand": Work, Culture, and Conflict in American Nursing* (Philadelphia: Temple University Press, 1982), 113–59.

28. John Duffy, "Social Impact of Disease in the Late Nineteenth Century," in *Sickness and Health in America*, ed. Judith W. Leavitt and Ronald L. Numbers (Madison: University of Wisconsin Press, 1985), 414–22; Kraut, *Silent Travelers*, 180.

29. District nursing, an innovation created in the second half of the nineteenth century, involved sending trained nurses to care for the indigent sick in their homes. See Karen Buhler-Wilkerson, *False Dawn: The Rise and Decline of Public Health Nursing, 1900–1930* (New York: Garland, 1989), 1–45.

30. For a description of America's first settlement house, located in Chicago, see Jane Addams, *Twenty Years at Hull House* (New York: Macmillan, 1910), 90–110.

31. Wald, born in 1867 and raised in an upper-middle-class German-Jewish home in Rochester, New York, epitomized Carroll Smith Rosenberg's Progressive Era "new woman." Carroll Smith Rosenberg, *Disorderly Conduct: Visions of Gender in Victorian America* (New York: Knopf, 1985), 176. A chronicle of Wald's life and work can be found in her autobiography, *The House on Henry Street* (New York: Henry Holt, 1915), and in biographies such as Doris Groshen Daniels, *Always a Sister: The Feminism of Lillian Wald* (New York: Feminist Press at City University of New York, 1989).

32. Bates, *Bargaining for Life*, 237–43.

33. Karen Buhler-Wilkerson, "False Dawn: The Rise and Decline of Public Health Nursing in America, 1900–1930," in *Nursing History: New Perspectives, New Possibilities*, Ellen Lagemann, ed. (New York: Teacher's College Press, 1983), 89–106. For several firsthand accounts of public health nurses' daily activities, see Caroline Bartlett Crane, "The Visiting Nurse in a Small City," *Charities and the Commons* 16 (April 1907): 25–28 (hereafter cited as *CC*, and Lillian Wald, "In the Day's Work of a Settlement Nurse," ibid., 34–44.

34. Perhaps the most famous postgraduate course for public health nursing was the program developed by Adelaide Nutting at Teacher's College, Columbia University. For a description, see M. Adelaide Nutting, "Education for Nurses for the Home and Community," *Modern Hospital* 6 (March 1916): 196–200. For a discussion of why nursing leaders believed TB public health nurses needed additional education beyond that acquired in their training programs, see F. Elizabeth Crowell's "Report of the

Special Committee on TB Nursing," presented at the Fourteenth Annual Convention of Nurses' Associated Alumnae of the United States, *American Journal of Nursing* 11 (August 1911): 973 (hereafter cited as *AJN*).

35. Elizabeth Stringer, "What Every Public Health Nurse Should Know," *AJN* 14 (August 1914): 976–79.

36. Karen Buhler-Wilkerson, "Bringing Care to the People: Lillian Wald's Legacy to Public Health Nursing," *American Journal of Public Health* 83 (December 1993):1778–86 (hereafter cited as *AJPH*). Johns Hopkins Hospital physician William Osler made one of the earliest calls for the home treatment of tuberculosis, arguing that the disease lurked in the home and was thus a "house disease." Osler also believed that home treatment was more cost effective than institutionalization. See Osler's "Home Treatment of Consumption," paper read in 1899 at the Medical and Chirurgical Faculty of Maryland. Archives of the Medical and Chirurgical Faculty, Baltimore, Md.

37. Hermann M. Biggs, "What Has Been Learned About Tuberculosis Since the International Congress of 1908, and What Modifications, If Any, Should This Have on the Constructive Program?" *Journal of the Outdoor Life* 13 (February 1916): 45–48 (hereafter cited as *JOL*).

38. Jessica Robbins, "Class Struggles in the Tubercular World: Nurses, Patients, and Physicians, 1903–1915," *Bulletin of the History of Medicine* 71 (Fall 1997): 412–34; Annie M. Brainard, *The Evolution of Public Health Nursing* (Philadelphia: W. B. Saunders, 1922; reprinted by Garland Press, 1985); Mary Sewall Gardner, *Public Health Nursing* (New York: Macmillan, 1932), 269–70.

39. Melosh, *"The Physician's Hand,"* 113–59,

40. Committee on the Prevention of TB of the Charity Organization Society, *TB Needs and the City Budget.* Community Service Society Archives, Box 109, Rare Book and Manuscript Library, Columbia University, New York. By 1910, New York City was divided into districts, each with a centrally located clinic. Each district was subdivided into sections with a nurse assigned to each section. The nurse visited homes for half the day and practiced in the clinic the rest of the time. Nurses' clinic duties included obtaining patient histories, weights, and temperatures, keeping records, and educating sufferers and their families about TB. For more on TB nursing in New York City, see Elizabeth Gregg, "The Tuberculosis Nurse Under Municipal Control," *Public Health Nurse Quarterly* 5 (October 1913): 15–25, and *General Description and Annual Report of the Tuberculosis Clinic, Bellevue Hospital, 1909* (New York: Martin B. Brown Press, 1909), 8–15.

41. M. Adelaide Nutting, "The Tuberculosis Exposition, Baltimore," *AJN* 4 (April 1904): 497–99; M. A. Nutting, "The Visiting Nurse for Tuberculosis," *CC* 16 (April 1906): 51–55; Robbins, "Class Struggles," 412–34; Bates, *Bargaining for Life,* 234–35.

42. Reiba Thelin, "Visiting Nurses and the Prevention of Tuberculosis," *AJN* 5 (August 1905): 743–56. Thelin, a 1902 graduate of the Johns Hopkins Training School for Nurses, was the first TB nurse in Baltimore. Thirty-two years old when she completed her training, she had no experience in public health nursing when she took the position. She worked in the role for only one year and then, desirous of more public health experience, left Baltimore to work at Wald's Henry Street Settlement. For an overview of Thelin's career, see Brainard, *Evolution,* 278, and Robbins, "Class Struggles," 417. For more on antituberculosis nursing efforts in Baltimore, see *Johns Hopkins Nurses Alumni Magazine,* vols. 2 (1903) to 14 (1915). See also Ruth Brester Sherman, "The Discussion on Tuberculosis," *AJN* 2 (October 1901): 24–27; Thelin, "Report of Results of Nursing Dispensary Tubercular Patients," *Johns Hopkins Hospital Bulletin* (May 1904): 171; J. S. Ames, "The Work of District Nurses Among Tuberculous Patients in Baltimore," *AJN* 4 (June 1904): 671–73; Ellen N. La Motte, "Tuberculosis Work of the Instructive Visiting Nurse

Association of Baltimore," *AJN* 5 (1905): 141–48; and Jane B. Newman, "The Public Health Nurses of the Baltimore City Health Department," *Public Health Nurse* 16 (July 1924): 339–41 (hereafter cited as *PHN*).

43. Gregg, "Tuberculosis Nurse, "15–25; Anonymous, "Visiting Nurses in Connection with the Phipps Dispensary, Baltimore," *AJN* 8 (1908): 541–42.

44. F. E. Crowell, "Standards of Nursing in Communities With TB Dispensaries," *PHN* 7 (April 1915): 14–21; Elsie Thayer Patterson, "The Visiting Nurse," *JOL* 4 (December 1907): 412–14.

45. Sara E. Shaw, "Social Activities of Bellevue Tuberculosis Clinic," *JOL* 9 (October 1912): 230–33; Winifred M. Allen and Elizabeth McConnell, "The Teachableness of the Consumptive Patient," *AJN* 15 (October 1914): 25–30; Ames, "Work of District Nurses," 671–73.

46. Sarah B. Stevens, "The Tuberculosis Nurse and Some of Her Problems," *PHN* 7 (April 1915): 35–41.

47. Ibid.

48. Ibid., 35–41; Crowell, "Standards of Nursing," 14–21.

49. Stevens, "Tuberculosis Nurse," 35–41.

50. Delores Gladys Spicer, "The Foreign Mother and Her Child," *Trained Nurse and Hospital Review* 92 (March 1934): 257–61 (hereafter cited as *TNHR).*

51. Karen Buhler-Wilkerson, "Public Health Nursing: In Sickness or in Health?" *AJPH* 75 (October 1985): 1155–60.

52. Shaw, "Bellevue Tuberculosis Clinic," 230–33.

53. Jane Delano, "Outline of TB Work in Connection With the Outpatient Department of Bellevue Hospital," *AJN* 4 (March 1904): 440–42.

54. Mabelle S. Welch, "Control of Tuberculosis Through Family Health Supervision," *PHN* 20 (August 1928): 413–15.

55. They characterized 18.1% as fairly intelligent, 69.5% stupid, and 12.4% intensely stupid or defective. Allen and McConnell originally defined three categories: (A) intelligent, (B) fairly intelligent, and (C) stupid, but acknowledged that they felt that their revised groupings better fit the characteristics of their patient population. Allen and McConnell, "Teachableness," 25–30.

56. Elsie M. Courrier, "Some Aspects of the TB Problem," *AJN* 9 (1909): 924–31.

57. Rose C. MacGowan, "The Attitude of the Various Nationalities Toward the Work of the School Doctor and Nurse," *Pacific Coast Journal of Nursing* 21 (August 1922): 490–92 (hereafter cited as *PCJN*).

58. Gregg, "Tuberculosis Nurse," 15–25.

59. Wald defined civic intelligence as the ability to plan and carry our comprehensive public health programs for a given community. Lillian D. Wald, "The Visiting Nurse and Tuberculosis Control," *JOL* 9 (December 1912): 306.

60. For example, the *Philadelphia Inquirer* trumpeted the life and career of Philadelphia TB nurse Mabel Jacques on February 18, 1909.

61. Reverby, *Ordered to Care,* 128–29.

62. La Motte was born in Louisville, Kentucky. She graduated from the Johns Hopkins Hospital Training School for Nurses in 1902, and soon joined the Instructive Visiting Nurses Association (IVNA). Vern L. Bullough, Olga Maranjian Church, and Alice P. Stein, "Ellen La Motte," *Dictionary of American Nursing Biography* (New York: Garland, 1988), 204–5; Obituary, "Ellen La Motte," *TNHR* 81 (September 1928): 312.

63. Mary Lent, a 1905 graduate of the Johns Hopkins Training School for Nurses, was employed as head nurse at Hopkins until 1898, when she went to work at the Baltimore IVNA. She became the IVNA superintendent in 1903 and held the post until 1916. Vern L. Bullough, Olga Maranjian Church, and Alice P. Stein, "Mary

Lent," *Dictionary of American Nursing Biography* (New York: Garland, 1988), 211–12; Brainard, *Evolution,* 238.

64. Ellen La Motte, *The Tuberculosis Nurse: Her Functions and Qualifications* (New York: Knickerbocker Press, 1915), and Grace M. Longhurst, *Tuberculosis Nursing* (Philadelphia: F. A. Davis, 1945).

65. Ellen N. La Motte, "The Unreachable Consumptive," *Transactions of the Sixth International Congress on Tuberculosis,* vol. III, sec. V (Philadelphia: Wm. F. Fell, 1908), 256–63; Mary E. Lent, "The True Functions of the Tuberculosis Nurse," ibid., 576–85; Mary E. Lent and Ellen N. La Motte, "The Present Status of Tuberculosis Work Among the Poor," *Maryland Medical Journal* 52 (April 1909): 147–63.

66. Mabel Jacques, "Saving the Home," *JOL* 6 (November 1909): 265–69. For an overview of Jacques's professional life and activities, see Bates, *Bargaining for Life,* 244–45; La Motte, *Tuberculosis Nurse,* 87–104.

67. Buhler-Wilkerson, *False Dawn,* 1–45, 85–129.

68. Lillian Wald, "Visiting Nurse," 306–7, 310; La Motte, *Tuberculosis Nurse.*

69. For the best overview of the early twentieth-century trend toward specialization in medical care, see Rosemary Stevens, *American Medicine and the Public Interest: A History of Specialization* (New Haven, Conn.: Yale University Press, 1971; updated edition by University of California Press, 1998), 132–48 (page references are to reprint edition).

70. Louis Hammond, *The Tuberculosis Nurse,* xi.

71. Theodore B. Sachs, "The Tuberculosis Nurse," *AJN* (May 1908): 597–98.

72. Benjamin Lee, "The Value of a Nurse in a Tuberculosis Dispensary," *Transactions of the Sixth International Congress on Tuberculosis,* vol. 3 (Philadelphia: William F. Fell, 1908), 554–55. Lee made this comment with regard to the nurse's role toward patients, but the subtext of the article shows that he believed nurses should structure their interactions with physicians in the same way.

73. Mary S. Gardner, Letter to the Editor, *PHN* 21 (February 1929): 66–67.

74. Linsley R. Williams and Alice M. Hill, "The Public Health Nurse and Tuberculosis," *PHN* 21 (January 1929): 4–7. Gardner was not the only nurse incensed by Williams's and Hill's conclusions. An editorial written by Violet H. Hodgson, assistant director, National Organization for Public Health Nursing, accompanied the article by Williams and Hill. Hodgson identified multiple flaws in the way in which Williams and Hill designed the study, gathered data, and interpreted their findings with regard to capturing the nursing contribution. For example, Hodgson noted that physicians often limited private patients' access to TB nurses so that nurses could not be held accountable when those patients were not evaluated by them. Further, she wondered if the 18 sanatoria and 1,499 patients reviewed could be considered representative of the 600 sanatoria and 60,000 TB sufferers in the United States. Williams and Hill reported that only two of 1,499 TB patients had been located by nurses. Hodgson argued that nurses may in fact have identified potential patients, but because it was the physician who made the diagnosis it was he who was given sole credit. Finally, she expressed surprise that the authors had not looked at nursing efforts for those under the age of 15 years, since nurses directed much of their time and energy toward TB prevention in children and adolescents. Violet H. Hodgson, "Some Remarks About the Study Which Follows," *PHN* 21 (January 1929): 2–3.

75. Editorial, *AJN* 8 (June 1908): 665.

76. La Motte, *Tuberculosis Nurse,* 88.

77. Delya Nardi, "The Special Training of the Tuberculosis Nurse," *Transactions of the National Tuberculosis Association* 22 (1926): 479–87; Margaret G. Weir, "Problems in Tuberculosis Work," *PHN* 12 (February 1920): 111–15.

78. Weir, "Problems," 111–115.

79. Grace L. Anderson, "Standards for Tuberculosis Work in a Generalized Nursing Program," *JOL* 24 (June 1927): 340–45.

80. Wald, "Visiting Nurse," 306–307.

81. Lavinia Dock, "The World's War Against Consumption," *AJN* 3 (1903): 160–61.

82. Editorial, "Consumption," *AJN* 5 (1905): 392; Arthur Hamilton, "Some Direct Relations Between the Science of Eugenics and the Nursing Profession," *AJN* 15 (1915): 475.

83. La Motte, *Tuberculosis Nurse,* 161.

84. Ellen La Motte, "The Neglected Tuberculous Child," *JOL* 7 (March 1910): 65–70.

85. Mabel Jacques, "Educational Leaflet for Mothers," *Transactions of the Sixth International Congress on Tuberculosis,* vol. I (Washington, D.C.: National Tuberculosis Association, 1908), 307–9.

86. Mabel Jacques, "Special Schools for Tuberculous Children," *TNHR* 41 (October 1908): 234–36.

87. Spaeth, "Public Health Nurse," 438–39.

88. Anne Sutherland, "Tuberculosis Nursing by a Generalized Staff," *Transactions of the National Tuberculosis Association* 17 (1921): 536–55; Mary A. Meyers, "The Public Health Nurse in Tuberculosis Work, Especially As It Touches Children in the Clinic," *Transactions of the National Tuberculosis Association,* 19 (1923): 434–38; Spaeth, "Public Health Nurse," 438–39; Van Zile, 508–11; and Grace L. Anderson," Standards for Tuberculosis Work in a Generalized Nursing Program," *JOL* 24 (June 1927): 340–45. Every one of these articles champions the idea, and all concur that nurses must play the central role in obtaining patients for, and managing the operations of, the preventorium.

89. Elizabeth Stringer, "What Every Public Health Nurse Should Know," *AJN* 14 (1914): 976–79. The Metropolitan Life Insurance Company operated a well-known visiting nurse service. For an overview, see Diane Hamilton, "The Cost of Caring: The Metropolitan Life Insurance Company's Visiting Nurse Service, 1909–1953," *Bulletin of the History of Medicine* 63 (1989): 414–34. The Framingham tuberculosis project, an epidemiologic study of TB morbidity and mortality based in Framingham, Massachusetts (and heavily dependent on the services of Metropolitan Life) also grew out of the liaison between the insurance company and public health leaders. See Diane Hamilton, "Research and Reform: Community Nursing and the Framingham Tuberculosis Project, 1914–1923," *Nursing Research* 41 (January/February 1992): 8–13. For other articles in the nursing literature supporting the preventorium concept, see Alice C. Bagley, "The Public Health Nurse in Tuberculosis Care," *PCJN* 27 (May 1931): 301–305, and Marcia A. Patrick, "Our Local Preventorium Camps," *PCJN* 16 (July 1920): 434–38.

90. Van Zile, 508–11.

91. Rest Haven Preventorium Manuscript Collection #6, San Diego Historical Society, San Diego, Cal.

92. Bagley, "Public Health Nurse," 301–5. Bagley not only gave examples of nurses' founding California preventoria, she also suggested that if the relationship between children and TB had been discovered earlier, child welfare and tuberculosis public health nursing might have developed as one specialty.

93. Ibid., 301.

94. Genevieve Parkhurst, "A Chance for the Borderline Child," *Good Housekeeping* 84 (May 1922): 143–46.

95. Maguire emphasized that she sought to select those children "who in the future will bring the greatest amount of good to the community." Presumably she believed the children she selected were those whose health she deemed salvageable. Maguire did not note whether factors such as race or ethnicity went into this determination. The hundred

children cared for at the San Gabriel Canyon preventorium resided there an average of 2 months. After discharge, follow-up was conducted by Los Angeles city and county public health nurses. Sidney M. Maguire, "Tuberculosis in the Southern Section," *PCJN* 17 (October 1921): 589–93.

96. Editorial, *New York Times,* April 25, 1912.

97. Letter to Marcus Marks from Alfred Fabian Hess, dated August 1, 1909. Straus papers, Box 16, NYPL.

98. Organizational Report of the TB Preventorium; First Medical Report of the Preventorium, July to November 1909. Straus papers, Box 8, NYPL. A man by the name of Sherburn Wheelwright, perhaps Ella Wheelwright's husband, is listed in the above records as an employee who taught industrial training to the boys at the preventorium.

99. Registration of nurses was an attempt to restrict nursing practice to only those nurses who had undergone some form of training. For history and analysis of the registration movement in one state, New York, see Nancy Tomes, "The Silent Battle: Nurse Registration in New York State, 1903–1920" in *Nursing History,* ed. Lagemann, 107–32.

100. First Medical Report of the Preventorium, July to November 1909. Straus papers, Box 8, NYPL; Hess, "Tuberculosis Preventorium," 666–68; J. Palmer Quimby, "The Tuberculosis Preventorium for Children, Farmingdale, N.J.," *Modern Hospital* 8 (1917): 177–79.

101. Transcript of radio interview with Rest Haven Preventorium board members Mrs. Osborn and Ekern, April 1947. Manuscript Collection #6, Box 3, File 4, San Diego Historical Society, San Diego, Cal.

102. First Medical Report of the Preventorium, July to November 1909. Straus papers, Box 8, NYPL.

103. Records of the Rest Haven Preventorium for Children, San Diego Historical Society Research Archives, San Diego, Cal.

104. Quimby, "Tuberculosis Preventorium," 177–79.

105. Preventorium Annual Report for 1912, 5–6. Straus papers, Box 8, NYPL.

106. The National Tuberculosis Association's *Directory* listed Quimby as superintendent in its 1916, 1919, 1923, 1926, 1928, 1931, 1934, and 1938 editions.

107. Quimby, "Tuberculosis Preventorium," 177–79.

108. Ibid.

109. Alfred F. Hess, "The Significance of Tuberculosis in Infants and Young Children," *JAMA* 72 (January 1919): 83–88.

110. Preventorium Annual Report for 1912, 6–7. Straus papers, Box 8, NYPL.

111. Quimby, "Tuberculosis Preventorium," 177–79; J. Palmer Quimby, Report of Nursing Activities in "The Tuberculosis Preventorium for Children," 15. New York Historical Society, 1928; Maguire, "'Tuberculosis," 593.

112. Maguire, "Tuberculosis," 589.

113. Spaeth, "Public Health Nurse," 438–39.

114. Weir, "Problems," 111–15.

115. Unlike sanatorium nursing, however, no record can be found of training schools for nurses at preventoria. For a discussion of sanatorium nursing and sanatorium nursing schools, see Bates, *Bargaining for Life,* 110–12, 197–213.

116. Buhler-Wilkerson, *False Dawn,* 87.

117. Patrick, 434–38; Spaeth, "Public Health Nurse," 438–39.

118. Buhler-Wilkerson, *False Dawn,* 48–49.

119. Ibid., 89–106.

CHAPTER 10

"The Steel Cocoon": Tales of the Nurses and Patients of the Iron Lung, 1929–1955

Lynne M. Dunphy

And now I see with eyes serene

The very pulse of the machine;

A being breathing thoughtful breath;

A traveler betwixt life and death.

William Wadsworth, "She Was a Phantom of Delight"

THE ARRIVAL OF AN INVISIBLE ENEMY

72,000 CATS KILLED IN PARALYSIS FEAR proclaimed the headline of the *New York Times* for July 26, 1916.[1] Tony Gould describes the first major polio outbreak to occur in the United States with particular eloquence: "In the summer of 1916, while European armies battered each other senseless, New Yorkers were engaged in a very different kind of struggle. An invisible enemy was killing and crippling children . . . quite

Originally published in *Nursing History Review* 9 (2001): 3–33. Copyright Springer Publishing Company.

as effectively as bullets and shrapnel killed and maimed infantrymen stumbling through the wire and mire of Somme."[2] The outbreak started in the Italian community; the immigrants became the scapegoats. Indeed, panic, hysteria, confusion, and chaos characterized the outbreak. Quarantine was the predominant response; dying children were refused care. Cats and dogs, suspected of being carriers of the disease, were slaughtered. There was a wholesale exodus of the children of the well-to-do from the city. In New York alone there were 9,000 cases during the summer of 1916 and 2,343 deaths. Nationwide, 29,000 cases were reported and approximately 6,000 deaths.[3] Polio would flourish in this country, as in no other, until the mid-1950s.

I would speculate that for a long time we have not been able to bear to look at the horror of those years. Kathryn Black, for example, reports how her memories of her mother's protracted struggle with and subsequent death from polio were ones she had kept buried for years. The polio vaccine in 1955 and the virtual eradication of polio in this country are another tale of American triumph over adversity, a salute to scientific and technological progress, and yet another sign of medical dominance over disease. With the advent of a polio cure, it became as though all memories of that frightening and painful time—of the suffering, dying, and, worse yet, crippled children—were stuffed into a big black box, taped up, and put away, somewhere out of sight, under the bed or in the back of the closet. However, the passage of time and the emergence of the postpolio syndrome plaguing many polio survivors have brought our collective memories of the polio epidemics of the first part of the twentieth century closer to the surface. Likewise, the reintroduction of the iron lung as a therapeutic option suggests that the time is ripe for examination of the development and use of these earlier mechanical ventilators, sometimes referred to as "steel coffins."[4]

Little attention has been paid in the nursing literature to the unique, heroic, arduous, and terrible nursing care involved in the care of polio patients, most of whom were babies and children. Although considerable examination has gone into the development of intensive care units (ICUs) and their associated technologies, little is known about the use of early cylinder respirators, the "iron lungs," and the unique nursing care they engendered.[5] These machines use negative pressure ventilation, as opposed to the positive pressure ventilation in almost exclusive use today. The nursing care of iron lung patients called for nurses to care concurrently for both patient and machine, and much can be learned from nursing's response to this early technology. I will provide an overview of the polio epidemics in this country in the first half of the twentieth century, describe the development of the iron lung and its use during the polio epidemics, and describe the nursing involved in caring for patients in iron lungs.[6] The time frame of 1929–1955 was chosen because these were the years in which the iron lung was most heavily used.[7]

THE POLIO EPIDEMICS

First called *infantile paralysis,* because of its tendency to attack small children, this fearful disease seemed to come out of nowhere, striking rich and poor, educated and ignorant, city and rural areas, and black and white alike. It came in waves, striking mainly in late summer and early fall, and no one was ever sure where it would strike next. Black writes of "the fear that hung like heat in the summer air. No one knew how you got it. Did you breathe it in, swallow it in contaminated milk, drink it down in a public fountain, or get it from flies on your picnic lunch?"[8] An ancient stele from Egyptian times depicts a priest leaning on a staff; one leg withered and shortened with the foot dropped in a way characteristic of paralytic polio, providing archaeologic evidence that the disease has been with us since 1500 B.C. However, prior to the latter part of the nineteenth century the polio virus was probably endemic, silently infecting infants through fecal contamination of water and food. No one associated the disease's vague and inconsistent symptoms with the occasional, surprising paralysis or even death of a child.

Polio, not being a disease of filth and poverty, flourished in highly developed countries. Viruses need a population of susceptible people to survive. As the United States, the Scandinavian countries, and Great Britain raised their standards of living, they began to experience polio epidemics of greater size and severity because their populations had not gained immunity through exposure. Epidemics occurred somewhere in the United States almost every year from 1900 to 1956. The age of onset of the disease increased as well as its severity.[9] In 1916, 95% of cases occurred in children under nine years of age; by 1955, 25% of the victims were over age twenty. The Swedish epidemics of 1908–1911 established that mortality was lowest in children under the age of five. Mortality and morbidity rose with age. Previously referred to as infantile paralysis, the disease was renamed *poliomyelitis* or "inflammation of the grey matter," *polios,* meaning grey, and *myelos,* meaning matter.[10]

The virus leapfrogged across the country unpredictably, coming into its full strength between the years 1942 and 1953. The years 1944 and 1945 saw outbreaks along the Atlantic seaboard; after 1946 epidemics spread from the Appalachians to the Rocky Mountains. Minneapolis, home of the world-famous Elizabeth Kenny Institute, had the worst outbreak of any U.S. city. One of its victims was the three-year-old daughter of the medical supervisor of the Kenny Institute, Dr. John Pohl. Dr. Richard

Aldrich was a resident at the University of Minnesota Hospital at the time. Having just returned from the battlefields of World War II, Aldrich likened the epidemic summers in the hospital to combat zones during wartime. The horror of those years is clearly apparent in his narrative:

> We admitted 464 proven cases of polio just at University Hospital which is just unbelievable. And this was a very severe paralytic form. Maybe two or three hours after a lot of these kids would come in with a stiff neck or a fever, they'd be dead. It was unbelievable. . . . At the height of the epidemic, the people of Minneapolis were so frightened that there was nobody in the restaurants. . . . A lot of people just took up and moved away, went to another city. It was really a disaster.

He recalled that the hospital cleared whole wards: "I remember there was a room 43, and another one, 33. They had nothing but polio there." The worst part, he remembered, was telling the parents: "Those were some of the worst experiences I ever had in my life; I've never forgotten them."[11]

By 1948, Los Angeles County Hospital was caring for 2,900 cases of polio, nearly one tenth of all the cases in the United States, and approximately one tenth of those patients needed iron lungs. The summer of 1952 saw a nationwide peak of the disease, with nearly 60,000 cases being reported. In the summer of 1955 the epidemic hit Massachusetts, resulting in almost 4,000 cases, the majority of whom were paralytic. Thomas Whitfield was a pediatric resident during that summer at Massachusetts General. He recalls "a feeling of ominous foreboding and fear that started towards the end of June, maybe mid-June."[12] The cases started early and kept going, with new patients arriving daily. William Tisdale, a second-year medical resident, recalls that the summer was hot and tempers were short; the twelve-hour shift work seemed endless. "We were running scared," he said. "We were exhausted, depressed by what we'd seen." Another doctor recalls "steeling" himself for what was a desperate situation. One "devastating night" several patients on the respiratory unit died.[13]

Not only did the doctors not know what to expect from the illness, which could range from mild and self-limiting to rapidly fatal, they feared getting it themselves or, worse, taking it home to their families, their wives and children. They washed their hands a lot, but they knew that that would not prevent their taking it home. Every day, doctors and nurses alike could look around at their patients and think, "There but for the grace of God go I." It was not unheard of for student nurses to become ill; some died.[14]

Doctors seldom touched the patients, and when they did, it was with gloved hands. Some doctors did not even enter the rooms of children with polio but stood in the doorway or waved through a glass partition. Whitfield recalled, "You wanted to pick them up and hold them [referring to the children], but you just didn't do that." When staff did enter the rooms, they came covered in gowns and masks, which they shed when they left. In 1949, at Willard Parker Hospital, in the midst of a Buffalo, New York, epidemic, Doris Seligman, a teenager at the time, lay "encased in an iron lung and isolated except for some rare contact with nurses . . . soaked in urine most of the time." Not until a night when the hospital lost electrical power and someone rushed to handpump her iron lung did she realize that she was not forgotten.[15]

Usually, the polio virus got no farther than the gastrointestinal tract, where it caused temporary discomfort. However, no one could predict why, or when, it would course through the blood, finding the central nervous system, destroying cellular chemical messengers, and causing paralysis—sometimes temporary, often permanent. Although never the leading childhood killer (a child under ten had only three chances in a thousand of becoming the victim of a severe attack of polio), it remained the most feared of diseases. Permanent paralysis occurred in only 3% to 4% of all cases. Over time, however, the number of persons disabled by the disease reached tremendous proportions.[16]

"Polio Nurses": Following the Epidemics

Nurses cared for patients throughout, in all kinds of circumstances, with varying degrees of knowledge and experience. Juanita Howell, RN, talked about her work as a polio nurse. Employed as a school nurse in Mississippi in 1946, she found herself without work when the school was closed down during a polio epidemic. She recalled, "Well, why don't I try the polio clinic? . . . They needed help, the patients were coming in from all around the state, nurses were coming from all over the country, it was just a very desperate time. . . . We had a lot of nurses who came back from the war in 1945 and followed the epidemics."[16] She remembers that all the nurses went to work in street clothes. They were concerned about the reaction of average citizens who observed them in uniform getting off the bus and going to work in the polio clinic. This was not an uncommon practice and was described in a number of sources.[17]

The National Foundation for Infantile Paralysis (NFIP), founded on the initiative of President Franklin D. Roosevelt, opened its doors in 1938. This nonprofit organization worked unceasingly throughout the epidemics to provide help and relief and, most important, to eradicate the disease. The organization raised money through the collection of dimes, the March of Dimes campaign being one of the most effective fundraising endeavors of the twentieth century. NFIP funded Jonas Salk's and Albert

Sabins' research and was instrumental in the implementation of the massive public health campaigns of the 1950s to ensure immunization of the population, which led to the eradication of the disease in this country.[18]

By the 1940s, along with the Red Cross, the NFIP held regular training sessions for nurses in the care of polio patients, especially those in iron lungs. Large numbers of nurses attended regional workshops, provided by the NFIP in conjunction with the Joint Orthopedic Nursing Advisory Service (JONAS), to bring expert instruction and the latest information to all nurses interested in learning the techniques of polio nursing. These nurses, often educators and supervisors, would return to their own communities and provide training for local nurses. Additionally, since predicting where the next outbreak would occur or its severity was impossible, any community in need would be given intensive, emergency training courses by representatives from JONAS sent to the area. NFIP, in conjunction with the Red Cross, also maintained an active registry of "polio nurses" and provided support, including housing for those nurses, when epidemics struck. Josephine Weligoschek, RN, provides this account of her experiences:

> San Antonio was my next assignment . . . the Red Cross official did very well finding us a delightful place to live. He said that the nurses' home was practically in shambles and he wouldn't like us to live there and after some scouting around he found us a tourist court with a swimming pool. All the nurses, physiotherapists and visiting interns shared these quarters. Living together made for excellent friendships and I don't believe any nurse had any occasion to become lonesome. [19]

In some locales the nurses lived in private homes secured by the Red Cross before their arrivals. They were welcomed by the communities they came to serve: "The citizens realized that the nurses might be lonely and called frequently" to invite them to dinner or sightseeing. Teas were given by local clubs to honor the nurses. Also,

> In traveling from one epidemic to another one often meets old friends from a previous epidemic . . . in San Antonio I met a nurse from Illinois whom I had met in Houston, Texas the previous summer. We both had vowed we would never go south again in the summer so it was amusing when we met in the South.[20]

As the number of patients who survived in iron lungs grew, respiratory centers popped up dedicated to the care and rehabilitation of chronic patients.[21]

The NFIP supplied grants on an annual basis to nursing organizations such as the National Organization for Public Health Nursing to assist accredited colleges and institutions to install centers where nurses could be sent to study and practice orthopedic nursing under supervision, to prepare manuals for the care of polio patients, and to provide grants to individuals to study how to care for these patients. Basil O'Connor, the vigorous and magnetic president of NFIP who is credited with many of the organization's achievements, described the activities of 1941. A grant was made to the National League of Nursing Education in 1941 for the purpose of establishing a joint orthopedic advisory service with the National Organization for Public Health Nursing. Scholarships were made available to prepare nurses for teaching and supervisory positions. Teachers College at Columbia University, Western Reserve University, and the University of Minnesota were all recipients of grants in the funding year of 1941.[22]

THE EMERGENCE OF THE IRON LUNG

A Dr. Steuart in South Africa in 1918 first constructed an airtight wooden box sealed at the shoulders and waist with clay and powered by a motor-driven bellows specifically for the treatment of polio. However, the first widely used mechanical respirator was developed by Philip Drinker in 1928.[23]

While watching a colleague measure the breathing of an anesthesized cat lying in a metal box with a rubber collar around its neck and its head exposed, Drinker had an idea. He paralyzed the breathing muscles of the cat, placed its body, again up to its neck, in a sealed box, and pumped air in and out of the box. He was able to keep the cat alive for hours! Drinker approached Consolidated Gas with his findings, and the company gave him $500 to pursue his ideas. Drinker and a colleague, Louis Shaw, constructed a man-sized respirator using the same principles as the cat box. It opened and shut like a drawer and had a rubber collar to fit around the head to prevent any escape of air from the box. Drinker's device was controversial. His brother Cecil, a Harvard professor of physiology, did not believe the device would work. He thought that any collar tight enough to prevent the outflow of air would impede cerebral circulation. However, Drinker demonstrated the apparatus on himself, proving it effective.[24]

Catherine Drinker Bowen, Drinker's sister and a well-known author, recounts the device's first use on a human in her 1971 book *Family Portrait*:

> On his way through the wards [of the Children's Hospital in Boston], Phil saw children dying of suffocation induced by polio; he could not

forget the small blue faces, the terrible gasping for air. The respirator had not been designed specifically for infantile paralysis. Yet when the machine was perfected, the first patient happened to be a little girl from Children's Hospital, suffering from severe polio and expected to be in respiratory difficulty very shortly. Phil had the machine moved into the ward near the child's bed so she could see it and get used to the loud whine of the motor. Early next morning, the hospital called Phil. By the time he reached the hospital the child was in the machine, unconscious. The staff had been afraid to turn on the power. Phil started the pump and in less than a minute saw the child regain consciousness. She asked for ice cream. Phil said he stood there and cried.[25]

The little girl survived only for a short time, however, succumbing by week's end to pneumonia, but it was clear that the machine worked and could save lives. When presented with these findings, the doctors at the Children's Hospital resisted on moral grounds. If the life of the patient were saved, would they have to remain in the machine forever? The experience of a second respirator patient, treated at Peter Bent Brigham Hospital, proved these fears groundless. The patient recovered the ability to breathe; at the end of a year he was walking again, although with calipers and a stick.[26]

Time would show that not all patients made such speedy recoveries. Agonizing questions persisted. There might be several patients with severe respiratory difficulties and only one machine. Who should get to use the machine? The patient with the severest distress, who might never recover, or the one who appeared to have the best chance of survival? Although doctors continued to feel conflicted about the saving of lives of such severely handicapped people, what choice did they have? Predicting the extent of enduring disability at the beginning of the illness was impossible.

However, the indisputable role of the iron lung, functioning on principles of negative pressure, a legacy of medical technology, was now established, and poliomyelitis had only begun to cast its terrifying shadow. The year 1931 saw a record high of 16,000 cases nationwide; by the 1940s, over 40,000 cases per year were documented. These numbers increased in the 1950s, and the nation could see no end in sight. Some fatal diseases were more prevalent, but none was more feared.

Whoosh-Whoosh-Whoosh

Negative pressure body ventilation (NPBV) uses the principles of normal breathing, producing a negative or subatmospheric pulmonary pressure (anything below atmospheric pressure [760 mm Hg]), which actively expands the chest and forces air through the nose and mouth into the lungs. When the pressure is released, the chest returns to a resting position, causing air to be passively expelled out of the lungs.

The Drinker respirator consisted of a cylindrical metal tank sealed at one end; the patient's entire body was surrounded by an airtight chamber with the head and neck protruding through an airtight collar at one end. The respirator was equipped with motor-powered blowers, also called bellows, and a control knob. When the bellows expanded, the air pressure in the tank was lowered, the chest expanded, and air flowed into the lungs. When the bellows contracted, the air pressure in the tank was raised, and the air was forced out of the lungs. By this method a movement of the chest was produced that simulated normal breathing. The expansion and contraction of the bellows was set to correspond with the normal number of respirations per minute; the depth of the respiration was also able to be controlled. The action of the bellows was what created the characteristic and distinctive *whoosh-whoosh-whoosh* sound of the iron lung.

June Opey, who spent two years in an iron lung, describes the lung as follows:

> Attached to the end of the lung was a long, fat, hose-like piece of tubing. Somewhere along this was a huge contraption, resembling fireside bellows, from which a further length of tubing led to an electric plug in the wall. With the turning of a switch the bellows worked in exactly the same manner as they would to create a fire draught. They pushed and sucked air in and out of the lung at intensely high pressure, sufficient to flatten the whole of my chest wall for expiration, and to release it for inhalation. As the air pressed down against my body my ribs were forced inwards, and air came rushing out of my mouth. As the pressure was released so my ribs and lungs expanded, causing air to be sucked into my mouth. Thus, I breathed.[27]

"Such Comfort!"

Although often initially terrifying to patients, the iron lung often became a significant source of comfort and relief. Regina Woods describes her feelings when first put into the iron lung: ". . . before I realized what was happening I was in a huge cylinder with only my head sticking out. A few adjustments were quickly made and it was closed. To my amazement, the cylinder had rolled open and it had not been necessary to stuff me through the small opening at the end. Such comfort! I was no longer struggling to breathe and the whole thing seemed simply wonderful. So wonderful that I cannot remember a night before, or since, of such sheer comfort. I did not know that these changes signaled a worsening of my condition and were viewed by my family with great alarm."[28]

Of course, Woods could not breathe. A nurse informant describes her sensation of negative pressure as follows:

> I never understood the concept of negative pressure until I volunteered one day as a student nurse to demonstrate an iron lung. I know that it would be breathing for me, so at the last minute I tried to take a breath in case it didn't work so I wouldn't be without air AND I COULDN'T TAKE A BREATH. It was worse than choking. I had no will of my own. It was the scariest feeling I've ever had.[29]

The problem was not in getting the patient *into* the lung, as it turned out. It was getting them out. One nurse informant said, "The lung comes to mean a place of security. It's almost as if it were a retreat back into the womb."[30]

"Yellow Caskets"

The iron lung remained the most effective ventilatory device throughout the polio epidemics, but it continued to engender fear and a variety of psychological repercussions virtually unexplored:

> Various ways were tried to get me and those like me out of the lungs that lined the halls like so many caskets, their motionless inhabitants filled with fear and rage. Fear they would not survive the next attempt to help them and rage that they could do nothing to strike back when their keepers went beyond the bounds of human decency.[31]

NURSING CARE

What the Literature Said

The specific nursing care of a patient with polio was dependent on many different factors. It changed significantly from the start of the epidemics to their end in the mid-1950s with the development of the Salk vaccine. For example, immobilization was a primary concept in the early treatment of polio and remained the conventional approach through the mid-1940s. Patients were put in plaster casts to "rest" the muscles. Challenged by Elizabeth ("Sister") Kenny, the Australian nurse who took the United States by storm and revolutionized the treatment of the polio patient in the late 1940s, immobilization gave way to "hot packs" and rigorous physical therapy.[32]

The acute, and what was considered infectious stage of the disease was thought to last anywhere between two and four weeks, and required different approaches than the more chronic care of polio patients. Each hospital that took patients with contagious diseases established its own quarantine periods. No one was really sure how long polio was contagious. Children lay on beds, or in oversized cribs, with signs above them stating in big letters **POLIO**. They were put in pajamas with big red dots on the backs to warn of contagion. Pain medication and sedation were used with extreme care, as respiratory collapse was a common fear. As late as 1945, Dr. W. H. Bradley, senior medical officer at the Ministry of Health, London, summed up our approaches to polio as characterized by "ignorance, impotence, and insecurity."[33]

Care of a patient with polio was challenging enough; care of a patient in an iron lung demanded a highly expert level of professional nursing care. The inability to see the patient, the potential for skin breakdown, the difficulties with feeding, the potential for aspiration, and the problems related to excretion posed daunting challenges for all involved. This is what led to the "portholes" fashioned from boat windows in the early days of respirator development.[34] Teamwork was essential. The problem of airway patency was ever present. Weaning from the lung also emerged as a prime issue.[35] In nursing journals in the 1930s, in articles frequently authored by physicians, the nursing care of the patients in the iron lung began to be addressed.

Nursing textbooks of the time are matter-of-fact in their approach. Bertha Harmer's 1934 edition of the *Textbook of the Principles and Practice of Nursing* (third edition) contained very little reference to poliomyelitis or the care of the patient with polio and no reference to the iron lung. In 1939 the fourth edition of this text noted that a complete revision of the earlier edition had been undertaken to make it "conform more nearly to the Curriculum Guide, published by the National League of Nursing Education in 1937." This text outlines the use of a respirator and provides a detailed diagram of the Drinker-Collins respirator as well as photos. By 1955 this text included an expanded section on managing the respirator patient and more detailed photographs outlining aspects of care. A section was also devoted to weaning the patient from the respirator, and examples of oscillating (rocking) beds as well as portable external respirators were included.

Margaret Tracy's 1949 text *Nursing: An Art and Science* devotes two pages (with two pictures) to the Drinker respirator. This source explains that the artificial respiration must be regulated for each patient so that "the patient's efforts of breathing are synchronized to the rhythm of the machine." The nurse is instructed to monitor the patient closely for cyanosis and any possible airway obstruction. The emotional needs of the patient are addressed as follows: "Throughout the entire period of treatment within the respirator, the patient needs encouragement and reassurance. Cheerful surroundings, someone to read to him, contribute to his happiness and lessen the tedium of his hospital stay."

The Art, Science and Spirit of Nursing by Alice L. Price was published in 1954. This text devotes several pages to the "The Mechanical Respirator" and notes that detailed instructions are provided with each respirator and in some models, instructions are posted on the side of the respirator for all to read. Photographs are included. This text also notes the need to monitor the patient for any sign of cyanosis. Certain forms of entertainment or diversion for the patient are recommended "to help maintain an optimistic state of mind."[36]

The NFIP published manuals on nursing care, some in conjunction with the National League for Nursing Education. These outline care of the contagious patient as well as care of the iron lung patient. Information and instructions were also available from the companies that built the lungs; Emerson Collins supplied detailed drawings of the lung and its respective parts as well as providing all information on the pressure settings and gauges.[37] Although these were usually set by the doctors and determined by the physicians ordering them, as is so often the case, the nurses were the ones who operated and made the machines "fit" the patient.

Emotional needs of patients and families were conceptualized in terms consistent with the times. The need for reassurance when placing the patient in the lung and the need for diversion when the patient was kept in the lung for an extended period were consistently mentioned in the nursing literature. Given the potentially long-term nature of the disease and its exceedingly uncertain outcome, people dealing with these patients seemed uncertain how to respond. For example, a 1943 British textbook on physiotherapy for polio patients has a brief paragraph on patient psychology, which states, "No crippled individual must be left to indulge in his own thoughts." At the 1948 First International Poliomyelitis Conference, held in New York City, a speaker acknowledged that "The psychiatry of polio is the least well understood segment of the problem." Another source states, "Nothing can be worse for both patient and parent than the constant hovering of an anxious mother of an irritable child."[38]

Nurses were cautioned not to be too sympathetic to the children and reminded that an "objective" (i.e., "professional") attitude was to be maintained at all times. In many settings, families were allowed to visit only once a week, usually on Sundays, especially during the acute phase of hospitalization. The idea was that complete separation from their parents would help the children make a "better adjustment" to their illness. One article states that the parents were allowed to call the hospital operator during a certain hour every day, to receive a terse report, such as either "good," or "fairly good," or "serious." Parents who appeared excessively anxious and distraught were viewed as "psychologically immature." An especially homesick or distraught child, who, today, might be viewed as having a psychologically healthy reaction to the trauma of hospitalization and immobilization, was viewed as having an "abnormal" attachment to his/her mother, or as unstable. Instituting "wholesome" activities for the child was recommended: Good books (not comics!), nature films (no cartoons—too stimulating!), and classical music were favored.[39]

An article on the hospitalization of children published in the *American Journal of Psychiatry* in 1937 suggested that the hospitalized child be surrounded by an atmosphere of "neutrality"; additionally, it noted the benefits of not having anxious friends and families nearby. A 1935 *New England Journal of Medicine* article noted that for a child who had completely recovered, "the disease seems to have no darker memories than an attack of measles."[40]

This all predated Benjamin Spock and the mainstreaming of profoundly different approaches to child rearing and child development that began in the 1950s. The stance of many child experts of that day was one of strict adherence to a by-the-clock routine. The regimented and mechanistic care of children in hospitals was encouraged by many authorities. John Bowlby's work on maternal deprivation and separation had not yet appeared. Ideas of interpersonal process and therapeutic communication did not begin to be brought into the nursing curriculum until the 1950s. In the early 1950s, but unfortunately near the end of the epidemics, new attitudes began to be expressed in the nursing and medical literature.[41]

Teamwork

One aspect of nursing care that emerges repeatedly from the professional literature, as well as from first-person accounts by nurses themselves, was the necessity of teamwork. The process of getting the patient into the lung was difficult. Pictures surveyed in nursing texts, as well as in reviews of procedures, all portray a team of workers, usually nurses, facilitating the movement of the patient into the lung. A nursing text of the time states, "A team of at least four persons is needed to move the patient in a supine position to the respirator either by the hand carry method or the use of a lifting sheet." When the patient can be removed from the respirator for only a very short time, another text suggests the following: "All articles and equipment should be assembled. Two to four nurses should be available to perform the necessary procedure. The doctor should hyperventilate the patient. The stretcher should be withdrawn quickly and the nurses should work together very rapidly and in unison to complete the nursing care in the shortest possible time."

... they told me they could put me in a machine to make me feel better, easier to breathe. They took me into a small room. I saw this giant machine. To me it was giant. And they had to slide it open. There was a tray inside. They put me on it, slid my head through. I thought it was silly at the time because it took three people to carry me.[42]

The epidemics, in general in late summer through fall and striking in a seemingly random fashion, called for teamwork. The following is a description by a nurse, of working in a respiratory unit during a 1952 epidemic:

We always had fifteen to twenty respirators in service. The Army and Navy flew respirators from center to center as needed. . . . Tracheotomies were done right in the unit . . . almost every patient in the unit was receiving oxygen; almost every patient had to be suctioned and each one had to have his own setup for this care. Most patients on this unit were unable to swallow properly, so most of them had feeding tubes or were being nourished intravenously or by clysis. The number of nurses available for this unit was not sufficient so each nurse had to be assigned as many as four patients daily. (Teamwork in this unit was a reality not a thesis!)[43]

Every nurse spoke of the mental stress of being prepared for power outages: "Once the current on three of the respirators failed. Until maintenance could restore it we had to man the respirator bellow by hand. This is extremely hard to do, the person pumping tiring within a minute or two." The teamwork in this situation was essential for the patient's survival: "The staff on duty (doctors, nurses, aides, orderlies), in short, everybody available and able, lined up and in relays we kept the respirators going." Another nurse recalled a similar sentiment, stating that her greatest fear was power failures: "And there was never enough help. Those were the days that I recall working twelve-plus hours per day. Without a day off for weeks on end." Another nurse states, ". . . someone had to provide manual power. The machines could be switched into manual and operated by hand. There was a crank on the back of it, and maintenance people, gardeners, sweepers, anybody who was available came to help do that."[44]

Technical Skill

Another theme that emerged in the nurses' narratives was the skill that was necessary to provide care to the patient in an iron lung. One nurse recalled, "One had to learn to quickly adapt to being able to put equipment into the machine and get it out properly. One had to be able to utilize linens for moving the patients properly." A nursing text of the time states, "The patient in the respirator is completely dependent on the nurse." The text goes on to note that treatments such as enemas, catheterization, and hypodermic injections may be done without removing the patient from the respirator, "although they may be difficult." Another nurse recalled, "You have a patient in an iron lung, you've got to be able to get in those portholes when you have zero pressure. And you have got to be skilled and time yourself so carefully, so that you don't disrupt the respiratory cycle if possible . . . not an easy task." One source noted:

> There were good-natured attractive nurses who were nonetheless dreaded by patients because they couldn't give a sponge bath without soaking the bed linens. And the worst of the caregivers were a disaster. Patients joked about the dim-witted helpers, like the one who threw a blanket over the iron lung when the patient inside complained about being cold. They joked, but they must have also been furious.[45]

Managing the Machine

One nurse provided us with a copy of a newspaper article featuring her in the early 1950s, explaining the functioning of an iron lung to a reporter. "The lung," she told the newspaper reporter, who also got inside the lung to experience its power, "you might as well face it, is going to be the *complete master* of the situation and there is no use arguing with it. You breathe as it dictates, speak when it permits, swallow according to its whims."[46]

The nurses came to know the machines intimately. One nurse describes the following incident:

> I recall having only one machine on standby and we had to use it. Which left us with nothing but a machine that was inoperable. And I recall saying to the engineer on a Saturday or a Sunday (I know it was a weekend) "You've got to repair the machine." He looked at me and he looked at the machine and he says, "I've never seen one before." I said, "OK." I rolled up my long sleeves, I put a sheet on the floor and I said, "let's take it apart." And I took it apart, I laid out every nut and bolt that we removed, I found the problem, and put everything back. And that was a sight to see! Me, crawling around under the machine in a white uniform, a cap on my head. But we did it. And it was operable.[47]

The manuals done by NFIP show an illustration of the physician setting the pressure gauges for the lung. However, this was not as straightforward as it appears. The machine had to be adapted to the individual needs of each patient. As one nurse said: "Each machine had to be adapted to the needs of the client. Even in the setting of the cycle for respiration . . . the positive and negative pressures, the changing of the collars. These are things that always had to be done."[48] Everything centered on observation of the individual patient, and settings had to be changed constantly.

Another nurse, in an article published in 1950 in *Trained Nurse,* called, "Personal Experience with Polio Nursing," recalls her introduction to polio in 1945. ". . . when I saw an iron lung in operation as I went on duty that night I was ready to run in the opposite direction. The isolation ward was filled to capacity."[49] She continues:

> My first night on duty was such that I have remembered it vividly. My assignment was with another nurse, experienced in polio nursing, who taught me the care of the patient in the respirator and explained to me the mechanism of the iron lung. . . .

She goes on:

> My second night I was on duty I worked alone with a patient. He was a boy of fifteen years, very, very restless, and at that time the doctors were reluctant to give the patients any sedatives. I kept an alert and constant vigil.

Make no mistake, though, the machine gave the nurses tremendous control over their patients. Stories like the following unfortunately abound:

> I had a cloth around my neck, to keep my neck from getting rubbed away by the collar . . . One day it slid . . . I couldn't breathe. I was crying and calling the nurse. You had to learn to really melt to get her attention. She came in and she seemed really frustrated, overworked, and just too busy. So I told her what was wrong and she told me to stop crying. She said she would turn my respirator off if I didn't stop crying. When she did I passed out immediately.[50]

This incident was recollected by Marilyn Rogers, 9 years old in 1949 and in an iron lung.

Total Care Around the Clock

Keeping the patient alive meant the maintenance of a patent airway. This was not as easy as it might seem. In cases of positive pressure ventilation, at least in the short run, this is accomplished by intubation. Maintaining airway patency for an acutely ill patient in a lung was much more challenging and was dependent essentially on good nursing care. Often, the pharyngeal nerves were paralyzed. These patients required frequent suctioning so as not to choke on their own secretions. As noted by Emma Manfreda, who nursed during polio epidemics:

When the mouth and secretions are welling or damming up, the nurse has to remember to suction regularly to prevent the patient from literally drowning in his own fluids. She must watch also for signs of oxygen supply loss due to bronchial plugging by mucous or blood clots and attempt to suction these out, thereby relieving the patient without need of a bronchoscopy.[51]

Even with the most constant vigilance and best nursing care, some patients would still need to have an emergency tracheotomy to survive. Black recalls her mother's tracheotomy:

During her first night in the hospital, when the virus raged through her body, deadening muscle after muscle but leaving her on fire with pain, the doctors had performed an emergency tracheotomy. The incision, a slice in the throat just below the Adam's apple, made a hole in her windpipe where the O_2 [oxygen] tube could be inserted and from which phlegm could be drawn, saving her from drowning on her own mucous . . . the tracheotomy signaled to all that Mother was among the sickest, highest-risk polio patients.[52]

The care of the acutely ill polio patient, especially one in an iron lung, was endless. Care was total. Responsibility was enormous:

The care of the polio respirator patient is a tremendous responsibility. It is physically exhausting in actual physical energy expended to care for the patient and it is a mental strain trying to imbue him with confidence and a hopeful outlook. It is a great mental strain also watching for signs indicating a change [adverse] in the patient's condition. One of the biggest mental responsibilities is remembering to check on the respirator pressure. Pressure may be lost from the smallest leak occurring around the head opening, a porthole door being left open, incomplete closure of the head and body parts of the respirator, or an unplugged opening. A patient's life could shortly be lost from pressure failure.[53]

Another nurse recalls caring for a "chronic":

She wasn't a one-to-one. I remember taking care of her one day . . . because she was a "chronic" . . . she had "hospitalitis." "Get me this . . . do this!" I had three other children to take care of that day and I couldn't get out of the room.[54]

Fear and Bravery

In retrospect, truly recalling the horror of the polio epidemics for all concerned, the ever-present backdrop of the nursing care of the patients of the iron lung, is difficult. One physician described his experience as a resident at the University of Minnesota Hospital during the epidemics of 1948 and 1949 in the following terms:

> It was like being in combat. You have to be on the ball and ready to go all the time. You were excited, exhausted, and frightened at the same time. We didn't want to get polio ourselves. We were all concerned as heck about it because we'd bring it home. . . . You couldn't avoid it. Because you were covered with saliva, you'd bring it with you.

Nurses recruited for "polio duty" had their salaries underwritten jointly by local hospitals and NFIP chapters. A slightly higher rate of pay was common in communicable disease settings; however, in setting up salaries for polio nursing, no differential was allowed "because the NFIP has insurance coverage for recruited nurses who contract polio. This covers medical and hospital expenses, as well as a salary stipend on a decreasing rate over a period of a year." Dr. Joseph Melnick, a scientist at Yale University who was central to the testing and development of the oral polio vaccine, likened the polio epidemics in the 1950s to the AIDS epidemics of today.

Informants were questioned as to their memories of fear:

Researcher: You mentioned that you had some fear of contracting polio?

Nurse: Yeah, I think everybody did in those days that was assigned to it . . . I mean, you had to gown up, you wore a mask, you did all this . . . I think there was greater fear of contracting polio than AIDS today . . . because you knew if you got it you could be crippled for life . . . during the infectious stage, nurses were afraid.

Researcher: Did you, or any of the nurses that you remember, ever refuse to care for a patient that had polio?

Nurse: That I really don't know about because as student nurses we didn't have much right to refuse . . . couldn't refuse . . . that was, it was like, you will learn isolation. It was a good lesson in isolation technique.

Yet, of course, nurses persevered. Nurses bravely, and often gaily, cared for acutely ill patients, many of whom were in lungs. A patient informant recalled the following:

> My primary nursing care was very good in the iron lung, especially. They kept me close to the nurses station . . . well, mostly the student nurses did most of the work . . . I really had a good time, I enjoyed the banter . . . I had a roommate and our room was very popular. In the

morning there would be six, seven student nurses in there having coffee with us.[55]

Wonderful tales of caregivers abound. When one patient was asked what was going through her head at age nine, being on the "machine," she answered:

> Staying alive. The staff was very, very nice to us. Some of the nurses they called "plague nurses"—they were from the National Foundation [NFIP]. They were the best. One of them brought peas in with straws so we could see if we could hit the ceiling to increase our vital capacity. I usually give everybody nicknames. She wore purple fingernail polish so I called her purple.[56]

The polio epidemics also provide an early example of patient triage and the grouping of very ill patients together to render more effective care. When asked about the number of patients cared for and how they were able to do it, one nurse responded, "We would have all eight respirator [patients] in the room if necessary. You see, they were rather large, and it made nursing care much more easy to do. You could stand there and see every patient."[57] The experience of caring for polio patients provided nurses with tremendous opportunities for ingenuity.

The Need for Caring

The need for new understandings rippled throughout the memories of all alike—nurses, patients, families, and physicians. No one knew what to do; no one had the answer. This affected different people in different ways. The following is a recollection by a nurse who was interviewed about a difficult patient that she cared for:

Nurse: She was probably 25 or 26 and it was just she wanted to be waited on constantly. And then I had the frustration of not being able to care for my other patients. And being a young nurse I didn't comprehend why she had to be so demanding.

Researcher: Do you think looking back, you see things differently?

Nurse: Oh, yes. I do. I mean I can comprehend her anxieties of being left alone, but at that time I didn't interpret it as anxieties . . . I just [thought she was a] . . . selfish individual . . . who was so used to being . . . everything being done for her that I couldn't . . . I wasn't mature enough to understand what she was going through . . . all I could see was that my other patients weren't being taken care of. And being at a hospital, supposedly learning my pediatric experience, and this being an adult, it was like this isn't fair! I'm not here . . . I'm being used! . . . and we really felt we were being dumped on! But, immaturity was part of our problem too.[58]

Another informant brought this up during the interview process:

Researcher: What else do you remember about the care of patients in a respirator?

Nurse: Their psychological needs were so vital, and yet we did not attach as much importance to those things in those years as we recognize today as an integral part of health care delivery. I don't think we paid as much attention to that [psychological needs] as we could have.

Researcher: Why do you think that is?

Nurse: We were rushed, keeping the patient alive and seeing to their physical needs, was paramount . . . we were in the same position as today . . . Who is going to be in control? The patient? Or the health care provider? And we [the health care provider] were in control. This poor, helpless, paralyzed individual really had no control. And I think some of us took advantage of that.

When asked in what way, she continued: "We weren't as understanding. We weren't as empathetic. We didn't meet their needs with far better understanding and treatment of their psychological needs."[59] This nurse went on to earn a master's degree and was in a variety of supervisory positions for much of her career. She shared at length her fight, over a period of years and in a variety of institutions, for longer visiting hours for patients and families.

SUFFERING AND GROWTH IN THE SHADOW OF POLIO

To revisit the polio epidemics of the first half of the twentieth century in this country is like visiting a foreign shore. Tales from nurses and patients alike are nothing short of horrific. Yet, similar to the crisis of war, out of the crucible of human suffering emerged tremendous advances, and nurses played a role in each one.

The most significant of these advances was the cure for polio, the development of the polio vaccine, the public health triumph of the 1950s that led to the virtual eradication of the disease. The extreme crisis of the epidemics rallied the nation to contribute and support the development of a vaccine, and nurses were as instrumental in the massive public health campaign of the 1950s for education and immunization of the populace as they were during the epidemics.[60]

The erratic and sporadic nature of the epidemics, spread across the country, unpredictable and frightening, called forth a network of organizations united in the fight against the disease. Nurses were a vital component of this effort, especially the "polio nurses," who traveled from epidemic to epidemic, providing education and leadership.

The development of the iron lung, an astounding piece of technology that was able to keep patients who otherwise would not have survived, alive, was another significant development to arise out of the polio epidemics. The use of this new technology raised new ethical issues not easily resolved. While saving the lives of the patients, the machines bred a hideous dependency, both physiologic and psychologic. Large respiratory care centers arose for the care of chronic patients, a situation which then led to further advances in the management of respiratory problems.[61] The technology called forth ingenuity in nursing management, as nurses grouped patients together for accessibility and close monitoring, foreshadowing the development of intensive care units. Although it was clearly designated to be the domain of medicine to "set" the particular pressure gauges on the machines, the nurses monitored the settings, adjusting and individualizing the settings to each patient and situation, and troubleshooting when problems arose.

The nursing care of patients with polio changed as understanding of the disease advanced. However, certain essentials remained the same, especially the care of patients in the iron lung. Every patient was "different" and, yet, the same. The nursing care provided these patients could make the difference between life and death, yet staffing was often poor, and pay was low.[62] Work during the epidemics was likened by some to doing "combat" duty. Teamwork was demanded as well as technical competence, speed, and skill. The nurse needed to be able to manage the machine as well as the patient. Care of the patients in the iron lungs was total; their dependency on the machine, and thus on the nurse who managed the machine, was complete. Patients were powerless, and in many situations, so were the nurses—powerless to meet the needs of their patients, to save the lives of some, and to stop the relentless spread of the disease. Care of patients with polio confined to iron lungs engendered fear. Nurses were afraid of catching the disease itself, of managing patients who could die at any time, and who depended on their every action and reaction. Care of the patients in iron lungs also fostered bravery, leadership, and ingenuity. Care of these patients made nurses realize that they needed to understand more, to care more. The iron lung created a shared technological bond between nurses and patients, a nexus for caring; and although some of the sounds now are different, the "hospital symphony" plays on:

> There was the perpetual humming of motors, loud, then soft, whoosh . . . Whoosh; teeth grinding, crunch . . . crunch; feet moving through the corridors, rubber shoes squeaking, from cubicle to cubicle, squish . . . Squish; the whispering of voices mouthing incomprehensible sounds beneath the infrequent shouts and cries of patients, "Nurse! Nurse!", the stretchers and wheelchairs, squeak . . . squeak; the clatter of bedpans and urinals at all hours; the tinkle and rattle of dishes and silverware at meals. All these sounds make up the hospital symphony.[63]

NOTES

1. "72,000 Cats Killed in Paralysis Fear," *The New York Times,* 26 July 1916.
2. Tony Gould, *A Summer Plague: Polio and Its Survivors* (New Haven, Conn.: Yale University Press, 1995), 3–4. The first chapter of this book details the New York City epidemic.
3. Naomi Rogers, *Dirt and Disease: Polio Before FDR* (New Brunswick, NJ: Rutgers University Press, 1992); John R. Paul, *A History of Poliomyelitis* (New Haven, Conn.: Yale University Press, 1971), 4–7.
4. Kathryn Black, *In the Shadow of Polio: A Personal and Social History* (Menlo Park, Calif.: Addison-Wesley, 1996); Nina Gilden Seavey et al., *A Paralyzing Fear: The Triumph Over Polio in America* (New York: TV Books, LLC, 1996), also a PBS video that provides an excellent overview of polio in this century, including the 1916 New York City epidemic. This work includes many pictures—almost all March of Dimes photos—and interviews with polio survivors, health care workers, and scientists; Gould, *A Summer Plague*; *Post-Polio Association of South Florida,* newsletter (June 1999); Marinos C. Dalakas, "The Post-Polio Syndrome as an Evolved Clinical Entity," *Annals New York Academy of Science* (1998): 68–79; Donald Mulder, "Clinical Observations on Acute Poliomyelitis," *Annals New York Academy of Science* (1998): 1–10, which provides an excellent overview of acute epidemics, with particular emphasis after 1940, the associated treatment, as well as the coping strategies utilized by patients with residual paralysis; Marita Widar and Gerd Ahlstrom, "Experiences and Consequences of Pain in Patients With Post-Polio Syndrome," *Journal of Advanced Nursing* 28, no. 3 (1998): 606–13; and Helen Zimmerman, "Ventilation Therapy Flashback," *RN* 59, no. 12 (1996): 26–31, which provides an excellent discussion of negative pressure body ventilation (NPBV) as it is used today.
5. Julie Fairman, "Watchful Vigilance: Nursing Care, Technology, and the Development of Intensive Care Units," *Nursing Research* 41, no. 1 (1992), 56–60; Margarete Sandelowski, "Making the Best of Things: Technology in American Nursing, 1870–1940," *Nursing History Review* 5 (1997): 3–22; and Julie Fairman, "Alternative Visions: The Nurse–Technology Relationship in the Context of the History of Technology," *Nursing History Review* 6 (1998): 129–146; Zimmerman, "Ventilation Therapy Flashback," 26–31.
6. A variety of primary and secondary data sources have been utilized, including the study of pictorial images, first-person accounts by patients, doctors, and nurses of the time, and a data set of interviews with patients and nurses conducted specifically for this study. The nursing and medical literature of these years was surveyed, including nursing

procedure manuals and social history accounts of the polio epidemic of the first half of the twentieth century. Accounts from both patients and nurses were included to provide a more rounded view; additionally, of interest were the often disturbing images sometimes encountered in the patient literature of the cruelties perpetrated by caregivers, some of whom were nurses. While analyzing this issue was not the intent of this chapter, it did warrant some exploration.

Originally, five interviews with nurses who cared for patients in the iron lung (solicited through the Florida Nurses Association Council of Retired Nurses, as well as through word of mouth contacts) and five interviews with patients who had spent time in iron lungs (solicited through post-polio support networks) were planned. The study received human subjects approval in May 1999 at Florida Atlantic University. Numerous personal accounts by patients were found in the existing literature; thus we cut back the number of patient interviews to one. The literature from patients, while often describing wonderful accounts of care by nurses, also contained a significant number of accounts of cruelty, as perceived by patients. The British literature surveyed seemed to contain the most accounts of this phenomenon. Early on, a Web site , from the UK, was discovered (http://members.xoam.com/_XOOM/html.lungmuseum [defunct]), which contained a large collection of reminiscences by patients as well as a variety of other historical photos and advertising brochures from iron lung companies from the 1930s and 1940s. This led to the identification of other useful sites and sources. An updated Web site is http://americanhistory.si.edu/polio/howpolio/ironlung.htm, from the Smithsonian's National Museum of American History.

7. Philip A. Drinker and Charles F. McKhann, "The Iron Lung: First Practical Means of Respiratory Support," *Journal of the American Medical Association* 255, no. 11 (May 1992): 1476–80 (hereafter cited as *JAMA*). Drinker developed the lung in 1928. The first documented usage was published in May 1929 in *JAMA* (cited elsewhere).

8. Black, *In the Shadow of Polio*, 31.

9. The most prominent example of this was Franklin Delano Roosevelt, who contracted polio at age 39 with severe resultant paralysis. The accounts of his struggle with infantile paralysis, as it was still called when he initially contracted it, can be found in numerous biographies of FDR, such as Geoffrey Ward, *A First Class Temperament: The Emergence of Franklin Roosevelt* (New York: Harper and Row, 1989). FDR was perhaps one of the most major influences on polio in this country through the establishment of Warm Springs, Georgia, a major site of rehabilitation for polio patients, his own example, and his involvement in the founding of the National Foundation for Infantile Paralysis (NFIP), a separate story in its own right. See also Hugh Gallagher, *A Splendid Deception* (New York: Dodd, Mead, 1985), a biography specifically about FDR's relationship with his disease and its aftermath. Gallagher is a "polio" himself, and a lengthy interview with him about his own experiences with the disease as well as a derailed account of life at Warm Springs during FDR's lifetime can be found in Seavey, *A Paralyzing Fear*, 51–64. Likewise, Seavey, "Politics, Hollywood and Money" in *A Paralyzing Fear*, 67–97, details the founding of the NFIP and the conception of the brilliant March of Dimes campaign. Seavey, *A Paralyzing Fear*, 85–96, provides a detailed interview with Charles Massey, who took his first job with the March of Dimes in 1948 and ultimately became its president from 1978 to 1989. Gould, *A Summer Plague*, 29–40, 41–53, 54–84, discusses FDR, Warm Springs, and the March of Dimes, respectively.

10. The history of the polio epidemics in this country has been abstracted from a variety of sources, notably: Black, *In the Shadow of Polio*; Gould, *A Summer Plague*; Paul, *History of Poliomyelitis*; Howard Howe, "Are You Afraid of Polio?" *Harper's* (June 1945): 646–53; Jane Smith, *Patenting the Sun: Polio and the Salk Vaccine* (New York: Morrow, 1990); Steven Spencer, "Where Are We Now on Polio?" *Saturday Evening Post*, September 17, 1949, 26–27, 87–93; and Roland Berg, *Polio and Its Problems*

(Philadelphia: Lippincott, 1948). Christopher J. Rutty, "'Do Something! Do Anything!' Poliomyelitis in Canada, 1927–1962," (PhD diss., University of Toronto, 1995), provides an excellent history of the epidemics in Canada. Additionally, contextual information was obtained from assorted sources, such as an oral history of Rhode Island in the postwar decade, written by tenth-grade students at South Kingston High School, *The Family in the Fifties: Hope, Fear, and Rock and Roll* (Providence: Rhode Island Historical Society, 1993). Time-Life Books, *The American Dream: The 50s* (Richmond, Va.: Time-Life Books, 1998), provides photographic images of the times.

11. Seavey, *A Paralyzing Fear,* 113–19, from an interview with Richard Aldrich, MD, who was a resident at the University of Minnesota Hospital during the epidemics of 1946–1949, a very heart-rending account of life during the polio epidemic.

12. Black, *In the Shadow of Polio,* 29. This book, subtitled *A Personal and Social History,* details the author's mother's horrifying descent into an iron lung and her subsequent death two years later, when Black was 6 years old. Seeking to reconstruct the memory of a mother and father and a family long lost, this anecdotal personal account provides an excellent, well-researched overview of 1940s and 1950s America and the impact of the polio epidemics. In her research for this book, Black corresponded with and interviewed survivors of the epidemics. The quote from Thomas Whitfield came from an interview with the author in January 1994.

13. Black, *In the Shadow of Polio,* 29. The quote from William Tisdale is from a tape recording to the author, December 1993.

14. Student nurses' deaths were alluded to in some literature, as well as in personal reminiscences from retired nurses (American Association for History of Nursing Conference, Newton, Mass., September 1999).

15. Black, *In the Shadow of Polio,* 67. The quote from Whitfield comes from an interview with the author, January 1994. The quotes from Doris Seligman come from a letter to the author, May 7, 1994.

16. Paul, *History of Poliomyelitis.*

17. Seavey, *A Paralyzing Fear,* 147–52, interview with Juanita Howell, RN, who was a polio nurse during the big epidemic in Mississippi in 1946. In 1948 she went on to be one of the three African American nurses who went to study the Sister Kenny treatment for rehabilitating muscles paralyzed by polio.

18. Basil O'Connor, "Leading the Fight on Poliomyelitis," *Public Health Nursing* 34, no. 1: 12–16. See also Seavey, *A Paralyzing Fear,* 163–230. This source contains a number of significant interviews with people intimately involved with the development of the vaccines: interviews with Donna Salk, ex-wife of Jonas Salk; Darrell Salk, Jonas Salk's son; John Troan, reporter for the Pittsburgh Press who covered the development of the Salk vaccine from its earliest beginnings; Don Wegemer, one of Salk's laboratory assistants (who was inoculated with the yet-to-be proven killed virus vaccine); and Dr. Robert Nix, pediatrician for Allegheny County, Pennsylvania in the early 1950s and chief pediatric officer at the D. T. Watson Home where Salk first tested the killed-virus vaccine beginning in 1951. See also Smith, *Patenting the Sun*; Richard Carter, *Breakthrough: The Saga of Jonas Salk* (New York: Trident, 1966); John Rowan Wilson, *Margin of Safety: The Story of the Poliomyelitis Vaccine* (London: Collins, 1963); and Saul Benison, "The History of Polio Research in the United States: Appraisals and Lessons," in *The Twentieth Century Sciences: Studies in the Biographies of Ideas* (New York: Harper and Row, 1972).

19. Josephine Weligoschek, "Personal Experience With Polio," *Trained Nurse* (February 1950): 68–69, 74 (hereafter cited as *TN*).

20. Ibid., 76.

21. Evelyn Hamil, "What Is Nursing in a Respiratory Center?" *American Journal of Nursing* 57, no. 1 (January 1957): 42–45. Respiratory centers are also discussed in

Seavey, *A Paralyzing Fear*, 135–46, which provides an interview with John Affeldt, MD, who became head of Rancho Los Amigos, one of the largest respiratory centers for patients. There is also a detailed account by Black, *In the Shadow of Polio*, 111–85, about her mother Virginia's experiences at a respiratory center.

22. O'Connor, "Leading the Fight"; see Trudy Whitman, "The Polio Nurse: A Personal Account," *TN* (June 1948); Weligoschek, "Personal Experience with Polio"; and Seavey, *A Paralyzing Fear*, 85–96, interview with Charles Massey.

23. Actually the construction of devices for artificial ventilation began much earlier. For a more detailed account of these fascinating early devices, see Paul, *History of Poliomyelitis*; Black, *In the Shadow of Polio*; and *A Summer Plague*. The Virtual Museum of the Iron Lung Website contains reproductions of *Short History of the Modern Iron Lung*, (Cambridge, Mass.: J. H. Emerson, n.d.) J. H. Emerson company was an early U.S. manufacturer of iron lungs; and Richard Hill, "'A Being Breathing Thoughtful Breath': The History of the British Iron Lung, 1832–1995," winner of the 1995 Lord Brock Memorial Historical Essay Prize, Guy's Hospital, London. The early nineteenth-century history of the development of ventilatory devices is another fascinating study in itself. For example, Hill notes that Alexander Graham Bell, the American inventor of the telephone, invented a "vacuum jacket" on a visit to England in 1882, which he improved in 1892 (copies of Bell's sketches of this device are also available at the Virtual Museum of the Iron Lung).

    Phillip Drinker was an engineer working in the Harvard School of Public Health in the Department of Ventilation and Illumination. Drinker's work centered on ways to improve methods of artificial ventilation. He served on a commission, funded by the Consolidated Gas Company of New York, intended to reduce the number of lawsuits brought against the company by people accidentally gassed from leaking pipes or by families of attempted suicides who had stuck their heads in gas ovens, a popular means of committing suicide at the time. Consolidated Gas Companies theorized that effective means of artificial ventilation might save lives, thus saving the company money.

    See also http://www.neoucom.edu/library/technologyandarchives.htm [defunct]). Additional pamphlets published by J. H. Emerson, Cambridge, Mass., 1963, are available there.

24. At the Virtual Museum of the Iron Lung Website a photo of Drinker standing over the anesthetized cat in the early box was available and quite fascinating (although perhaps traumatic for cat lovers!).

25. Catherine Drinker Bowen, *Family Portraits* (Boston: Little Brown, 1970): 237–43. See also Philip Drinker, "The Use of a New Apparatus for the Prolonged Administration of Artificial Respiration: A Fatal Case of Poliomyelitis," *JAMA* 92 (May 18, 1929): 158–60. This report details the case of the first little girl.

26. Dr. James L. Wilson, "Memoirs of the respirator"; Paul, *History of Poliomyelitis*, 328: "The first patient was a little girl treated in a tank with household vacuum cleaners as pumps. One could hear it running for a quarter of a mile away because it was summer and all the windows were open. All the residents, including myself, took turns sitting up with this little child day and night until she died. . . .

    "He seemed totally paralyzed. . . . use of the respirator demonstrated several things. One, the great difficulty of caring for a big man. The thing was closed with multiple clamps on a hard rubber gasket so there was no access to the mans body to clean him, or do anything to him. To bathe him took an heroic effort with six men and nurses in an organized team."

27. June Opey, *Over my Dead Body* (New York: E. P. Dutton), 41. This book is an excellent description of the author's struggle with polio, two years of which were spent in the iron lung. As noted earlier, numerous patient accounts of their experiences in the lungs are available in the existing literature.

28. Regina Woods, *Tales From the Iron Lung and How I Got Out of It* (Philadelphia: University of Pennsylvania, 1994), 5.

29. Jill Winland-Brown, personal communication, September 20, 1999.

30. Nurse 1, interview by author, June 30, 1999.

31. Woods, *Tales From the Iron Lung*, 34. Woods alludes here to inhumane care. Patient accounts of their experiences often include memories of mistreatment by various health care providers.

32. T. Campbell Thompson, MD, stated, "In no disease, except perhaps pneumonia, is expert nursing care so essential. Rest, complete and prolonged, mental and physical, is by far the most important single factor in aiding the poisoned motor cells in the spinal cord to recover." T. Campbell Thompson, "The Essential Features of Poliomyelitis," *Public Health Nursing* (March 1938). Sister Kenny called iron lungs "torture chambers," objecting to the use of respirators because, she reasoned, they interfered with natural recovery and created dependency, much the same reasons she had used when objecting to immobilization and plaster casts. Nonetheless, ever the pragmatist, even she had to resort to respirators in cases of bulbar poliomyelitis. In these cases the virus damaged cranial nerves in the upper spinal cord, severely affecting breathing and swallowing. For these patients the iron lung was their only hope. No amount of hot packs could restore those functions. See Victor Cohn, *Sister Kenny: The Woman Who Challenged the Doctors* (Minneapolis: University of Minnesota Press, 1975); Ralph Ghormley, "Evaluation of the Kenny Treatment of Infantile Paralysis," *JAMA* 125 (June 17, 1944):466–69; Wallace H. Cole and Miland E. Knapp, "The Kenny Treatment of Infantile Paralysis: A Preliminary Report," *JAMA* 116 (June 7, 1941): 2257–80; H. A. T. Fairbank et al., "Report on the Kenny Method of Treatment," *British Medical Journal* (October 22, 1938): 852–54; Basil O'Connor, "The Story of the Kenny Method," *Archives of Physical Therapy* XXV (April 1944): 233–36; and Roland Berg, *Polio and Its Problems* (Philadelphia: J. B. Lippincott, 1948).

33. Gould, *A Summer Plague.*

34. Wilson, "Memoirs of the Respirator," 329: "Very early on the inaccessibility of the patient bothered me and I remember, with Phil Drinker's advice, buying some portholes made for boats and having them welded on to the machine so that we could open them, fit them with rubber collars through which we could put our hands and so manipulate our patient without taking him out of the tank, not interrupting the respirations."

35. Eva-Marie Pfeiffer and Mary Stevens, "Weaning the Respirator Patient," *The American Journal of Nursing* 56, no. 4 (April 1956): 454–57.

36. The following nursing texts of the time were reviewed: Bertha Harmer, *Textbook of the Principles and Practices of Nursing*, 3rd ed. (New York: Macmillan, 1936); Bertha Harmer and Virginia Henderson, *Textbook of the Principles and Practices of Nursing*, 4th ed. (New York: Macmillan, 1939); Bertha Harmer and Virginia Henderson, *Textbook of the Principles and Practices of Nursing*, 5th ed. (New York: Macmillan, 1955); Margaret A. Tracy, *Nursing: An Art and Science* (St. Louis: C. V. Mosby, 1949); and Alice L. Price, *The Art, Science and Spirit of Nursing* (Philadelphia: W. B. Saunders, 1954).

37. These manuals, as well as the detailed pamphlets available from companies of the time, seemed to provide the most detailed information on nursing care of the patient. The following manuals were provided by one of our nurse informants; some were without dates: "Isolation Techniques and Nursing Care in Poliomyelitis," the National Foundation for Paralysis (New York, 1952); "Nursing Care in Poliomyelitis," Division of Professional Education, National Foundation for Infantile Paralysis, and the National League for Nursing. Other pamphlets available at the time included *Orient the Nurse Recruited for Polio* (National League for Nursing, 1952) and *Suggested*

Outline of Nursing Care of the Poliomyelitis Patient As an Integral Part of the Basic Nursing Curriculum (National League for Nursing, 1952).

38. D. B. Kidd, *The Physical Treatment of Poliomyelitis* (London: Faber and Faber, 1943); International Poliomyelitis Congress, *Papers and Discussions Presented at the First International Poliomyelitis Conference* (Philadelphia: J. B. Lippincott, 1949); and Thompson, "Essential Features of Poliomyelitis," 145.

39. Edward Barbour, "Social Aspects of Poliomyelitis," *New England Journal of Medicine* 207 (1932): 1195–96; Mary Westbrook, "Early Memories of Having Polio: Survivors' Memories Versus the Official Myths" (paper presented at the First Australian International Post-Polio Conference, "Living with the Late Effects of Polio," Sydney, November 1996), 1–16.

40. William Barraclough, "Mental Reaction of Normal Children to Physical Illness," *American Journal of Psychiatry* 93 (1937): 865–77; Edward Barbour, "Adjustment During Four Years of Patients Handicapped by Poliomyelitis," *New England Journal of Medicine* 213 (1935): 563–65.

41. John Bowlby, *Child Care and the Growth of Love* (Harmondsworth: Penguin, 1953). See Marguerite Lucy Manfreda, *The Roots of Interpersonal Nursing* (Cromwell, Conn.: Cromwell, 1982), which discusses early ideas of the therapeutic nurse–patient relationship; Evelyn Bacon, "Curriculum Development in Nursing Education, 1890–1952," *Journal of Nursing History* 2, no. 2 (April 1987): 50–66; Jane E. Murdock, "Evolution of the Nursing Curriculum," *Journal of Nursing History* 2, no. 1 (November 1986): 16–35; Ina Madge Longway, "Curriculum Concepts—An Historical Analysis," *Nursing Outlook* 20, no. 2 (February 1972):116–19; and Beatrice Kalisch and Philip Kalisch, "Slaves, Servants, or Saints? (An Analysis of the System of Nurse Training in the United States, 1873–1948)," *Nursing Forum* XIV, no. 3 (1975): 223–63. This set of articles describes various attitudes and ideas that dominated nursing education during the time that most nurses who nursed during the polio epidemics in this country were educated. Murdock's and Longway's articles describe the integration of a more humanistic approach in the 1950s as well as the person-centered curriculum, with the inclusion of psychosocial concepts hitherto ignored. Morton Seinfeld, "Psychological Considerations in Poliomyelitis Care," *American Journal of Nursing* 47, no. 6 (June 1947): 369–70 presents an unusual and more humane perspective for its time. Seinfeld was a Ph.D. and director of psychological services, for the National Foundation for Infantile Paralysis. He encouraged nurses to see the "whole patient," not just the disability, and counseled listening to patients, especially when "he needs to let his hair down." This approach would prevent the buildup of tensions. He also emphasized the need to prevent a "vegetative" attitude. As late as 1956, however, the *New England Journal of Medicine* was reporting that the role of the physician in the care of the patient with polio is "a somewhat remote gatekeeper." See H. A. Robinson et al., "Psychiatric Considerations in the Adjustment of Patients With Poliomyelitis," *New England Journal of Medicine* 254, no. 21 (May 1956): 975–80.

42. Harmer and Henderson, *Principles and Practices of Nursing*, 4th ed.; Harmer and Henderson, *Principles and Practices of Nursing*, 5th ed., 789; Tracy, *Nursing*, 568; Seavey, *A Paralyzing Fear*, 25–34 from an interview with Marilyn Rogers, who was nine years old when she came down with polio in 1949. She has lived either in an iron lung or on a respirator since.

43. Emma Manfreda, "Polio Nursing, 1952," *American Association for the History of Nursing* 30 (spring 1991): 6–8 (hereafter cited as *AAHN*). This was a personal memoir submitted by Emma Manfreda's sister, Marguerita Manfreda.

44. Ibid.; Nurse 1, interview; Seavey, *A Paralyzing Fear,* 151, from an interview with Juanita Howell.

45. Nurse 1, interview; Price, *The Art, Science and Spirit of Nursing,* 683; Black, *In the Shadow of Polio,* 173.
46. Betty Garnet, "You Just Can't Argue with the Iron Lung," *The Miami Herald,* n.d.
47. Nurse 1, interview.
48. Nurse 2, interview by author, July 19, 1999.
49. Weligoschek, "Personal Experience," 68–69.
50. Seavey, *A Paralyzing Fear,* 27, from an interview with Marilyn Rogers. Numerous accounts such as this have been found throughout the patient literature. Gould, *A Summer Plague,* has a number of patient accounts, as did our patient interview. See also Judith Walzer Leavitt, "'Strange Young Woman on Errands': Obstetric Nursing Between Two Worlds," *Nursing History Review* 6 (1998): 3–24, for her ideas on the often bitter accounts of nurses by obstetrical patients who delivered during the 1930s to the 1950s.
51. Manfreda, "Polio Nursing," 6.
52. Black, *In the Shadow of Polio.*
53. Manfreda, "Polio Nursing," 7.
54. Nurse 2, interview.
55. Seavey, *A Paralyzing Fear,* 115, from an interview with Dr. Aldrich; Trudy Whitman, "Polio Nurse," *TN* (June 1949); Gilden, *A Paralyzing Fear,* 227; Nurse 3, interview by author, July 24, 1999; patient informant, interview by author, August 3, 1999.
56. Seavey, *A Paralyzing Fear,* 26, from an interview with Marilyn Rogers.
57. Nurse 1, interview.
58. Nurse 3, interview.
59. Interview. Nurse 1 went on to get a masters degree and fight for longer visiting hours; her research was on the need to have telephones available for hospitalized kids. See D. W. Smith, "A Study of Power and Spirituality in Polio Survivors using the Model of Martha E. Rogers" (PhD diss., New York University, 1992) for perceptions of power and spirituality in polio survivors.
60. See Smith, *Patenting the Sun;* Paul, *History of Poliomyelitis;* Rutty, "Do Something! ... Do Anything"; Gilden, *A Paralyzing Fear;* Wilson, *Margin of Safety.*
61. John Affeldt M.D. describes his pioneering efforts in weaning patients from the lungs at Rancho Los Amigos outside of Los Angeles as a ". . . warehouse of patients. It was a custodial program. There was no hope. When I came in, the staff was very skeptical of my ability to do anything different than they were doing. The key test was when the rocking bed arrived and I said, "We're going to get a patient out of the respirator here." And the staff gathered around with a look on their faces. "You're going to fail, this patient's gonna die [if you take him out]." Real tension and anxiety. We took the patient out of the respirator, put him on the rocking bed, and he started rocking. The patient was breathing with the bed. And the patient became so animated. "I can scratch my face! I can touch my nose!" The staff just turned on. I mean it was a turning point." Paul, *A Paralyzing Fear,* 140–41.
62. Victoria T. Grando, "A Hard Day's Work: Institutional Nursing in the Post–World War II Era," *Nursing History Review* 8 (2000): 169–84.
63. Woods, *Tales From the Iron Lung,* 1.

CHAPTER 11

Blood Work: Canadian Nursing and Blood Transfusion, 1942–1990

Cynthia Toman

Jean Milligan was a new graduate nurse when the Ottawa Civic Hospital (OCH) became the site of the first regional blood bank for civilians in eastern Canada in 1942. She was on duty the night of the Almonte train disaster on December 27, just six weeks after the blood bank was established. A military train crashed into the back of a passenger train at the small town located 42 kilometers west of Ottawa, killing 36 persons and injuring more than 150. Most of the victims were admitted to the OCH, where the new transfusion service was used for the first time. Newspapers heralded the role of the hospital and the use of blood as a "life-saving fluid" during the event. Events on the night of December 27, 1942, did not constitute a "first time" occurrence or a "great discovery" in the history of blood. Rather, these events illustrated in a very visible and public manner that blood transfusion technology was now readily available for use in general hospitals. The extension of blood use to civilian populations would require increased numbers of health care workers, available continuously, with the knowledge and skills necessary to assume the associated responsibilities. Nurses were well situated for these (and other)

Originally published in *Nursing History Review* 9 (2001): 51–78. A publication of the American Association for the History of Nursing. Copyright Springer Publishing Company. Reprinted with permission.

technological roles. According to Milligan, nurses during the early 1940s were prepared and "ready to take on more."[1]

Recognition of nursing as a science was an important step toward the achievement of professional status, which held educational, economic, and power implications for nurses. Nurses needed to distance themselves from their domestic roots in order to claim this scientific credibility, and in the process they increasingly assumed roles related to medical technology. These technologies grew in number and consumed an ever larger proportion of health care costs and nurses' work over the course of the twentieth century. Yet typically, nurses did not perceive themselves as having or using technology.[2] A variety of ways are needed to understand relationships to both past and present technologies, in order to raise serious questions regarding what is gained and lost as professional nurses take on and let go of technological roles in changing practice environments.

One approach is to examine what nurses did (and still do) at the bedside: what technology nurses' work comprised, how the technology became nurses' work, and how technology both shaped and was shaped by those who used it. Blood transfusion provides an example of one technology that was introduced into medical practice during the mid-twentieth century. Nurses were involved from the beginning, in a variety of ways that changed over time. While previous transfusion histories focused on chronological narratives from medical and institutional perspectives, the understanding of transfusion's social context and its evolution as a technology is limited. Little is known about its adoption, and no studies have examined nurses' involvement.

This chapter examines hospital nurses' roles and responsibilities related to "blood work" in the historically situated context of postwar Canada, using a social history framework, oral history, and a feminist approach. Nurses engaged in blood work on a variety of levels: both incorporating it into nursing practice and incorporating the work physically through the use of their bodies as part of the larger technological system around transfusion and within hospitals as health care factories.[3] I suggest that nurses enabled the extension of transfusion to the civilian population through their constant presence, their understanding of the hospital milieu, and their readiness to take on more for a variety of reasons; they also "embodied" the technology by becoming a physical part of the system; and in the process, blood work became "engendered" as dirty work and women's work, with a resulting loss of the power and status that was initially associated with the expanding technology.

Primary sources for this chapter consisted of hospital, city, and national archival records; photos and artifacts; records of professional organizations; contemporary professional and popular literature; and oral history interviews. The eight oral history participants were students, practitioners, and/or educators who graduated between 1942 (when transfusion became a relatively common medical therapy at the OCH, administered by physicians) and 1972 (when the change from student to professional nurse staffing facilitated transfusion as a basic competency of all nurses). Participants were identified from class lists, in consultation with the alumnae association. Interestingly, none of these nurses thought she would have any memories about blood transfusions. Yet, as they shared from a wealth of experiences, it became clear that nurses were involved with transfusion and participated in its social construction from its introduction into patient care.

Who are these women? Four of the participants are retired nurses. Jean Milligan graduated in 1942 and worked as a staff nurse, as an educator in the OCH School of Nursing, and then as director of nursing education, administrator of nursing, and finally as the assistant executive director of the hospital until her retirement in 1979. Margaret Henricks graduated from the Belleville General Hospital in 1947 and taught for two years prior to coming to the OCH, where she remained in nursing education until retirement in 1990. Isabel Simister came into nursing as a second career (having worked for the Hudson's Bay Company in Winnipeg until age 28). She graduated in 1950 and went into public health after several years. Patricia Crossley spent her entire career associated with the OCH, as a student who graduated in 1958, as a staff nurse, as a nursing instructor, and, finally, as a community college instructor who supervised students at the OCH site.

The remaining four women continue to practice at the OCH, although their careers have evolved in diverse directions. Gwen Hefferman graduated in 1960, worked as a staff nurse and an instructor in the school until it closed in 1973, and then became a staff nurse educator. She is presently director of nursing education. Florence Kinsella has worked continuously as a staff nurse on the same unit since her graduation from the school in 1967. Wendy McKnight Nicklin graduated in 1970 and at the time of the interviews was the chief operating officer of the Ottawa Hospital (formed by the merger of the OCH with two other Ottawa hospitals). She practiced as a staff nurse, a clinical nurse specialist in the Emergency Department, a supervisor, an educator, and an administrator, almost all at the OCH. Kathy Slattery graduated in 1972, one of the last classes of the hospital diploma program. She continues to practice there as the emergency department clinical nurse educator, after having been a staff nurse and manager of the department.

HISTORIOGRAPHY OF TRANSFUSION

The historiography of transfusion indicates that except for accounts of very early experiments with the ingestion of blood and animal-to-human transfusion, the history of blood is remarkably young. Development and acceptance of blood for transfusion required the ability to resolve three main challenges: immunological compatibility, coagulation problems, and practical methods for performing transfusions. Only when these problems were addressed by the recognition of blood grouping and type crossing, by anticoagulation methods, and by convenient and aseptic devices for conducting the transfusion did the technology gain increased acceptance as a therapy.[4]

By 1935 the basic knowledge and techniques existed for the collection and storage of blood, meaning that the donor and recipient could then be separated from one another by time and space.[5] Norman Bethune demonstrated the efficacy of using previously stored blood products during the Spanish Civil War (1936–1939), and World War II provided the opportunity and impetus for increased blood use.[6] The Canadian Red Cross (CRC) operated the National Donor Service between 1940 and 1945, but its responsibility was only to supply military needs. Since blood was required in vast amounts for the war effort, both the public and nurses viewed it as a scarce commodity to be preserved for use in North America for extreme cases only.

In the 1930s a few physicians transfused patients at home and in hospitals by direct syringe methods. Table 11.1 illustrates the frequency of very early attempts with transfusion at the OCH. These are the only

Table 11.1   Number of Transfusions and
Transfusion-Related Deaths, OCH
Annual Reports, 1925–1933

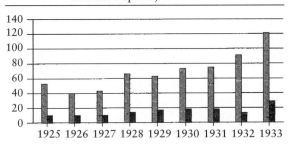

Transfusions

Transfusion-related deaths

data identified at the hospital that referred to transfusion deaths, and the reports did not differentiate between possible causes of death (such as incomparability versus nosocomial infections). Physicians were also quite aware that blood carried a risk of transmissible diseases such as syphilis, malaria, and hepatitis. Dr. H. J. G. Geggie was one physician who practiced in rural Quebec (near Ottawa) during the 1920s and 1930s. He later became head of the first blood bank at the OCH. When he attended to a woman with a postpartum hemorrhage, Geggie typed the eight potential donors assembled in the home and determined that only one had an acceptable blood type. He described that donor as "a bandit-looking brother-in-law, but his blood suited. We had to run the risk of venereal infection; he denied it of course. . . . That all happened in the lean part of the 20s. Last winter, our patient finished her course; third-stage syphilis, or general paresis of the insane. Perhaps we saved her life in the 20s; did we lose it in the 50s?"[7]

Beyond the physical capability to transfuse blood was the important issue of related costs and who would pay them. Some hospitals operated small, private blood banks referred to as "walking blood banks"; There were lists of potential donors who had been typed and could be called upon as needed. Like other hospitals, the OCR preferred that patients' families and friends replace any blood received on a "two for one" basis, thereby building up the total supply available. If they were unable to meet this expectation, the hospital billed for the cost of the transfusion. For comparison, patients were charged $15 in 1940 and $35 in 1950 for a unit of blood. The hospital experimented for a brief period with paid donors. This created competition between the hospital blood bank and the CRC for professional donors and led to complaints against the hospital regarding this practice. There was also a volunteer veterans' group in Ottawa, the Red Star Service, which attempted to supply blood for patients who could not pay for it. As well, various work groups and social clubs organized their members to donate blood voluntarily to the hospital's private blood bank as a type of credit, against which they or a family member could draw if blood was subsequently needed.[8]

Through strategies such as these, large hospitals in urban centers could potentially meet their requirements for blood, but smaller hospitals in outlying areas lacked the resources and population base to be self-sufficient. The Canadian government, on the basis of a national survey of transfusion needs, established a four-way partnership that began operation in 1947. Under the auspices of the National Blood Transfusion Service, provincial departments of health would supply the premises for laboratories; participating hospitals would contribute by administering the transfusions free of charge; the CRC would furnish the equipment, the medical and technical personnel, and the transportation, and would operate the service; and the public would contribute the blood on a volunteer basis forming an important difference between the American and Canadian blood services. Health insurance plans (such as the Hospital Insurance and Diagnostic Services Act of 1958, the Medicare Act of 1968, and the Canada Health Act of 1984) became increasingly comprehensive and universal, which influenced the social construction of blood utilization and delivery services.[9] Individual patients no longer had to bear the burden of costs of blood, hospitals no longer had to deal with financing them, and professionals began to use blood in greater quantities for diverse purposes.

Viewed initially as life giving and miraculous, transfusion was available throughout most of Canada by the end of the 1940s. The CRC developed new recruitment messages that advocated peacetime uses of blood to increase donations for civilian blood needs. Typical of these strategies were documentary films such as *Miracle Fluid* (1954), *Great Also in Peace: The Role of the Red Cross in Peace* (1950), and *Emergency Blood Transfusion* (1970). Meanwhile, the frequency of transfusion increased steadily over the next decades as new applications were found, such as treating Rh incompatibilities during the postwar baby boom. The film *Miracle Fluid* used pictures of babies receiving exchange transfusions for the treatment of erythroblastosis fetalis as a strategy to encourage donation. Saving babies was (and still is) motivational.[10] Other applications during the 1950s included the use of blood products for polio and hemophilia patient populations. Each innovation and new application brought challenges for nurses related to the type of products used, infection control, supportive care requirements, and decision making. Crossley suggested that as nurses "we got smarter with what we could do with our blood."[11]

By the 1960s and 1970s, nurses commented that blood was ordered routinely and seemed to flow freely. They recalled it being used for "building up" or "topping up" patients. One journal article described this view of blood as "cosmetic transfusions," referring to those "given only to bring a little color to the cheeks." While blood was generally known to carry some risk of infection, it continued to be predominantly perceived as miraculous and lifesaving until the 1980s and 1990s when the association between blood and fatal iatrogenic illnesses such as hepatitis C and acquired immunodeficiency syndrome (AIDS) led to a changed perception of blood as "tainted," "filthy," and "the gift of death." Crossley illustrated that nurses' changed their perceptions as well: "When the scare of HIV came . . . you looked at blood in an entirely different light."[12] Infection-control concepts focused on all persons as potentially infected, with the implementation of universal precautions and alternative technologies to avoid transfusion. AIDS and hepatitis C irrevocably changed the way blood was understood and used.

THE INCORPORATION OF BLOOD WORK

One interesting and potentially useful way to examine issues related to medical technology, transfusion, and nurses is to consider how blood work was both incorporated and "in-corporated" into nursing practice. Nurses engaged in blood work as they expanded previous roles and accepted new roles related to transfusion through a variety of motivations. In the 1940s they accepted these additional responsibilities with few, if any, questions. Henricks said: "[Nurses] had to do it and I guess it was part of the time—when they were told to do it, they did it. So it was part of their looking after the patient." In the 1950s, a perceived obligation to take on roles existed because "there wasn't anybody else to do it." During the alternating shortages and oversupplies of nurses after the mid-1970s, however, nurses commonly expressed the view that if they did not take on emerging technological roles, some other care provider would be introduced to the system and would contribute to job loss.[13] In addition to subsuming blood work into nursing activities, nurses also "in-corporated" the work through the use of their bodies as part of the larger technological system surrounding transfusion.

I suggest that nurses were a necessary link which enabled the extension of transfusion to the civilian population through their constant presence, their understanding of the hospital milieu, and their readiness to take on more for a variety of reasons. They also "em-bodied" the technology by becoming a physical part of the system. In the process of enabling and embodying, blood work became "en-gendered" as dirty work and women's work.

Enabling the Extension of Blood to Civilians

As military needs for blood declined toward the end of World War II, transfusion became a technology in need of an application. A convergence of complex influences resulted in a scientific capability to transfuse blood, an accumulated war experience in blood techniques, changing postwar economics that affected health care, an infrastructure to collect and distribute blood, and a ready source of labour to administer it. Nursing students comprised a flexible, constantly present, inexpensive source of labor. They learned the principles of asepsis and antisepsis through repetition of assigned procedures, which often involved a long series of elaborate steps in particular sequences. They were also socialized as women and as students to a work culture of obedience, precision, routine, and accountability, all essential conditions for the successful management of transfusion.

Table 11.2   Number of Transfusions Based on Blood Bank Statistics, OCH
            Annual Reports, 1944–1972

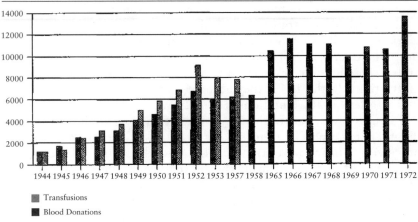

■ Transfusions
■ Blood Donations

Table 11.2 illustrates the increased frequency of transfusions at the
OCH between 1944 and 1972 on the basis of data available from hospital records. Until 1958 (when the CRC took over the blood supply) the
hospital continued to operate its own private blood donor clinic, which
explains why the number of donations was also reported. Where the
number of donations exceeded the number of transfusions, the imbalance can feasibly be explained as loss through wastage and outdated
units that became unusable. Records included transfusion statistics only
sporadically after 1958 and not at all after 1972. Interestingly, during
this period nurses took over responsibility for transfusions. At least three
explanations for this lack of record keeping may be posited: First, the
technology had become routine and no longer a valued indicator of hospital efficiency and efficacy; second, as nurses took on the roles, blood
assumed a lower profile appropriate to the hierarchical status of those
who now implemented it; and third, the need to report the statistics no
longer existed after the CRC assumed responsibility for the blood
supply, which seemed to be limitless. Likely, all three explanations were
operative.[15]

   Just as the frequency and application of transfusion changed over
time, so did nurses' work in relation to it. Initially, physicians (who
were most often interns) administered blood assisted by the nursing
workforce (who were most often students). Nursing roles in early transfusion procedures involved preparing the equipment and the patient,
assisting during the procedures, and cleaning up after the procedure.

This categorization of these roles is simplistic, however, because a great deal of complexity was involved in the management of two patients (a donor and a recipient).

Transfusion was a surgical procedure initially performed in the operating room, where blood was directly transferred from the donor to the recipient through venesection and suturing either their own arteries to one another or suturing cannulae in place between them. Patients lay next to each other, usually head to foot. The procedure for the semidirect or syringe method of transfusion required three physicians, working as rapidly as possible, to transfer syringes of blood between patients. The rate of coagulation of the blood within the syringe limited the volume that could be managed, and speed was a definite asset. By the late 1930s, blood was collected in open funnels and flasks, which presented challenges for sterility, transport, and storage.[16] Each of these stages of development required skilled labor to prepare for the procedure, assist during it, clean up after it, and provide patient care throughout it.

Blood work was labor intensive and time-consuming for nurses. The procedure involved two sets of equipment, two physicians to assist, and two patients to manage at the same time. It called for blood to be collected into glass beakers which were set in basins of warm water as a type of holding tank until the recipient was ready to receive the transfusion. The beakers were stirred continuously with a glass rod to prevent the blood from clotting; little wonder the first procedures called for one ounce of brandy though it did not indicate who was to consume it![17]

Another labor intensive aspect of early transfusion was the imperative for cleaning the equipment (needles, glass containers, and rubber tubing). Nurses completed this cleaning on the wards before returning the articles to the blood bank for sterilization and subsequent reuse. Antisepsis and asepsis formed the primary line of defense against bloodborne bacterial and viral infections, and septicemia brought grave consequences during this period prior to antibiotics. Students vividly recalled the difficulty of cleaning small areas, especially needles, tubing, and tall cylinders, as well as the rigor of inspection by the supervisors. Milligan will never forget the effort it took before the job was finished:

> The big job (that we all just loved) . . . was cleaning these sets afterwards to send them up to get them ready for the next one . . . cleaning the tubing and these long flasks. You couldn't even get your hand into them, they were so narrow. There couldn't be a mark on them anywhere. They [the night supervisors] used to hold these [flasks] up to the light, and look at them before they'd roll them up to go to the O.R. to be autoclaved for the next person. And you just had to wash and shine these, and make sure there was nothing left around.[18]

If the availability of nurses facilitated the initial expansion of transfusion to civilians prior to World War II, then the rapid introduction of
new technologies, the shortage of 2,000 physicians in Ontario, and the
increased use of blood after the war would require a differentiation
between novice and experienced nurses to facilitate further application of
the technology. Hospitals requested permission from the College of
Physicians and Surgeons of Ontario (CPSO) to delegate the administration of intravenous fluids (including blood) by specially trained nurses
only, as "doctors did not believe these responsibilities should be included
in the regular duties of a nurse."[19] Transfusion was the first officially recognized act delegated to Ontario nurses in 1947. It was followed by
blood pressures and intramuscular injections in 1954. By 1972, 22 acts
had been delegated, plus another 11 for nurses in specialty areas.

Delegation was not a one-way process. When the CPSO approved
tuberculosis tests and immunization injections for administration by
nurses in 1957, the Registered Nurses Association of Ontario (RNAO)
officially protested that they had not been consulted. Their argument centered on lack of training, lack of legal protection for the act, and that they
were being asked to take on procedures considered outside the field of
nursing. They also argued that with the continuing nursing shortage these
added acts were an unacceptable burden. The CPSO assured the RNAO
that they would be consulted in future decisions. A year later, the RNAO
opposed the delegation of the administration of intravenous medications
as a nursing role and issued warning notices that emphasized that the
procedure was a medical act. The two professional organizations compromised, however, with the decision that nurses would accept this role
only in hospitals without interns, in public health units, and in industrial
medicine settings.[20]

When the College of Nurses of Ontario (CNO) became the regula-
tory body for professional nurses in 1961, it emphasized that delegation
from medicine to nursing should be a consultative process—in other
words, acts could be delegated but would also require the recipients'
willingness to accept a particular responsibility. They applied the term
"sanctioned medical acts" to indicate an act that had been both delegated and accepted (or sanctioned).[21] Through this mechanism, nurses
exercised a degree of agency at the policy level and participated in shaping their work.

At the OCH, the Medical Board delegated transfusion to the "Blood
Team" in 1947. Two nurses (Louise Gourlay and Gladys Moorhead)
comprised the team, and according to Hefferman they "ruled the roost"
for the rest of their long careers in this position. Initially, delegation of
transfusion contributed a measure of power and enhanced status to these
nurses within nursing's work culture. The Blood Team commanded

respect and was able to create a separate occupational space for itself. It had more independence in scheduling and in the hours worked, better conditions of employment, more independent decision making in patient care, and more collegial nurse–physician relationships.[22]

Delegation also facilitated the development of a practice expertise not commonly found during the first half of the twentieth century, as graduate nurses were not employed in hospitals except in very limited numbers as supervisors and educators. In place of novice care providers (both interns and nursing students) the Blood Team remained at the bedside building experience, expertise, and knowledge. One unanticipated result was that interns and residents lost valued skills related to venipuncture. To compensate, interns subsequently rotated through a month's experience with the Blood Team; an example of where physicians learned from nurses.[23]

While blood work partially shaped nurses' practice, the availability of experienced nurses also shaped blood work. As noted by Anselm Strauss, increased frequency and routinization of particular tasks contributed to negotiation in the division of labor, mediated by shifting relationships among workers, concurrent work assignments, and the visibility or invisibility of the work itself. Not only did the physician and intern shortage shift work relationships after the war, but so did patient care conditions, which were changing rapidly in the hospital setting. The public also had expectations for a certain level of care. Following an 86% staff turnover in 1948, patient complaints about medical and nursing care at the hospital reached the media and the law courts by way of a judicial inquiry in 1949.[24] During the inquiry, conditions at the hospital revealed a rapid expansion of facilities and services following the war, a shortage of both interns and nurses, and an inexperienced student workforce unable to keep up with expanded requirements for increasingly technological care. The hospital responded to the inquiry's recommendations with more graduate nurses and increased use of delegation.

The widespread use of blood during the 1950s and 1960s provided ample opportunity for all nurses to become familiar and comfortable with the equipment and procedures. Also, as the Blood Team took on more and newer technologies, certain aspects of transfusion (such as patient assessment and monitoring) shifted to bedside nurses, who responded to the added responsibility in a variety of ways.

Although transfusion was no longer a surgical procedure, it commanded a great deal of vigilance and respect because of its unpredictability and the limited range of interventions nurses were permitted to use. Both as a student and later as an educator, Crossley remarked how blood "had to be watched because it was very unpredictable." Students were required to check patients frequently, to make sure the flow did not stop and the rate was accurate, to keep the needle positioned in the vein, and above all, to call the team at the first sign of problems. If a unit of blood did not transfuse within the designated time period (usually four hours for an adult), nurses had to fill out incident reports explaining circumstances and actions taken because it was considered a medication error: "It was a med error . . . an error you know, if you didn't get it [in] . . . you did everything that you could. If you didn't get it in on time you needed to fill out an incident report."[25]

Crossley reiterated the importance of surveillance: "You didn't go for a break and not tell somebody to watch your blood! And woe betide those persons if the blood was a way ahead or a way behind or even stopped . . . because you know it had to be done the way it should be done." In spite of procedural strictness, Henricks recalled the difficulty of shifting responsibility from the team to the nurse at the bedside: "As soon as the Blood Team left, [the patient] became [the nurse's] responsibility. That was one of the hardest things to get nurses to realize . . . [Nurses] thought, 'oh, this is something I don't have to look after.' But they really did have to look after it and you had to keep telling them." As Kinsella summarized her experience from the 1960s: "Making sure the patient got it—that was our responsibility."[26]

During the 1960s and 1970s, transfusion technology became even more "rooted in the practice of nursing" as a basic competency for practice. Several conditions facilitated this transition: Graduate staff nurses increasingly replaced the student labor force until 1973 when the hospital closed its School of Nursing; these graduate nurses developed a greater level of experience and technological confidence; and blood work rapidly proliferated beyond the workload constraints of a small core of designated nurses. As Slattery stated regarding this generation of nurses, "We had grown up respecting blood and what it could do and knowing that we have to be so careful with our surveillance."[27]

With the onset of new issues related to AIDS and hepatitis C in the 1980s, however, both health professionals and the public developed heightened awareness and suspicion toward blood as an infectious agent. New precautions and procedures were implemented to reduce the risks of exposure; where risks could not be reduced, liability was transferred to the patient by way of informed consent processes. By 1990 the concerns related to blood were so great that both medicine and nursing turned their attention to alternatives such as bloodless surgical techniques, autologous donations, and alternatives to blood products.[28] Throughout these decades, nurses not only learned to use new equipment and new forms of old equipment (as disposables replaced reusable items), but they also enabled the extension of a variety of blood products and techniques into patient care areas such as hemophilia, oncology, dialysis, and cardiology.

Increasingly, independent and interdependent roles involved problem solving, critical thinking, patient and family education, supportive care, patient advocacy, and decision making related to blood.

Technology continued to complicate caregiving through new issues related to infection control, patient information requirements, and informed consent. Henricks commented that prior to AIDS, "I can't recall having permission . . . they just said this patient needs blood. It was a life-saving device and it was something that the patient just had to have." By the mid-1990s, however, there was a requirement that patients had to be fully informed by their physicians of the risks in receiving a transfusion, that they had to give consent, and that they had to receive written notification of transfusions received during the hospital stay. Nurses were expected to ensure that the notification went home with the patient or family and to document the process on a variety of forms either retained in the chart or returned to the blood bank. Nurses were also the frontline caregivers to whom patients addressed their concerns and of whom patients asked advice "what would you do?"[29]

The use of alternatives to blood transfusions presented a second set of complications to nursing care. Limited alternatives were available prior to AIDS, but the research and innovations dramatically increased through the 1970s and 1980s. Nurses were involved in the administration of and patient teaching related to drug therapies that would increase clotting factors and/or the production of red blood cells (such as aprotinin, erythropoietin, and desmopressin) in the 1990s. In critical care areas such as the cardiac surgical unit they learned to work with cell salvage equipment. Autologous donation was available in the 1960s but not encouraged by the physicians or the collection agencies, who claimed it was more expensive to segregate a donor's blood and ensure that it was given back to her or him when needed. Autologous transfusions required additional logistics and surveillance by nurses as well: "That's another area of vigilance . . . that this person has donated blood and it's available in the blood bank and that is the only blood that person gets! And there again, you have more pieces of paper and forms in this institution . . . that have to be placed on the chart."[30]

Nurses enabled the extension of transfusion to the civilian populations through their constant presence and socialization to the hospital environment. They assumed a variety of roles and responsibilities as the frequency of transfusion increased. The delegation of transfusion to two nurses began a process by which blood work eventually became a basic nursing competency. This process also provided the template by which other technologies (such as the administration of intramuscular injections, blood pressure measurement, and intravenous infusions) were delegated to nurses on a limited basis initially and then transferred into nursing's scope of practice.[31] Throughout the transition, not only did technology complicate and shape patient care, but nurses and patients participated in shaping the technology.

Embodying Blood Work

The second way in which nurses incorporated transfusion in practice was by literally and figuratively embodying blood work as they became part of the equipment and delivery process, as they participated in blood donation campaigns, and as they used their knowledge of the larger contexts surrounding transfusion on behalf of the patients. Nurses not only used a range of tools and equipment, but they also became part of the technology when they used their bodies to provide suction, to be the pump, or to become the product itself, becoming, in reality, part artifact. In early transfusions, nurses acted as part of the equipment when they applied suction by mouth to the blood collection bottles. Blood was collected into glass flasks and bottles that were typically open at the top or loosely capped, lacking a vacuum seal. Photos from the 1940s featured equipment in which a second glass tube was inserted through the cap of the collection bottle as an air vent for the system that nurses then used to apply negative suction for the collection bottle, facilitating the blood flow, thus becoming the suction device. At other times the nurse became a human (manual) pump for infusing blood at a more rapid rate than was provided by gravity flow. Nurses even supplied the product when prevailed upon as a convenient emergency blood donor for the patient.[32]

Early transfusions were collected and distributed in large flasks. One of the nurse's jobs was to make sure that the bedside containers of blood were maintained with the proper volume as per physicians' orders. Milligan described the challenge of monitoring and filling these tall flasks when she was in charge of a large ward and it seemed that patients receiving blood were at opposite ends of the twenty-bed ward. After World War II the rapid expansion of hospital insurance programs made it difficult for nurses to maintain this constant observation of blood. As semiprivate and private rooms became affordable to more people, hospital architecture changed. Crossley recalled: "You had a large room with maybe twenty patients in it, . . . you could go into a room and at a glance you could see [the blood]. But as [there were more] semi privates and privates, you really had lots of walking to do to make sure that blood was alright."[33]

Tricks of the trade were practical solutions to problems that nurses encountered in assisting, maintaining, and monitoring transfusions, the result of accumulated, embodied wisdom. Tricks could only come with experience in dealing with the technology. Some of the blood tricks included "squeezing the rubber port (which we weren't supposed to do, it might dislodge a clot)" and "calling the technician to come and needle it." Crossley described strategies such as "how to gently rotate the blood . . . don't shape it, you will break the cells . . . the higher it is, the better it runs . . . tricks of the trade. . . . We learned to use saline [with] whole blood. You cleared your tubing with saline before and after; but it was never mixed with the blood."[34] She was especially proud of her taller-than-average height and used her body to advantage when transfusions needed to infuse rapidly during emergencies.

Although blood was refrigerated to prevent the growth of bacterial contaminants and to prolong its storage capability, the procedures of the 1940s required the nurse to warm it prior to transfusion. Milligan recalled: "We used to set them in a basin of warm water. . . . You knew it couldn't get it too hot. . . . So you just put them into warm water and let them sit there for a little while. You were trying to get them to room temperature." As late as the 1970s, Slattery confirmed: "Warming was always an issue then and so what we did was—we just took a basin, a wash basin and put warm water in it and just put the tubing in there, and so that was initially how we did it." In these examples, nurses became blood-warming machines as well as human thermometers, for actual thermometers were not used as part of the procedure. Finding ways to warm blood and prevent hypothermia was a recurring issue for nurses. When mechanical blood-warming devices became available in the 1970s, however, nurses resisted their introduction in the emergency department. As the primary users, they avoided a technology that appeared to come between them and their patients while requiring more complexity and removing familiar ways of controlling the process. In this example, nurses partially shaped the technology by avoiding it. As Slattery stated:

> We had a machine that was purchased for here (a Fenmore blood warmer) which everybody hated. . . . Even though we received in-service on it and knew how to use it, it was something that we didn't use frequently. None of us liked change and none of us liked being uncomfortable, particularly because it was a critical patient and we needed to get this on there. . . . And so we had this machine that we had purchased and spent money on, and it was not used for anything. So consequently, it gathered dust in a corner. Which is a real shame.[35]

On a second level, nurses also embodied the technology by becoming part of the larger technological system around transfusion, by participation in public relation campaigns for the CRC, and by their personal endorsement of blood donations. As noted earlier, the expansion of transfusion throughout the civilian medical population required a structured network. This network included scientific and medical innovations, but also an infrastructure for collection and distribution, an economic system to fund it, a regulation system, and a labor system. While the CRC provided the collection and distribution services, they needed an ever-increasing supply of donors. Nurses were already involved with blood work in patient populations; now, they would also be involved with its promotion and public relations.

An excellent illustration can be found in a 1954 *Canadian Nurse* article wherein CRC director Dr. W. Stuart Stanbury appealed to nurses to do their "duty as citizens" and use their influence over public opinion to increase the number of blood donations to meet the requirements for the production of gamma globulin. The project would "necessitate the collection each year of vast quantities of blood from the Canadian public, a task which will not only strain the resources of our [CRC] Society but will require the assistance of every public-spirited citizen . . . I can think of no more influential group in Canada than its professional nurses, not only in allaying the fears of timorous prospective blood donors but in disseminating authoritative information. . . ." In these cases, nurses were called upon to use their professional reputations and public image to promote blood work. CRC posters for blood donor campaigns during the 1940s and 1950s portrayed nurses predominantly as patriots, sisters, angels, and mothers.[36]

On a third level, nurses embodied blood work through the construction of knowledge around the technology. Over a relatively brief time span, nurses gained experience and constructed knowledge related to transfusion technology as they moved from managing equipment and following procedures to clinical judgments about patient status and needs for certain interventions. As patient advocates in the 1980s and 1990s, nurses increasingly questioned the amount of blood needed and the rate at which it should be given on the basis of the impact of adding volume over time: "We had a time limit of when the blood had to be hung. A doctor would write how long a period to give the blood over, and if we had any questions—for instance, this was a very small person . . . this was a person with a bad heart—then we would contact him and ask: 'How long do you want this to run?' because we were concerned about the overloading of this person."[37]

Nurses also used their knowledge to teach patients and to respond to their questions regarding blood. Crossley pointed out that in the 1980s and 1990s, "they pulled back from blood and the patient was started on iron. You taught as part of your discharge planning. You either had the nutritionist come or you got out the book yourself and you did a lot of teaching. . . . We have given way more [emphasis] to nutrition to build up people, than we did years ago." Teaching also included treatment rationale and medications related to blood: "We ha[d] some explaining to do, as to the fact that they had surgery and there was blood loss and this [was] a replacement . . . I think they let the hemoglobin go lower and sent [the patient] home with a bag of ferrous sulphate . . . in fact, it was started right after surgery."[38]

Thus nurses embodied blood work in a variety of ways. They literally used their bodies as part of the equipment, as suppliers of the product, as flow monitoring devices, as troubleshooters who knew tricks of the trade, and even as early warming devices. They lent their reputations as trustworthy angels and patriots to promotional material for blood donor campaigns in support of the larger technological system surrounding transfusion. They also embodied knowledge around blood work, which they used to teach patients and families and to advocate for patients' best interests related to blood.

"Engendering" Blood Work

The delegation of transfusion to nurses also en*gendered* blood work as women's work: easy enough for nurses to do, physically distasteful, routinized and therefore no longer challenging for interns or physicians, time-consuming, and associated with few rewards. Many of the components associated with transfusion can be labeled "dirty work," a socially constructed phenomenon that may be literally or symbolically dirty, as described by E. C. Hughes and further elaborated by Strauss.[39] The division of labor in blood work resulted in nurses gradually assuming all aspects except patient diagnosis and prescription (or ordering) of blood products, which was reserved for physicians. As in the case of Gourlay and Moorhead, blood work initially borrowed enhanced status, power, and autonomy (traditionally associated with maleness and physicians) based on a skill that differentiated them from the majority of nurses. When greater numbers of nurses engaged in the skill, however, it lost that associated power and status. It even disappeared visibly from statistical records (see Table 11.3); it no longer counted as a specialized role (nor was it apparently counted) after 1984.

On one hand, delegation was contingent on the availability of nurses to extend the technology on a large scale into civilian hospitals and for a wide variety of applications. On the other hand, the nature of this student workforce constrained the complete transferral of blood work into the nurses' domain. As well, the gendered construction of the workforce meant that nurses would remain at novice levels of knowledge and experience because of relatively brief careers—as women were expected to leave paid employment upon marriage (euphemistically referred to as "retirement"). Finally, as hospitals employed very few graduate nurses, most of them worked primarily in private duty until they "retired."

Table 11.3   Number of Transfusions, Nurse Technician Team Statistics, 1962–1984

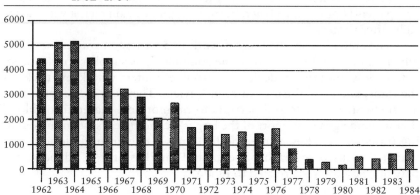

For these reasons, nurses' roles in blood work were initially restricted to traditional, domestic type of work (such as preparing and cleaning equipment), which in turn shaped decisions regarding what type of knowledge was appropriate for nurses.

As women and as students, and despite composing the majority of hospital staff (75–80% of the staff in 1924 and 69% of the staff in 1944), nurses experienced a double subordination to male physicians, and to nursing supervisors and educators.[40] The School of Nursing never did admit male students. Both gender and student status influenced decisions about their education. During the 1930s and 1940s, nursing lectures were taught typically by male physicians who focused on the cellular (or physiological) level of information. Traditional ideologies prevailed concerning what constituted gender-appropriate education for nurses. In 1930 for example, E. Stanley Ryerson (a physician and faculty member at the University of Toronto) wrote in the *Canadian Nurse* that "by gaining too great a scientific knowledge of diseases, the nurse has a tendency to become too professional in her attitude to the detriment of her services in a nursing capacity." Accordingly, "most lectures . . . should be inspirational, rather than to impart knowledge."[41] As previously described, Milligan recalled lectures on how to set up blood trays, assist the doctor, and clean equipment while physicians were expected to administer the transfusion and stay with the patients.

By the mid-1960s, according to Hefferman, nursing science instructors decided "they could do it themselves and more satisfactorily." She noted that most instructors had completed either a degree or certificate in nursing education; they considered themselves not only qualified in the content but better prepared in educational theory and strategies than physicians. The difficulty seemed to be that "doctors either talked over the students or they talked as if they didn't have a brain in their heads. So it was gradually just that we stopped inviting them to present."[42] Part of the instructors' growing confidence came from their educational preparation and longer-term clinical experience, but early influences of the women's movement were also felt by this generation of nurses. There was a rising awareness of the constraints of conventional, gender-based roles in medicine and nursing through the 1960s. While the resistance expressed by these nursing instructors was subtle and gradual, instructors could shape nursing knowledge development by gaining control over lectures.

Clinical instructors (who were also called "follow up" instructors at the OCH) supervised students in the patient care area to reinforce what was learned in classes and demonstration labs. While the classroom (or nursing science) focus was primarily on the cellular level and closely associated with anatomy and physiology content, clinical instructors focused on the procedural level (or nursing arts). Here routinization of procedures not only provided boundaries of safety for patients but also contributed to the process of shaping the technology through consistent performance. Mastery of techniques was essential, and students were very focused on the equipment and the procedures, at least in respect to blood work. Henricks commented, "The big thing was the necessity to observe, observe and observe . . . and there were so many things that you didn't know in the beginning. . . . You were so absorbed in that needle."[43]

As long as hospitals relied primarily on students for patient care, the delegation of specific technologies was restricted to a small number of nurses who met training and testing criteria and who seemed likely to remain in long-term careers. The hospital board argued that training was expensive, that the learner needed to use the technique frequently enough to maintain proficiency, and that staffing had to be stable enough to make it cost-effective.[44] Beyond economic arguments, as the judicial inquiry made clear in 1949, and as both physicians and nurses realized, a critical need existed for experienced nurses to replace the student workforce as the primary caregivers in order to respond to the increased use of technology and to the need for an expanded body of knowledge, and no longer just to deal with an intern shortage.

Experienced nurses, however, were not easily found nor easily convinced to continue their careers in the postwar context. Social expectations for married women combined with wartime opportunities for nurses and unsatisfactory working conditions contributed to a chronic shortage of nurses that lasted from the late 1930s into the 1970s. During World War II, Canadian women had mobilized to staff military units and replace hospital nurses who enlisted. In contrast to other women who experienced job losses when the war ended and men who returned to resume previous careers, nurses experienced pressure to remain in the workforce, even though they were married and had children. The OCH experimented with flexible hours and split shifts to meet the needs of married nurses who otherwise refused to work.[45] Milligan suggested that part of the problem underlying the patient-care conditions in 1949 was related to the hospital's inability to attract and retain married, graduate nurses. In these situations, women were able to use their absence (or refusal to work) partially to negotiate better conditions of employment. Even with improvements, the chronic shortage of nurses (partially constructed by the need for a critical mass of nurses who could accept increasingly technological roles) continued into the 1970s.

When the School of Nursing closed in 1973, the hospital was forced to hire over 400 graduate nurses to replace the student workforce. These newly hired nurses were recruited from "retirement"/marriage, from private duty, and through immigration. They found themselves in a rapidly changing environment with an increasing number of delegated skills that became standard competencies within a few years, while administrators found themselves struggling to implement education programs without the structure of a school of nursing or instructors. As assistant executive director of the hospital, Milligan recalled that "there was this explosion of knowledge. . . . The hospital was left to find out how to look after [the patients] . . . you had to set up in-service programs to teach them and it was difficult . . . for the nurses wanted to do it, but they were worried sometimes because they didn't know how to do these things."[46] Two strategies used by the OCH were refresher courses and the development of specialty units in which technology and nurses would thrive.

In contrast to the previous chronic nursing shortage, the late 1970s to 1990s experienced periodic cycles of oversupply and shortage. Through the cycles, nurses used their continual bedside presence to take on additional technological roles as a form of job security. Nurses were frequently the ones with more familiarity and practical knowledge pertaining to the equipment, procedures, and associated impact on the system. Nurses also used their expertise to gain entry to specific practice areas, such as specialty units in which technological competence was key: "You always knew that would get you in the critical care areas because critical care areas are about machines and equipment." One nurse who worked on the intravenous/transfusion team recalled that although she was required to resign from her position with each of her pregnancies, she was always rehired when she was ready to return to work because there were never enough experienced nurses. She lost tenure through the resigning/rehiring cycles, but her experience and knowledge provided a measure of power and control over her work life. As one author argued in 1974, nurses experienced little competition as care providers and "had the power that accrues to persons or groups who are essential to the maintenance and functioning of a system."[47]

If delegated skills and technological competence offered a measure of security and advancement opportunities for some, still others likely felt undervalued, limited in their roles, and forced away from bedside practice by the constraints placed on their practice. As Nicklin described her clinical nurse specialist role in the emergency department during the early 1970s, she shared her personal ambivalence over her choice to leave the position for a career in administration: "I was being stifled . . . I have always looked back and thought, 'You never know what your career might have done, eh?' And I thought what it could have been."[48]

Historians are always challenged to locate those missing voices— nurses whose experiences could contribute alternate perspectives on blood work and medical technology in general. Nurses who left the profession also shaped nursing practice by their absence as much as the nurses who remained did by their presence. Did the engendering of blood work (and other technological roles) contribute to their dissatisfaction as nurses? Did they perceive delegated medical technologies as unsatisfying, routinized, dirty work that did not conform to their professional goals? Does nursing gain more than it loses when it incorporates an increasing number of medical technologies into its domain? Our understanding remains incomplete.

SUMMARY

The extension of blood transfusion to civilian populations was contingent on the availability of a nursing workforce capable of taking on increasingly responsible roles. Nurses assumed a variety of roles as they incorporated blood work into patient care and, in the process, enabled, embodied, and engendered it as nurses' and women's work. Initially, the student workforce facilitated transfusion through roles that were congruent with nursing's domestic roots. Later, it constrained the expansion of blood work because of its perpetually novice nature. Delegation constituted one strategy by which a limited number of persons could become experienced and autonomous in a particular role. As long as the skill remained limited, nurses shared its associated power and status, which differentiated them within the work culture. A few women were able to shape blood work to their advantage, using their expertise either as job security or as a bargaining point to negotiate better working conditions. However, when the skill was routinized and dispersed among many nurses, it became dirty work. The examination of one specific technology that shifted from medicine into nursing contributes insights to current issues of expanded roles and delegated skills. Nurses need to question seriously what is gained and lost as they take on and let go of technologies. They need to consider what kinds of knowledge will be needed and how best to develop it. Finally, they need to reflect how changes might complicate caregiving and nurses' work.

ACKNOWLEDGMENTS

This chapter is based on my unpublished Masters thesis, "Crossing the technological line: Blood transfusion and the art and science of nursing, 1942–1990," University of Ottawa, Nursing, 1998. I would like to acknowledge my supervisor Dr. Meryn Stuart and the support of the Canadian Association for the History of Nursing and the Ottawa Hospital Interdisciplinary Research Committee.

NOTES

1. Hospital Annual Report (hereafter cited as HAR), 1942, Ottawa Civic Hospital Archives, Ottawa, Ontario (hereafter cited as OCHA). The disaster accounts are recorded in a variety of sources. Institutional perspectives are documented in the annual reports for 1942 and 1943 as well as in the national nursing journal: E. Gertrude Ferguson, "The Almonte Disaster," *Canadian Nurse* 39, no. 2 (February 1943): 117–8, (hereafter cited as *CN*). Headlines from *Ottawa Citizen*, December 28, 1942, read: "Arnprior Man is Tossed Through Window of Train," "Death Toll in Almonte Wreck Now, 33," "Injured Passengers Relate Vivid Stories of Tragic Wreck," "Troop Train Crashed into Standing Local"; "Fear Almonte Wreck Death Toll May Go Higher" (*Ottawa Citizen*, December 29, 1942);: "36 Dead in Almonte Train Wreck, 118 in Hospitals, 15 are Critical" and "Almonte Folk Heroically Toil Through Night" (*Ottawa Journal*, December 28, 1942); "Paratrooper and His Fiancee Badly Hurt in Train Crash" and "Valley Town Becomes Morgue" (*Ottawa Journal*, December 29, 1942); "Scene of Train Crash One of Horror and Confusion," and "Child's Body Dressed in Snow Suit Found in Debris at Almonte" (*Toronto Star*, December 28, 1942). Additional coverage of personal anecdotes was extensive for the two Ottawa news journals over the initial two days after the disaster. Jean Milligan, interview by author, audiotape, Ottawa, Ontario, October 29, 1997.
2. For an analysis of the domestic roots of nursing, see Patricia D'Antonio, "Legacy of Domesticity," *Nursing History Review* 1 (1993): 229–46 (hereafter cited as *NHR*), Diane Hamilton, "Constructing the Mind of Nursing," *NHR* 2 (1994): 3–28; Margarete Sandelowski, "'Making the Best of Things': Technology in American Nursing, 1870–1940," *NHR* 5 (1997): 3–22; and "Irreconcilable Differences? The Debate Concerning Nursing and Technology," *Image: Journal of Nursing Scholarship* 29, no. 2 (1997): 169–74.
3. I would like to thank the reviewers for suggesting this analytical concept. As a beginning discussion of hospital work, Anselm Strauss and his colleagues contribute a valuable sociological framework that describes categories of work, each socially constructed and

interactively negotiated with other components in the hospital system (e.g., physicians, nurses, patients, and families). What is missing, however, is an historical perspective that considers the specific context (persons, place, and time) in understanding the fluidity of the division of labor and perceptions of work. See Anselm Strauss et al., *Social Organization of Medical Work* (Chicago: University of Chicago Press, 1985). Thomas P. Hughes, "The Evolution of Large Technological Systems," in *The Social Construction of Technological Systems,* ed. Wiebe E. Bijker, Thomas P. Hughes, and Trevor J. Pinch (Cambridge, Mass.: MIT Press, 1989), 53–54. Canadian sociologist George Torrance described hospitals as health factories, building on eighteenth-century work by French hospital analyst J. R. Tenon, who referred to hospitals as machines that cure ("un instrument qui facilite la curation"). See George M. Torrance, "Hospitals as Health Factories," in *Health and Canadian Society: Sociological Perspectives,* ed. David Coburn et al. (Don Mills, Ontario: Fitzhenry and Whiteside, 1981). The original reference to Tenon can be found in Dora B. Weiner, *The Citizen-Patient in Revolutionary and Imperial Paris* (Baltimore: John Hopkins University Press, 1993), 373.

4. Peter Hutchin, "History of Blood Transfusion: A Tercentennial Look," *Surgery* 64, no. 3 (September 1968): 685–700. See also Pauline M. Mazumdar, *Essays on the History of Immunology, 1930–1980* (Toronto: Wall and Thompson, 1989), and Pauline M. Mazumdar, *Species and Specificity: An Interpretation of the History of Immunology* (Cambridge: Cambridge University Press, 1994).

5. Beginning references for traditional history of blood accounts include Maxwell M. Wintrobe, *Blood, Pure and Eloquent: A Story of Discovery, of People, and of Ideas* (Toronto: McGraw-Hill, 1980); William H. Schneider, "Blood Transfusion in Peace and War, 1900–1918," *Social History of Medicine* 10, no. 1 (April 1997): 105–26; Geoffrey Keynes, ed., *Blood Transfusion* (London: Simpkin Marshall, 1949); Camille Dreyfus, *Some Milestones in the History of Hematology* (New York: Grune and Stratton, 1957); John Boyd Coates and Elizabeth M. McFetridge, eds., *Blood Program in World War II* (Washington, D.C.: Office of the Surgeon General Department of the Army, 1964); C. C. Bowley, K. L. G. Goldsmith, and W. Maycock, eds., *Blood Transfusion: A Guide to the Formation and Operation of a Transfusion Service* (Geneva: World Health Organization, 1971); George Milles, Hiram T. Langston, and William Dalessandro, *Autologous Transfusions* (Springfield, Ill.: Charles C. Thomas, Publisher, 1971); Richard K. Spence et al., "Transfusion and Surgery," *Current Problems in Surgery* 30, no. 12 (December 1993): 1103–71; and Norman Miles Guiou, *Transfusion: A Canadian Surgeon's Story in War and in Peace* (Yarmouth, Nova Scotia: Stoneycroft Publishers, 1985).

6. Guiou, *Transfusion;* Richard W. Kapp, "Charles H. Best, the Canadian Red Cross Society, and Canada's First National Blood Donation Program," *Canadian Bulletin of Medical History* 12, no. 1 (1995): 27–46; William H. Schneider, "Blood Transfusion in Peace and War, 1900–1918," *Social History of Medicine* 10, no. l (April 1997): 105–26.

7. Guiou, *Transfusion,* 90–95; and H. J. G. Geggie, *The Extra Mile: Medicine in Rural Quebec, 1885–1965,* ed. Norma Geggie and Stuart Geggie (1987): 107–9.

8. Schneider, "Blood Transfusion"; Guiou, *Transfusion.* W. Stuart Stanbury conducted a national survey on the state of hospital blood banks which he summarized in *A National Blood Transfusion Service: What it Means to You* (radio address and monograph of the Canadian Red Cross Society, January 25, 1949); G. Harvey Agnew, *Canadian Hospitals, 1920–1970: A Dramatic Half Century* (Toronto: University of Toronto Press, 1974); Guiou, *Transfusion;* Kapp, "Charles H. Best"; "Civic Hospital May Supply Blood Free," Mary Lamb Collection, OCH School of Nursing Files, Box 30, City of Ottawa Archives, Canada (hereafter referred to as COA). Refer also to the memo from Dr. W. Douglas Piercey (superintendent of the OCH), "Schedule of Fees and Services: Blood Bank Policy," COA, MG 38, box 10, 2. Letter from the Canadian Red Cross (CRC) to the

Ottawa Civic Hospital (OCH) on December 20, 1947, contained in the files of the Finance and Properties Committee, COA, MG 38, box 10, file 38-1-3-11. E. H. A; Watson, *History of Ontario Red Cross, 1914–1946* (Toronto: Division Headquarters, n.d.); Kapp, "Charles H. Best," 3; Guiou, *Transfusion*, 98–101. The HAR, 1940, OCHA, contains a note of thanks to James Potter for blood donated free to patients in the public wards. A scrapbook of newspaper clippings and photos was maintained by Mary Lamb, one of the early graduates of the school of nursing at OCH. Among these clippings are "Start DVA Blood Bank," *Ottawa Journal*, April 18, 1957, in which members of the Ottawa and District Branch of the DVA Employees Association are pictured during donation, an entry simply dated 1951, in which Willis Kuhns is pictured after a donation for the Employees' Blood Bank at the OCH; and "Civic Hospital May Supply Blood Free" (source unidentified), 1958, which contains a description of how the volunteer blood banks work. Mary Lamb Collection, COA, Box 30.

9. Stanbury, *A National Blood Transfusion Service*; see also CRC *Despatch 5*, no. 7 (November 1946). Letter from W. Stuart Stanbury to the Honourable Paul Martin, Minister of National Health and Welfare, February 24, 1951, National Archives, Ottawa, Ontario, RG 29, 20–C-4, vol. 4 (hereafter cited as NA). For more comprehensive discussions regarding the Canadian health care system, refer to C. David Naylor, *Private Practice, Public Payment: Canadian Medicine and the Politics of Health Insurance, 1911–1966* (Kingston, Ontario: McGill-Queen's University Press, 1986); Malcolm G. Taylor, *Health Insurance and Canadian Public Policy: The Seven Decisions That Created the Canadian Health Insurance System* (Montreal: McGill-Queen's University Press, 1978); Jacalyn Duffin, "The Guru and the Godfather: Henry Sigerist, Hugh MacLean, and the Politics of Health Care Reform in 1940s Canada," *Canadian Bulletin of Medical History* 9 (1992): 191–218; and Juanne Nancarrow Clarke, *Health, Illness, and Medicine in Canada*, 2nd ed. (Toronto: Oxford University Press, 1996).

10. *Emergency Blood Transfusion* (Montreal: National Film Board, 1970), filmstrip; *Miracle Fluid* (Associated Screen Productions, 1950), filmstrip; *Great Also in Peace: The Role of the Red Cross in Peace* (Associated Screen Production, 1950), filmstrip. Each was produced in collaboration with Dr. W. Stuart Stanbury and the CRC, and is available from NA. Illustrations of the baby-saving themes in the news media include: "Blood To Save Babies' Lives," *Toronto Star Weekly*, February 28, 1948; Marjorie Earl, "Red Cross Scheme Can Save Rh Babies," *The Toronto Telegram*, May 13, 1949; and "Race Death With Rh Baby," *The Toronto Telegram*, May 11, 1949.

11. HARs, 1924–1975, OCHA. Patricia Crossley, interview by author, audiotape, Ottawa, Ontario, January 26, 1998.

12. F. B. Bowman and Sidney Katz. "Three Blood Transfusions Out of Four are More Likely to Harm Than to Heal," *Maclean's* (August 26, 1961): 19 (available from CRC Archives, Ottawa, Ontario); "Krever on Trail of Tainted Blood—2," *The Ottawa Citizen*, February 26, 1996; and "Krever on Trail of Tainted Blood—3," February 27, 1996; Michael Grange," Blood is 'Filthy,' Inquiry Told," *The Globe and Mail* (Toronto), December 11, 1996. Andre Picard, *The Gift of Death: Confronting Canada's Tainted Blood Tragedy* (Toronto: HarperCollins, 1995); and Crossley, interview.

13. Margaret Henricks, interview by author, audiotape, Ottawa, Ontario, February 2, 1998; Gwen Hefferman, interview by author, audiotape, Ottawa, Ontario, January 29, 1998; and Florence Kinsella, interview with author, audiotape, Ottawa, Ontario, February 24, 1998. See also Rita Maloney, "Technological issues," in *Canadian Nursing Faces the Future*, 2nd ed., ed. Alice J. Baumgart and Jenniece Larsen (Toronto: Mosby Year Book, 1992).

14. HARs, 1924–1975, OCHA.

15. Similarly, Margarete Sandelowski argues that when tasks were considered easy enough for nurses to perform them, the skill was degraded. She suggests delegation constituted

an ideological device to maintain power over nurses. See both "Venous Envy: The Post–World War II Debate Over IV Nursing," *Advances in Nursing Science* 22, no. 1 (1999): 52–62, and "The Physician's Eyes: American Nursing and the Diagnostic Revolution in Medicine," *NHR* 8 (2000): 3–38.

16. One of the interview participants, Patricia Crossley, had a direct transfusion from her father when she was three years old. Guiou, *Transfusion;* Hutchin, "History of Blood Transfusion," 685–700.

17. Blood procedures such as this one were described in the procedure books used by students, educators, and staff at OCH. The earliest procedure book is simply noted as "in use prior to 1948," and with each revision over the ensuing years the procedures related to transfusion became more involved and lengthy (OCHA).

18. Milligan, interview.

19. Dr. H. William Henderson, "Delegation of Special Procedures: The Current Situation" (address to the Session for Chiefs of Staff, Ontario Hospital Association Convention, December 1, 1981), from the files of the College of Nurses of Ontario, Toronto.

20. Ibid., 3.

21. This material has been summarized from Henderson's "Delegation of Special Procedures." The Registered Nurses Association of Ontario (RNAO) disseminated current information on these acts through the *RNAO News Bulletin,* often with a focus on the self-protection strategies nurses should use when participating in delegation; see, for example, "Medical Procedures—Important New Notice," *RNAO News Bulletin* 18, no. 1 (January–February 1962): 1, and "Medical Procedures by Nurses," *RNAO News Bulletin* 21, no. 5 (September-October 1965): 11.

22. Hefferman, interview; and Donna Martin, personal communication with author, Ottawa, Ontario, April 1, 1998.

23. Elizabeth Fenton, retired chief technologist of the OCH Blood Bank from 1943 to 1985, personal communication with author, May 22, 1998.

24. Strauss et al., *Social Organization,* 268–72. The precipitating events were documented in two editorials of the *Ottawa Citizen,* February 28, 1949, and March 4, 1949. Three volumes of court evidence offer insight to the care received and concerns of these patients; refer to the files on "Judicial Inquiry, vols. I–III," City of Ottawa Archives, MG 38, vol. 36, and to the final report as "Civic Hospital," Minutes of the City Council, August 2, 1949, City of Ottawa Archives, 662–76.

25. Crossley, interview; Kathy Slattery, interview by author, tape recording, Ottawa, Ontario, February 10, 1998. These expectations and penalties were also described in the Henricks interview; Kinsella, interview; Crossley, interview.

26. Crossley, interview; Henricks, interview; Kinsella, interview.

27. Hefferman, interview; Slattery, interview.

28. *Blood Transfusion Alternatives: What You Should Know,* Monograph Series EPXSUR-9637 (North York, Ontario: Ortho Biotech, n.d.); "Bloodless Surgery," interviews by Joan Leishman, *Sunday Morning Program,* Canadian Broadcast Corporation, November 17, 1996; Jean-Yves Dupuis, "An Analysis of Transfusion Decision Making in Cardiac Surgery: Comparing Patients Who Predonated Autologous Blood to Matched Controls" (presentation at Loeb Research Institute, Ottawa, February 21, 1997).

29. Henricks, interview; and personal experience of the author.

30. Results of a meta-analysis of the published professional literature on alternatives to blood transfusions from ten countries during the timeframe of 1966–1994, were presented by Ian Graham, "Bibliometric Analysis" (paper presented to the International Study of Perioperative Transfusion, [ISPOT], Ottawa, Ontario, May 25, 1996). Some 8707 articles were identified, and the data were analyzed for frequency by the blood technologies studied: autologous transfusions, cell savers, aprotinin, erythropoietin, desmopressin (DDAVP), and hemodilution. The number of documents remained fewer

than 10 per year from 1966 until 1986, when sharp rises in publication were noted in all ten countries. These increases continued through 1994. For example, in the United States alone, there were 5 documents in 1986, 10 in 1987, 24 in 1988, 35 in 1989, and 58 in 1990. Dupuis, "An Analysis of Transfusion"; T. Gwynford Jones, personal communication with author, April 12, 1998; Hefferman, interview.

31. Milligan, interview; Hefferman, interview; and Crossley, interview, described these technologies and the process of delegation as parallels to transfusion, in the manner of transferral to nurses' domain. They are also described in the procedure manuals and in various minutes of the Medical Advisory Board, as physicians discussed what, when, and how to delegate each.

32. See photograph in Guiou, *Translation,* 114. Photographs included in Guiou's *Translation* were taken at the OCH by the National Film Board of Canada. One of these shows the nurse "being" the suction force to create a vacuum in the blood collection bottle. See also photos in the CRC news bulletin, *Despatch* 5, no. 7 (November 1946) and the description in Frances Brown, "A Blood Donor Service in Halifax," *CN* 38, no. 11 (1942): 872–74. The CRC produced an audiotape for circulation in Canada as part of a campaign for blood donations during World War II in which radio reporter Bill Herbert described his experience during an actual donation of his own blood. Part of the description elaborated on the process as the nurse provided the suction during the entire procedure. Refer to "Our Blood for Their Lives," narrated by Bill Herbert, Canadian Broadcasting Corporation, Documentary Art and Photography Division, NA. Two student nurses were the blood donors in Helen Marie Caraher, "An Emergency Splenectomy," *CN* 37, no. 3 (1941): 185–86.

33. Crossley, interview.

34. Hefferman, interview. The technician was allowed greater discretion to "needle" the transfusion line. This procedure involved using a syringe to clear a sluggish needle or tubing by flushing it with saline. Crossley, interview.

35. Milligan, interview; Slattery, interview.

36. W. Stuart Stanbury, "Gamma Globulin," *CN* 50, no. 6 (1954): 466; and loose poster collection, uncatalogued, CRC archives, Ottawa, Ontario.

37. Crossley, interview.

38. Ibid.

39. E. C. Hughes, *The Sociological Eye* (Chicago: Aldine, 1971), as cited in Strauss et al., *Social Organization,* 246–51.

40. These statistics are constructed from the HARs, 1924–1973, OCHA.

41. E. Stanley Ryerson, "The Preparation of a Curriculum," *CN* 25, no. 9 (1929): 535–40.

42. Hefferman, interview.

43. Henricks, interview.

44. Loose papers dated March 1, 1976 and contained in the SMA binder on delegated acts, OCHA. Letter from B. Jean Milligan to Shirley Kerr, February 5, 1975, OCHA.

45. Kathryn McPherson, *Bedside Matters: The Transformation of Canadian Nursing, 1900–1990* (Toronto: Oxford University Press, 1996); Milligan, interview.

46. A fuller understanding of immigration and racial construction in Canadian nursing contexts is needed. An important beginning point is Agnes Calliste, "Women of 'Exceptional Merit': Immigration of Caribbean Nurses to Canada," *Canadian Journal of Women and the Law* 6, no. 1 (1993): 85–102; Milligan, interview.

47. Slattery, interview; Donna Martin, personal communication, April 1, 1998; Katherine B. Knuckolls, "Who Decides What the Nurse Can Do?" *Nursing Outlook* 22 (1974): 627.

48. Wendy McKnight Nicklin, interview by author, audiotape, Ottawa, Ontario, April 21, 1998.

CHAPTER 12

Blurring the Boundaries Between Medicine and Nursing: Coronary Care Nursing, Circa the 1960s

Arlene W. Keeling

This chapter is part of a larger historical research project describing the inception and proliferation of coronary care units (CCUs) in the United States in the 1960s and analyzing the roles of nurses within these units. I argue that the artificial disciplinary boundaries between medicine and nursing were blurred when nurses assumed the technological skills of cardiac monitoring and cardiac defibrillation in the early coronary care units— skills that were accompanied by an expanded knowledge of cardiology.

The role of the nurse was one of the most significant areas of change in the coronary care units of the 1960s. On 15 March 1966, four years after the institution of the CCU, cardiologist Carleton B. Chapman summarized what had transpired during a New York Heart Association conference on coronary care:

> If there is a single thread around which most of the discussion has ranged itself in this conference, it is the role of the nurse. Nurses are present in the CCU 24 hours a day. It is inescapable that in most

This chapter was originally published in the *Nursing History Review* 12 (2004):139–165. Copyright Springer Publishing Company. Reprinted with permission.

instances, it will be a nurse who will save the patient's life by recognizing a potentially fatal arrhythmia and by operating the complex equipment that will convert the arrhythmia to normal. . . . The only alternative to this is to assign experienced physicians to the units around the clock. This is not possible in any hospital I know of.[1]

Recognizing "a potentially fatal arrhythmia" and *operating* the complex equipment that will convert the arrhythmia to normal can be translated as *diagnosing* lethal arrhythmias and *defibrillating* the patient to cure him of the arrhythmia and save his life. These two acts were major changes from nursing's traditional caring role in the "care versus cure" dichotomy. Indeed, in the coronary care units in the 1960s, the invisible boundary separating the permissible from the non-permissible in the practice of medicine and nursing was blurring. To understand what happened, we need first to examine the historical setting in which the high profile changes occurred.

THE SETTING: POSTWAR AMERICA

The "coronary problem" in post-World War II United States was a significant one. As President Harry Truman noted in a 1949 address to the nation, "The tremendous toll of the heart diseases must be of deep concern to all our citizens. Combating the Nation's leading cause of death has become our most serious national health problem. . . . The heart diseases, I am informed, now account for one out of every two deaths after the age of forty."[2]

For the most part, the patients dying from acute myocardial infarction were white middle-class men in the prime of life. As such, they played an important role in the American economy. Moreover, they included prominent national leaders whose medical conditions warranted national press coverage. Senate Majority Leader Lyndon Baines Johnson experienced a massive heart attack in July 1955 and was hospitalized in the U.S. Naval Hospital in Bethesda for six weeks, during which time members of the press were in constant attendance. Then, while Johnson was convalescing at his Texas ranch, on 24 September 1955, President Dwight D. Eisenhower also suffered a coronary thrombosis.[4] The press coverage was immediate, and it continued throughout Eisenhower's seven-week stay at Fitzsimmons Army Hospital in Denver and subsequent convalescence at home in Gettysburg.[5] Moreover, Eisenhower's cardiologist, Paul Dudley White, MD, used the historic opportunity provided by the president's illness to educate the American public about coronary disease.[6] In fact, soon after he examined President Eisenhower in the Denver hospital,

White held a national press conference in which he explained in detail the process and treatment of coronary thrombosis, referring to it as the "commonest important illness that besets a middle-aged man in this country today."[7] Heart disease was indeed receiving national attention.

THE POSSIBILITIES OF SPACE-AGE TECHNOLOGY

In the period following World War II, optimism about the possibilities of space-age research and scientific knowledge permeated the United States. In 1961, the press provided extensive coverage of astronaut Alan Shepard's first venture into space, and in 1962, *Life* magazine covered John H. Glenn's orbit around the world.[8] Both events were also covered on national television. In their reporting, newscasters included information about the new technology used to monitor the astronauts' vital signs during the missions. Americans were fascinated. If science and technology could provide solutions to complex medical problems in space, then they held promise for finding solutions to the more mundane problems on earth. The popular opinion was that scientific research should be supported. "Space-age technology" would soon be expected to solve all manner of problems. One of the most significant was heart disease, the number one killer of Americans.

THE NEW TECHNOLOGY AND SCIENTIFIC ADVANCES IN CARDIOLOGY

Scientific and technological advances in the field of cardiology also played a significant role in setting the stage for the changes in coronary care that would occur in the 1960s. From the early twentieth century, physicians had been receptive to the incorporation of new machines and medical treatments to diagnose disease and cure patients. In the 1910s and 1920s, they adopted both the x-ray and the electrocardiogram (EKG) as diagnostic tools.[9]

By the 1950s, the new radiological technique of cardiac catheterization offered great promise for the diagnosis of coronary artery disease. Cardiac pacemakers were invented and perfected, and cardiac drugs such as quinidine gluconate, potassium salts, and procainamide hydrochloride were available to treat ventricular arrhythmias.[10] Most important, there was groundbreaking research about the technique of cardiopulmonary resuscitation (CPR), experimental equipment for continuous monitoring of the electrical activity of the heart, and new portable cardiac defibrillators and external pacemakers.

External Cardiac Massage

The widespread acceptance of external cardiac massage as a treatment for cardiac arrest in 1960 was of particular importance to the changes that would take place in the care of coronary patients in 1962. Although a German physician had made some of the earliest reports of closed chest cardiac massage in 1891, it was not until more than fifty years later, in 1959, that the procedure was rediscovered by physicians William B. Kouwenhoven, James R. Jude, and G. Guy Knickerbocker at the Johns Hopkins University School of Medicine. Experimenting on dogs, these physicians developed a safe and effective method of "massaging the heart without thoracotomy"[11] and immediately implemented the technique in the clinical area, resuscitating twenty patients in a ten-month period. Reporting the results in 1960, Kouwenhoven and his colleagues concluded:

> Closed chest cardiac massage has been proved to be effective in cardiac arrest. It has provided circulation adequate to maintain the heart and central nervous system, and it has provided an opportunity to bring a defibrillator to the scene if necessary. Supportive drug treatment and other measures may be given. The necessity for thoracotomy is eliminated.[12]

External Cardiac Defibrillation

The success of external cardiac defibrillation in saving lives after cardiac arrest was another advance in cardiology that would provide the backdrop for the inception and growth of the coronary care unit and the specialty of cardiac nursing. In 1941, Claude Beck, MD, a surgeon at Case Western Reserve School of Medicine in Cleveland, Ohio, reported the first two attempts of cardiac defibrillation during surgery. His conclusion, that "the heart can be defibrillated . . . a coordinated beat can be restored," was groundbreaking and laid the foundation for future research.[13] Publishing again in 1947, Beck and his colleagues emphasized the necessity of knowing precisely and immediately whether the underlying cardiac mechanism responsible for the death was cardiac arrest or a fatal arrhythmia:

> Since cardiac arrhythmias cannot be diagnosed by inspection alone, easy access to an electrocardiograph is necessary. Precise knowledge of the cardiac mechanism is of utmost importance if successful restoration of a normal rhythm is to be intelligently planned.[14]

Thus the unique interaction of complex social forces in the late 1950s and early 1960s provided the setting in which changes could occur in the care of the patient with acute myocardial infarction. In the 1950s, death from coronary artery disease was the number one health problem in the United States. The occurrence of heart attacks in famous leaders called the nation's attention to the problem of heart disease. Americans were infatuated with experts and specialists. Experimental drugs and technologies became available to treat heart disease, and new knowledge about cardiac resuscitation was being published in prestigious medical journals. The 1960s saw even further emphasis on technology as "space-age research" became the norm.

NURSING CARE OF THE PATIENT WITH MYOCARDIAL INFARCTION, 1950s

Despite the advances in science and technology, the role of the nurse caring for heart attack patients in the postwar period remained relatively unchanged from the prewar years. Essentially, her job included the traditional "caring" tasks of putting the patient to bed and making him or her comfortable. Mildred Crawley, chief of the Heart Nursing Service, National Institutes of Health, described the nurse's role in the care of the acutely ill MI patient in a paper published in the *American Journal of Nursing* in 1961:

> During the first hour of a patient's hospitalization, the doctor must make an initial examination, an electrocardiograph will be taken, blood may be drawn for analysis, probably oxygen will be started, and medication will be given for pain. During all these activities, the nurse or aide is expected to admit the patient, care for his belongings, undress him and get him settled as comfortably as possible in bed, [and] care for the needs and questions of the family. . . . Rather than yield to her desire to keep the room straight or the bed neat, she can delay rearranging the covers until after all the examinations, and she can quietly place the used equipment or instruments aside to be cleaned or put away after the essentials have been done and the patient is at rest.[15]

The boundaries between medicine and nursing were clear. The physician would examine the patient, take the ECG, and draw blood. The nurse would settle the patient comfortably in bed, manage his or her belongings, and answer the family's questions. In the course of the patient's illness, only the physician would diagnose cardiac arrhythmias and decide on the proper intervention. The nurse would take the pulse, check the blood pressure, and count respirations. In addition, she would make observations and record facts in the nurses' notes.

By the early 1960s, however, it was becoming apparent that these clearly delineated boundaries of medical and nursing practice were not always in the best interest of the patient. Cardiac arrhythmias often presented life-threatening emergencies in which prompt diagnosis and treatment could be lifesaving. Observing and reporting a cardiac arrest without attempting to intervene did little good.

THE GENESIS OF THE CCU: BETHANY HOSPITAL, KANSAS CITY

In 1961, Bethany Hospital in Kansas City, Kansas, was the site of one of the first coronary care units in the United States. In many ways, Bethany was not unlike the 6,000 other community hospitals in America. Established in 1892, this midwestern hospital, located on the fringes of the downtown area, provided services to the residents of Kansas City. It was operated by a Board of Trustees who set policy for the hospital and governed its financial affairs. Moreover, its physician staff exerted considerable influence over both medical and nursing policies in the hospital.[16]

During the 1950s Bethany had experienced phenomenal growth, subsidized by funds supplied by the federal government 1946 Hill-Burton Act. In fact, the construction of a large west wing in 1957 provided the 90-bed hospital with an additional 110 beds, doubling both its size and the community's expectations for services.[17] Along with the expansion came changes in the way nursing care was delivered. Instead of the traditional open wards, the renovated Bethany had multiple private and semiprivate rooms opening off long corridors, providing privacy for patients but decreasing visibility and accessibility to the nurses.

The new configuration stressed a system already short of nurses because it required them to walk long distances up and down hallways to care for patients in separate rooms. The configuration of the new private and semiprivate rooms also blocked the nurses' view of critically ill patients. Consequently, patients who needed 24-hour-a-day observation were either placed near the nurses' station or assigned a private duty nurse. A private duty nurse was not, however, assigned to care for cardiac patients considered to be in "stable" condition. Instead, the hemodynamically stable patient recuperating from a heart attack was often assigned to a private room near the end of a hall where he or she could rest quietly. Nurses would check the patient periodically. Aides would take blood pressure and pulse at regular intervals, usually every four hours.[18] However, even hemodynamically stable, pain-free cardiac patients could have a sudden cardiac arrest. In that case, assignment to a private room could be life-threatening.

In an attempt to rectify the situation and respond to sudden cardiac deaths, Hughes W. Day, a forty-six-year-old general practitioner who practiced internal medicine and cardiology at Bethany, implemented a "Code Blue" procedure in which a team of physicians and nurses responded to these cardiac emergencies and began cardiopulmonary resuscitation, defibrillating the patient's heart if necessary. A diligent and caring physician, Day was both concerned about the sudden deaths of his middle-aged cardiac patients and aware that the cutting-edge research reported in the medical literature might have the answer he was looking for.[19]

The idea was an excellent one—at least in theory. In reality, the success of the Code Blue protocol at Bethany was less than optimal. The protocol was used for about ten months without a significant decrease in mortality after cardiac or pulmonary arrest. Initial delays in recognizing that a patient had suffered a cardiac arrest and subsequent delays in getting the equipment and the Code team to the bedside often meant that it was too late to save the patient. As a result, of those in whom resuscitation was attempted, only 4 percent survived. Moreover, the lack of an effective alarm system to alert the nurse to initiate a Code Blue resulted in a persistent pattern of cardiac patients dying unobserved in their private rooms.[20]

Frustrated by the poor success rates of the Code Blue procedure, Day decided to try a new approach. He would monitor all MI patients by attaching them to the same type of continuous cardiac monitoring equipment being used in space. Furthermore, he would place the cardiac monitor outside the patient's room and set the arrhythmia alarms. That way, theoretically, the nurse caring for the patient could immediately observe an arrhythmia or respond to alarms signifying cardiac arrest or changes in heart rate. In reality, the solution eluded him. Judith Stuart, a Bethany nurse in 1961, recounted what happened:

> One of the engineers at Bethany, Johnny Walker, rigged up a cardiac monitor for Dr. Day. Originally the cardiac patients were just put in a room out on the floor and hooked to a monitor that sat outside the room. When the patient's heart stopped, the alarm would go off and the nurse would call Dr. Day at home so he could come to the hospital and try to resuscitate the patient. Usually it was too late because more than ten minutes had elapsed.[21]

It was becoming apparent that the electronic equipment Day had installed could not be used to its fullest capacity without specially trained nurses who could operate it effectively and interpret the arrhythmias. According to Day,

> Several discouraging facts soon emerged. The hearts that were "too young to die" eluded us in our cardiac resuscitation program, and the electronic gear attached to patients proved of little value. The reason

was obvious. We had no nurses who could correctly interpret the f EKG patterns or fathom the alarm systems. . . . This was especially true at 3 a.m. . . . It was apparent that our crying need was for a group of specially trained nurses working in a specific area, who could give the patient with coronary disease expert bedside attention, interpret signs of impending disaster, and quickly institute CPR.[22]

Having reached this conclusion, Day collaborated with hospital administrator Walter Coburn and requested funding from the John A. Hartford Foundation, proposing to develop a Cardiac Unit in which specially trained nurses could provide care for MI patients. The Hartford unit, with its seven-bed ICU and four-bed CCU, opened to receive patients on 20 May 1962.[23] Almost simultaneously, Lawrence Meltzer conducted a similar experiment at Presbyterian Hospital in Philadelphia.

THE PRESBYTERIAN NURSING EXPERIMENT

Apparently unaware of Day's work in Kansas City, Lawrence E. Meltzer, MD, a seasoned research physician at Presbyterian Hospital in Philadelphia, applied to the Division of Nursing, United States Public Health Service (USPHS) in 1962, requesting funding for a research project in the newly established cardiac research unit at Presbyterian. Working with the chief of cardiology, J. Roderick Kitchell, MD, Meltzer proposed a nurse-focused study in Presbyterian's recently completed two-bed cardiac unit to determine whether nurse monitoring and intervention could reduce the high incidence of arrhythmic deaths from acute myocardial infarction (MI).[24]

Like Day, Meltzer was determined to find a way to reduce the high mortality from AMI. Hypothesizing that he could prevent sudden unexpected deaths from AMI by careful monitoring and the cardiac defibrillation procedures described by Paul Zoll in the January 1960 issue of the *New England Journal of Medicine*,[25] Meltzer proposed the following research plan:

> The intensive care that the investigators believe could reduce the fatality rate from acute myocardial infarction (and particularly those deaths that occur suddenly from arrhythmias) involves a specially trained scientific team of nurses, cardiologists and resident physicians functioning in a hospital unit planned solely for the treatment of acute myocardial infarction in which (a) patients will be continuously observed for the critical 72 hour period after admission by a professional nurse member of the team, (b) patients will be continuously monitored by advanced electronic means which will immediately alert the nurse observer by

auditory and visual alarm systems of the onset of arrhythmias or changes in the heart rate beyond predetermined danger limits. When these events occur, a specific planned program of treatment is immediately instituted, (c) complete therapeutic means (electric pacemaker, defibrillators, resuscitators, etc.) will be available (and ready for use) at the bedside to interrupt would-be catastrophic arrhythmias. (d) All necessary drugs, intravenous solutions, plasma etc., will be on hand in this self sufficient unit to treat congestive heart failure and shock, the next major causes of death from myocardial infarction.[26]

Key to the plan's success was the new two-bed cardiac research facility, to which physicians could admit patients diagnosed with acute myocardial infarction. There, they could be monitored with high tech space-age equipment. The problem: there were no nurses trained to work in the pilot facility.

Meltzer was cognizant of the fact that a team approach to the care of cardiac patients would be necessary if he and his research colleagues were to reduce mortality from acute myocardial infarction. "Team nursing," as defined by Lambertsen in 1953, was already in place at Presbyterian;[27] however, Meltzer's concept of a new specialized cardiac team was different. The proposed team would include registered nurses who had specific skills in caring for cardiac patients being monitored by the new machines. These highly specialized RNs would provide round-the-clock comprehensive, direct patient care themselves rather than supervising licensed practical nurses (LPNs) and aides. Moreover, the specialized RNs would also take on a responsibility heretofore assumed only by research cardiologists or anesthetists: they would interpret the heart rhythms displayed on the cardiac monitors and initiate emergency treatment for life-threatening arrhythmias. According to Meltzer's proposal, "the nurse, by definition of her responsibility, will be the vital member of the scientific team."[28]

A few years later, in a 15 July 1966 symposium on the "Status of Intensive Coronary Care," Meltzer discussed his original idea, noting:

It was clear to us that physicians could not remain with patients constantly, nor could they reach the bedside from elsewhere in the hospital in time to prevent an arrhythmic death. . . . For this reason, we decided that the nurse would be the key to the system and that she would be responsible not only for electrocardiographic monitoring, but more significantly, the nurse herself would initiate the treatment program of defibrillation and pacemaking.[29]

In 1962, Meltzer proposed that the role of the nurse would be central to the system of coronary care. The nurse would be present in the

CCU 24 hours a day. In contrast, the physician would come and go. By 1965, in the first edition of his book for CCU nurses, Meltzer diagrammed and labeled his scientific team approach, demonstrating how the physician (labeled D in his diagram) would be based outside the unit, away from the patient, while the nurse (labeled C) would be the link between the patient, the monitor, the treatment (labeled E), and the physician.[30] Rose Pinneo, in a 1967 publication, wrote:

> The nurse (C) is in constant attendance and is continually aware of the clinical and cardiac status. In the event of an emergency situation, the nurse notifies the physician (D) and then initiates the planned treatment program. The treatment program (E) involves a variety of equipment necessary to terminate potentially fatal arrhythmias, devices to assist respiration, and drugs to combat cardiac emergencies.[31]

In 1962, however, the CCU nurse's role was not so fully articulated and was still to be determined. According to Meltzer's original proposal, the long range goal of his research was "a detailed consideration of the role of the professional nurse in an intensive care unit of this type, including her needs for specialized knowledge and skills."[32]

Meltzer was interested in determining "whether or not nurses could be trained for this exacting work" (recognizing and treating cardiac arrhythmias).[33] In fact, his nursing experiment was much like the experiment conducted by the character Henry Higgins in Shaw's play *Pygmalion* and Jay Lerner's Broadway production *My Fair Lady*. Like the snobbish phonetics professor Higgins, who taught proper English grammar to a cockney flower seller (Eliza Dolittle) in the hope that she could pass for a duchess, Meltzer trained nurses in acute cardiology to see whether it was possible to improve their clinical skills. And just as Professor Higgins expected that Eliza Dolittle would attain social status by improving her grammar, Meltzer predicted that the coronary care nurses' status in the profession would be similarly affected. According to Meltzer, "If nurses are capable of performing these exacting tasks and assuming this degree of responsibility, the role of the nurse will be materially different than her present day status."[34] As he would later write in the preface to his *Intensive Care: A Manual for Nurses,* "it was apparent that a separate, higher division within the nursing profession must be established for this purpose in the form of nurse specialists."[35]

To his credit, Meltzer's intentions in performing the nursing experiment were admirable. Unlike the fictional Professor Higgins, who wanted to trick European aristocrats into thinking Eliza Dolittle was a royal duchess, Meltzer's purpose in training the CCU nurses was to save

American lives. Thus nurse training would be a major focus of the project. An enthusiastic Meltzer reasoned:

> The purpose of this uninterrupted nursing care and continuous monitoring of the patient becomes obvious with the realization that in fatal arrhythmias the time between onset and death is no more than a minute or so. For this plan to succeed, the nurse observing the patient must be trained to interpret changes in the rhythm of the heart or other catastrophic event, and institute planned measures to combat these happening, often by herself, at the instance of their occurrence.[36]

Meltzer's enthusiasm not withstanding, his proposed nursing experiment could not be implemented without administrative support. That support was forthcoming. Carl L. Mosher, executive administrator of the hospital, enthusiastically approved of the idea.[37] Moreover, Mary Ellen Brown, director of nursing, not only agreed to serve as the nursing consultant on the innovative project, but also offered to pay 20 percent of the salaries for five nurses to work in the unit.[38] Thus, as was the case with Hughes Day at Bethany Hospital, who had the backing of hospital administrator Walter Coburn and director of nursing Ruby Harris, Lawrence Meltzer had the cooperation he needed from Presbyterian's administration.

Meltzer's proposal also made sense to the grant reviewers in the USPHS Division of Nursing. Based on his own scientific research and the most recent medical literature, Meltzer's hypothesis was credible. If nurses were trained to observe AMI patients using the new cardiac technology and were permitted to implement emergency treatments on their own, perhaps mortality from AMI could be reduced. It was a commonsense argument. Furthermore, the chief of the research grants branch of the Division of Nursing was Faye Abdellah, PhD., a well-known nurse researcher whose own published ideas on "progressive patient care," particularly her ideas about using intensive care units, could be implemented in Meltzer's project.[39] In this case, patients who were diagnosed with AMI would be grouped together in a small intensive care unit where both nursing resources and the new technology could be maximized.

Altogether, given Meltzer's research interests and experience, the national problem of mortality from MI, the recent medical literature advocating cardiac defibrillation, the technological support available at Presbyterian, the approval of hospital administration, and Abdellah's interest, it is not at all surprising that the USPHS Division of Nursing awarded Meltzer and Kitchell $26,900 to implement the project.[40] Funding a physician as the primary investigator on this project focusing on an experimental role for nurses may have been unprecedented. It was not without stipulations, however. Abdellah insisted that a nurse project director be hired for the coronary care unit study. Moreover, Abdellah herself would personally visit Presbyterian to assess the study's progress.[41]

THE CCU

The small cardiac research unit at Presbyterian Hospital was self-contained rather than connected to a general intensive care unit, as was the case at Bethany. Having been designed and constructed at the expense of the hospital, the unit, already in operation at the time Meltzer and Kitchell submitted their proposal to the USPHS, was adjacent to the bustling Maximum Care Unit, a general ICU used for patients undergoing heart surgery, but it was isolated from the larger intensive care unit.[42]

The physical structure of the Presbyterian CCU facilitated nurses observing patients continuously. The unit consisted of two patients' beds and a nurses' station from which the nurse had direct vision of each patient through a window.[43] In addition, each patient was connected to cardiac monitoring equipment located centrally in the nurses' station. As Rose Pinneo later described it:

> When the monitor is turned on, it sets in action the continuous visual electrocardiogram which the nurse can observe as it proceeds from left to right on the oscilloscope on her desk. For every heartbeat, a light flickers and a faint "beep" sound is heard. The nurses could hear the beeps; the patients could not.[44]

Given the combination of a small isolated unit and the fact that the heartbeats were only heard in the central nurses' station, the Presbyterian CCU was much more peaceful than the combined ICU/CCU at Bethany Hospital in Kansas City.[45] The dilemma was that sometimes it was *too* quiet and *too* isolated. In fact, several nurses would later recommend that the unit be more closely connected to an intensive care unit so that staff could be shared and the monotony of caring for MI patients could be relieved.[46]

RECRUITMENT OF STAFF

When the research project began on 15 January 1963, about eight months after the Hartford CCU opened in Kansas City, Meltzer immediately faced the challenge of staffing it. According to Janice Lufkin, a recent graduate who was working in the Maximum Care Unit (MCU):

They didn't have nurses at first in the CCU, so we had to rotate there from the Maximum Care Unit [MCU]. Some of the other MCU nurses hated to go there. They would get so upset about doing it. I liked it, so they would ask me to take their rotations. I kept taking their turns until I finally just worked in the CCU fulltime.[47]

While he had solved the staffing problem temporarily, Meltzer found no one "in house" to serve as the nursing director for the coronary unit. He would need to find a qualified nursing administrator outside Presbyterian. A logical starting place was the University of Pennsylvania School of Nursing, which had a prestigious nursing faculty. Therefore, Meltzer contacted the dean of the School of Nursing, Dorothy Mereness, and asked whether any of the Penn nursing faculty might be interested in directing the nursing aspects of the research program. Dean Mereness, aware that one of her medical-surgical faculty, Clinical Instructor Rose Pinneo, had written her master's thesis on patients with myocardial infarction, asked her to consider the opportunity. Pinneo, a graduate of both Johns Hopkins School of Nursing and the University of Pennsylvania, agreed. The job matched her interests in the care of patients with myocardial infarction. Furthermore Pinneo, recently prepared to conduct nursing research in her graduate program at Penn, was excited about the prospect of participating in a study. Finally, the timing was right; she welcomed the challenge to try something new and agreed to begin after the spring semester. In July 1963, six months after agreeing to accept the job, Pinneo, a small-framed, unassuming professional, took on the nursing leadership role in the new unit.[48]

Pinneo's first task was to recruit a full-time nursing staff to work exclusively in the two-bed research unit. Presbyterian Hospital was already understaffed and she had to stop pulling nurses from the MCU, so she advertised in the local newspapers and recruited nurses from out-side the hospital. Like the Bethany nurses, the ones who responded to the advertisements and were subsequently hired for the Presbyterian CCU were young. Karen Campbell, Miki Iwata, Lynn Warner, and Janice Lufkin were all recent diploma graduates from the Presbyterian Hospital School of Nursing. Each had about one year of experience as a nurse before taking on the position in the CCU. They were in their early twenties; all were female.[49]

Others who followed them were also young and female. In fact, the median age of the 31 nurses employed in 1963-1967 was 22.9 years.[50] Not surprisingly, given the demographics of the nursing profession in the early 1960s, they were also female.[51] Both their age and their gender would influence their new status and professional relationships as they worked with young interns and residents as well as middle-aged attending physicians who were predominantly male.

It is clear that the CCU recruits shared some characteristics in addition to age and gender. They were a new breed of young professionals eager to accept a challenge, learn about the new technology used to monitor patients, and step outside the traditional role of nursing. Moreover, as Pinneo noted, they were carefully selected for their intelligence and their reputation for providing excellent nursing care.[52] According to Miki Iwata, a twenty-two-year-old registered nurse who began working in the Presbyterian CCU in September 1963:

> We were really nervous at first. No one knew about these arrhythmias and as they popped up we got nervous. But then, later, we got used to looking for the lethal arrhythmias and not worrying about the others.[53]

Those recruited were also willing to participate in research. In fact, collecting research data was to be a major component of the nurses' job. Not only would the CCU nurses provide care for patients, but they would also be expected to collect data every hour of the patient's stay and record these data on flow sheets. According to Pinneo,

> An hourly status report that included 75 columns was completed by the nurse for each hour the patient was in the CCU. The nurse recorded the patient's study number, the day of observation, the report number, the time of day, her own assigned number, the patient's pulse, BP and the code number for any arrhythmias present during the proceeding hour. . . . Whenever an arrhythmia developed during the hour, the nurse stated what her action was in regard to it.[54]

In addition to noting their actions in relation to arrhythmia, the nurses in the Presbyterian CCU documented their interpretations of the cardiac rhythm by attaching the ECG printout to the status report.[55]

The time and energy involved in these protocols for data collection were enormous. Hourly recordings were no easy feat, and the nurses had to collect data on both the experimental group (patients admitted to the CCU) and the control group (those admitted to the general units). All the data pertained to the patient; some were physiological, while other data dealt with the "emotional progress of the patients."[56]

For the nurses, there was no escaping the fact that they were involved in an important research study having to do with cardiac patients, cardiac arrhythmias, and the effect of the coronary care unit on patients' physical and emotional states. They knew that they were a select group and that they were developing specific skills that enabled them to save lives in a highly specialized clinical setting. They may have been less cognizant of the fact that data were being kept about them as well.[57] While they expressed an understanding that the new role for nurses was a part of the study, the nurses were clearly focused on the patients. Only one expressed her thoughts directly. Miki Iwata noted: "I think the nurses were also in an experiment to try a new role."[58]

CREATING SPECIFIC KNOWLEDGE FOR NURSES

The key to the entire coronary care project was, by necessity, the advanced training of the nurses to work in this highly specialized area. According to nursing director Rose Pinneo, "It became obvious that specialized training beyond basic nursing education was essential in order for nurses to fulfill their role in CCU."[59] Meltzer was at first of the opinion that this specialized training should include complex knowledge of 12 lead EKGs, but later decided that the principles of cardiology, pared down to the essential knowledge needed for safe practice, were all that was required for the nurses. In his opinion, the nurses needed to learn to recognize the patterns of the basic cardiac arrhythmias. They also had to know the emergency treatment for the arrhythmias that were life-threatening.[60]

After the brief introductory course and a few weeks of orientation to the monitoring equipment and the unit procedures, the CCU nurses learned on the job, practicing their newly acquired skills as they cared for patients.[61] Even the technique of cardiac defibrillation, in which nurses learned to shock the patient with 400 watt-seconds of electricity, was taught in the clinical setting rather than in a laboratory.[62] At first, some of the nurses defibrillated patients after simply observing how it was done by the physicians. Miki Iwata gave the classic example, stating:

> At first they wouldn't let nurses defibrillate. They didn't think nurses could do it. But then, later, we did. One time, a patient was in ventricular fibrillation and I just defibrillated him. I was one of the first to do it. I just did it! There was no doctor around. I was making rounds on the patients and saw him in V-fib and just did it . . . and the patient survived![63]

Later, Meltzer himself supervised this training exercise using the high-tech equipment. As Pinneo described the process:

> The way we taught our nurses to defibrillate was when we were doing elective cardioversions in the unit. Dr. Meltzer would allow the nurse to hold the paddles and defibrillate the patients. So, we knew where to place the paddles, how to lubricate the paddles, and to avoid touching the bed. That helped give the nurses confidence that they could do it.[64]

Organized clinical conferences occasionally supplemented nurse-to-nurse or physician-to-nurse training. Every month or so, Meltzer met with the nurses to review cases in which the patient had had a cardiac arrest and "would point out areas in which the nurses might have done something different."[65] In general, the atmosphere in the CCU was one that supported ongoing education.[66]

It wasn't long before Meltzer and his colleagues also identified the need for a textbook for the nurses. In 1964, Meltzer, Kitchell, and Pinneo collaborated to construct specific cardiac knowledge for nurses in *Intensive Coronary Care: A Manual for Nurses*. This textbook of more than 200 pages was a far cry from the twelve-page booklet on arrhythmias mimeographed at Bethany.[67]

AN EXPANDED ROLE FOR NURSING

Having received advanced training, these "cardiac specialist nurses" were expected to assume new responsibilities heretofore considered outside their scope. As described by Pinneo, "The nurses' role is more complex than that of the usual hospital nurse. By means of cardiac monitoring, and bedside observation, the nurse identifies complications at their onset and initiates stipulated emergency treatment for those which are life-threatening."[68]

Equipped with their new knowledge and skills, the young nurses enhanced their usual care for cardiac patients. But they did not discard what they already knew and practiced. Particularly, they did not change the routine protocols they had been instituting for MI patients for many years. Like the Bethany nurses, CCU nurses at Presbyterian enforced doctors' orders for complete bed rest for MI patients. In addition they withheld caffeinated coffee and iced beverages (thought to cause arrhythmias and vasoconstriction). During the patient's entire hospital stay, the nurses also provided psychological support for both patient and family.[69] "Skin care," historically a primary concern of nurses, was also a focus of CCU nursing. According to Janice Lufkin, "The first EKG monitoring leads were the round metal ones. We had to clean the skin and apply tincture of Benzoin and tape them onto the patient. The skin would get irritated, so we would have to do skin care."[70]

However, the new environment with its high tech equipment, combined with the expectations outlined in Meltzer's research project, demanded that the nurses expand their traditional role. In the early days of the unit's existence, the primary purpose of the CCU project was to determine if an immediate response by the nurses to medical emergencies, particularly cardiac arrest, could save lives. Since each minute of delay could be life-threatening, autonomy in decision making during those emergencies was essential. So was the authority to treat the patient. As Pinneo would later explain:

> Utilizing this unique combination of clinical assessment and cardiac monitoring, the nurse makes independent decisions. She determines those situations requiring her immediate intervention to save life prior to the physicians' arrival or those situations that warrant calling the physician and waiting for his evaluation. It is in these precious moments that the patient's life may literally be in the hands of the nurse.[71]

What was new was the fact that nurses had to move from simply collecting data and reporting their findings, as they had long been doing when they took temperatures and blood pressures, to acting on their own assessment of the data when necessary, prior to reporting it to a physician. In essence, the nurses expanded their role to include curing as well as caring. Meltzer clearly understood the implications of extending the responsibilities of the nurse from the caring to the curing role. Discussing the change in 1970, he identified it as critical to the new "scientific team approach," noting: "That the physician delegates unusual authority to the nurse in this team approach to care is one of the most distinguishing characteristics of the system of intensive coronary care."[72] Later, reflecting on what had occurred he stated in the introduction to the second edition of his *Textbook of Coronary Care* in 1972:

> Until World War II even the recording of blood pressure was considered outside the nursing sphere and was the responsibility of a physician. As late as 1962, when coronary care was introduced, most hospitals did not permit their nursing staff to perform venipunctures or to start intravenous infusions. That nurses could interpret the electrocardiograms and defibrillate patients indeed represented a radical change for all concerned.[73]

STANDING ORDERS

In addition to the cardiac monitoring and emergency CPR, nurses also assumed other tasks formerly performed by physicians, as they worked in the CCU. Some of the responsibilities were documented in "standard order sets," a list of medical procedures written ahead of time to cover foreseeable circumstances in which the nurse might have to initiate treatment in the absence of a physician. Based on such "standing orders," nurses attached patients to EKG machines, inserted intravenous lines to provide fluids, performed venipunctures to draw blood samples, dispensed emergency medications, and administered oxygen. In addition, they conducted ongoing physical assessments of the patient's condition and explained the care to the family.[74] In a 1965 presentation, Rose Pinneo described the nurse's role during the process of admitting a patient to the CCU:

> Mr. J., a 75-year-old man, was brought to the coronary care unit after a myocardial infarction attack at home. He was dyspneic on admission and had severe chest pain accompanied by anxiety. In evaluating Mr. J., while making him comfortable, the nurse realized that his chest pain must be relieved before she proceeded with any other measures. Therefore, she administered an ordered narcotic. Since dyspnea was another obvious problem, she started oxygen therapy by nasal canula and evaluated its effectiveness in relieving the dyspnea. As soon as possible, she applied chest electrodes and connected them by wires to cardiac monitors, meanwhile explaining the monitoring concept to Mr. J and his family in understandable terms. After turning on the monitor, she could see the electrocardiogram pattern on the oscilloscope and in written form on a rhythm strip. Mr. J. was in sinus tachycardia on admission. Since the rate was not dangerously high, the nurse decided to observe this arrhythmia further before calling the doctor. When the doctor arrived, one hour later, the nurse conferred, with him concerning her observations and assisted him with the physical examination She then carried out his orders by drawing specimens for blood chemistry determinations, taking a full 12 lead EKG and starting the drug program.[75]

AFTER MIDNIGHT

What nurses could do after midnight was clearly different from what they could do at times when physicians were present in the CCU. Defibrillating patients was a classic example. During the day and in the evening, there was usually a physician available who could defibrillate a patient whose cardiac rhythm had degenerate to ventricular fibrillation. After midnight, defibrillating a patient was often up to the nurse. Presbyterian Hospital did have interns and residents on call during the night. However, they did not sleep in the CCU but "catnapped wherever they could find an empty bed. Sometimes this was in the intensive care unit, and sometimes in a bed across the hall from the CCU."[76] As a result, there was often a delay in a resident's arrival in the unit in response to a Code. According to Lynn Warner, "I defibrillated many patients. I worked at night of course, so I was there first." Janice Lufkin agreed, noting, "mostly I defibrillated at night when no one was there right away. Sometimes the doctor was away from the unit, in the ER admitting a patient or in the ICU."[77]

Even when a resident or intern was present, the nurse might have to take the lead in treating the patient because some of the CCU nurses soon knew more than the house staff about the interpretation of cardiac arrhythmias and the necessary treatments. Head nurse Janice Lufkin recalled:

> We soon got experience with the rhythm strips. The interns would even come up the stairs from the ER and ask if we could read the rhythm strip of an ER patient or interpret their EKG. They would ask if they should admit the patient. We were good at the rhythms, but just ok with the 12 lead EKGs. We could recognize the basics, like ST elevation in some leads . . . the obvious MI. And then we would tell them what to do.[78]

Sometimes the house staff's inexperience was a problem. CCU nurse Lynn Warner recalled one instance: "We were giving Dilantin IV for ventricular tachycardia . . . the residents would try to help, but they would forget to use Normal Saline to mix it in, and the medications would precipitate in the IV line."[79]

By 1970, Meltzer did not mince words when discussing the relationship between house staff and CCU nurses, writing:

> The unique role of the CCU nurse and her status on the team should be carefully explained to the house staff. As might be anticipated, the traditional physician–nurse relationship may become distorted in this setting when the nurse is assuming duties and responsibilities beyond those generally expected of nurses . . . the wise house officer will recognize their judgment and expertise.[80]

JUSTIFYING THE NEW SKILLS

The CCU nurses at Presbyterian readily accepted the new cardiac technology but explained it as an extension of their powers of observation. Lynn Warner recalled: "The monitors were just another piece of clinical information . . . that was how Rose presented it to us. I thought it was exciting—especially when you checked an apical pulse and you could see on the monitor just what you'd heard with your stethoscope!"[81] Rose Pinneo captured the essence of how they used the equipment in a 1972 article in which she discussed the nurses' relationship to the monitors:

> As valuable as they are, however, cardiac monitors will never supplant the well prepared nurse, but they serve as tools that extend human

observations of the heart's activation. By deliberately and systemati-
cally seeking clinical signs and symptoms of cardiac problems through
direct observations, the nurse is able to correlate these findings with
those obtained from the cardiac monitor.[82]

THE BLURRY LINE

These first units were as much an experiment on nurses—to see if they
could do it—as they were about decreasing mortality in AMI patients.
The experiment about nurses' roles was a success. It was clear that nurses
could and would learn new skills and expand their scope of practice.
They could also be assertive, take responsibility for their actions, and
acquire medical knowledge. In so doing they did in fact elevate their
status from physicians' handmaidens to emerging nurse specialists. But
despite claims of collegial status in the literature, and despite the fact that
they were indeed members of the scientific team, they were not really
equals. Their gender, age, and socioeconomic status as nurses would
influence their ability to be accepted by physicians as colleagues.
Nonetheless, the professional relationship between CCU nurses and
physicians was quite different in some respects from the traditional
nurse/physician relationship. These young nurses made independent decisions in emergency situations. They experienced a new level of autonomy
and gained a new level of respect. If the physicians did not like the nurses'
new role, they either did not express their feelings or perhaps only discussed them in private with their colleagues. The nurses reported no
problems and in fact felt that their new role was well received.[83]

Some aspects of their role did not change. In fact, the boundary lines
between medicine and nursing remained blurry. Even though the nurses
worked from standing order sets, and even though they diagnosed cardiac arrhythmias and selected the appropriate treatment, they did not
have the legal authority to prescribe medications. Instead, during the
night when no physician was available, the nurses made treatment decisions for life-threatening arrhythmias based on the standing orders,
administered drugs, and wrote verbal orders for them in the patient's
record, relying on the fact that the doctors would sign the orders when
they made rounds in the morning.

Undeniably, the implementation of the cutting edge technology and
the new knowledge brought a shift in responsibilities for nursing, expanding the boundaries of what was considered within their scope of practice.
That shift occurred gradually and unsteadily as the decade of the 1960s
progressed. Conflicting expectations coincided as new duties were combined with traditional ones. CCU nurses who still needed a physician's

order for a specific diet for their post-MI patients were entrusted with the authority to identify a fatal cardiac arrhythmia. On the other hand, the staff nurse who had never before dared call a physician directly during the night was now not only calling him, but reporting that she had defibrillated his patient or given a bolus of lidocaine intravenously. Nurses who had been "ordered to care" now stepped over the nursing practice domain line into the realm of scientific medicine and "cured" the patient's arrhythmias—in dramatic lifesaving moments.[84] In so doing, they set the stage for continued expansion of nursing's scope of practice.

NOTES

1. Chapman was past president of the American Heart Association (AHA) and Professor of Medicine, Texas Southwestern University Medical School, Dallas. Carleton B. Chapman, "Conference Summary," paper presented at the New York Heart Association Conference "Impact of a Coronary Care Unit on Hospitals, Medical Practice and the Community," March 15, 1966. *USPHS Proceedings of the New York Heart Association Conference: Impact of a Coronary Care Unit on Hospitals, Medical Practice, and Community* (Arlington, Va: Heart Disease Control Program, National Center for Chronic Disease Control).

2. Harry S. Truman, "Statement by the President on the Toll Taken by Heart Diseases," 7 February 1949; www.whisclestop.org/50yr_archive/50yr020749_state- ment.htm.

3. "Lyndon Johnson: Out for This Session," headline, *New York Times,* 3 July 1955.

4. "Eisenhower Is in Hospital With 'Mild' Heart Attack; His Condition Called 'Good'," headline, *New York Times,* 25 September 1955.

5. See, for example, Clarence G. Lasby, *Eisenhower's Heart Attack: How Ike Beat Heart Disease and Held on to the Presidency* (Lawrence: University Press of Kansas, 1997); "President's Attack Found 'Neither Mild nor Serious': Condition Satisfactory," *New York Times,* September 26; "Eisenhower Is Improving; Chance of Full Recovery Called 'Reasonably Good,'" *New York Times,* September 27; "President Spends Day Without Use of Oxygen Tent," *New York Times,* September 29; "Physicians to Let President Initial Two Papers Tonight," *New York Times,* September 30; "A Look at the World's Week: The President's Sudden Illness," *Life,* October 3, 32; "Eisenhower's MI," *Life,* October 19, 35–43; "The World Watches a Window," *Life,* October 10; "President Flies Back to Capital; Shows No Fatigue," *New York Times,* November 12; cover story (Ike in wheelchair), *Life,* November 14, 71–74.

6. Paul Dudley White, MD, "the most famous heart specialist in the world," was called to Denver on 25 September 1955 to examine the president. "President's Specialist Top Man in His Field," headline, *Life,* 10 October 1955, 157; "Heart Attack: The President's Ailment, Coronary Thrombosis, Is the Worst U.S. Killer, Deadlier Than Cancer," Life, 10 October 1955, 150.

7. Lasby, *Eisenhower's Heart Attack,* 87.

8. For Shepard, see, for example, *Life,* 19 May 1961; for Glenn, see *Life,* 9 March 1962.

9. Joel D. Howell, *Technology in the Hospital: Transforming Patient Care in the Early Twentieth Century* (Baltimore: Johns Hopkins University Press, 1996).

10. James Jude, William B. Kouwenhoven, and G. Guy Knickerbocker, "Cardiac Arrest," *Journal of the American Medical Association* 178, no. 11 (16 December 1961): 1063–70 (hereafter cited as *JAMA*).

11. William B. Kouwenhoven, James R. Jude, and G. Guy Knickerbocker, "Closed Chest Cardiac Massage," *JAMA* 173 (9 July 1960): 1064.

12. Kouwenhoven et al., "Closed Chest Cardiac Massage," 1067.

13. Claude S. Beck, "Resuscitation for Cardiac Standstill and Ventricular Fibrillation Occurring During Operation," *American Journal of Surgery* 54 (October 1941): 273; Claude S. Beck, E. C. Wechesser, and F. M. Barry, "Fatal Heart Attack and Successful Defibrillation," *JAMA* 161, no. 5 (2 June 1956): 434-36.

14. Claude S. Beck, W. Prithard, and H. Feil, "Ventricular Fibrillation of Long Duration Abolished by Electric Shock," *JAMA* 135, no. 15 (1947): 985-86.

15. Mildred Crawley, "Care of the Patient With Myocardial Infarction," *American Journal of Nursing* 61, no. 2 (February 1961): 68 (hereafter cited as *AJN*).

16. Hughes W. Day, "History of Coronary Care Units," *American Journal of Cardiology* 30 (1972): 4057; Judith Stuart, "Hartford Coronary Care Unit, Bethany Medical Center, Twenty Years Later," unpublished manuscript, 1982, Keeling Collection, Center for Nursing Historical Inquiry, University of Virginia (hereafter cited as KC, CNHI).

17. "History of Bethany Medical Center," photocopy, Public Relations Department, Bethany Medical Center, KC, CNHI.

18. Judith Stuart, RN, BA, CCRN, interview by author, Kansas City, Missouri, 22 July 1999; transcript KC, CNHI.

19. Hughes W. Day, "An Intensive Coronary Care Area," *Diseases of the Chest* 44, no. 4 (1963): 423–27.

20. Day, "Intensive Coronary Care Area," 424.

21. Judith Stuart, "Hartford Coronary Care Unit". KC, CNHI.

22. Hughes W. Day, "History of Coronary Care Units," *American Journal of Cardiology* 30 (1972): 405.

23. Judith S. Jacobson, *The Greatest Good: A History of the John A. Hartford Foundation* (New York: John A. Hartford Foundation, 1984).

24. Presbyterian was a 325-bed institution. Approximately 170 patients were admitted each year with AMI. Lawrence E. Meltzer and J. Roderick Kitchell, Grant Proposal NU 00096-01, Division of Nursing, Bureau of Sate Services-Community Health, 1962, 11 (hereafter cited as "Grant"; Pinneo Collection, CNHI (hereafter cited as PC, CNHI).

25. Paul M. Zoll, Arthur J. Linenthal, and Leona R. Norman Zarsky, "Ventricular Fibrillation: Treatment and Prevention by External Electric Currents," *New England Journal of Medicine* 262, no. 3 (21 January 1960): 105-12.

26. Meltzer and Kitchell, "Grant," 6.

27. Eleanor Lambertsen, *Nursing Team Organization and Functioning* (New York: Teachers College Bureau of Publications, Columbia University, 1953); Carl Mosher, *Presbyterian Medical Center Annual Report, 1966*; box 94/02, Main Presbyterian Medical Center Collection, 1841–1996, University of Pennsylvania Archives (hereafter cited as PMC Collection), 13.

28. Meltzer and Kitchell, "Grant," 6.

29. Lawrence E. Meltzer, in *The Current Status of Intensive Coronary Care: A Symposium Presented by the American College of Cardiology and Presbyterian-University of Pennsylvania Medical Center, Philadelphia, July 15, 1966* (New York: Charles Press, 1966), 4.

30. Lawrence E. Meltzer, Rose Pinneo, and J. Roderick Kitchell, *Intensive Coronary Care: A Manual for Nurses* (New York: Charles Press, 1965).

31. Rose Pinneo, "A New Dimension in Nursing: Intensive Coronary Care," *American Association of Industrial Nurses Journal* (February 1967): 7–10.

32. Meltzer and Kitchell, "Grant," 7.

33. Meltzer and Kitchell, "Grant," 9.

34. Meltzer and Kitchell, "Grant," 11.
35. Meltzer et al., *Intensive Coronary Care*, preface.
36. Meltzer and Kitchell, "Grant," 6.
37. Carl Mosher, folder 5, box 47, PMC Collection.
38. Meltzer and Kitchell, "Grant," 12.
39. Faye Abdellah and E. Josephine Starchan, "Progressive Patient Care," *AJN* 59, no. 5 (May 1959): 649–55; Faye Abdellah, personal interview by author, 30 October 2000, USPHS Graduate School of Nursing, Bethesda, MD.
40. "Highlights of 1963: Presbyterian Hospital in Philadelphia," box 64, 63/1, PMC Collection.
41. Rose Pinneo, RN, MSN, interview by author, Sebring, Florida, 19 November 1999; transcript in PC, CNHI.
42. Karen Campbell, a 1963 diploma graduate of Presbyterian Hospital School of Nursing, worked in the CCU about 1964 and 1965, after working in the new Wright Wing II (a general medical-surgical unit). She received her BSN from PSU and subsequently worked in research at the University of Pennsylvania Children's Hospital testing Merck vaccines. Telephone interview author, August 2001; transcript in KCCNHI. Lufkin, a 1962 diploma graduate from Presbyterian Hospital School of Nursing, worked for a few months after graduation in the eye and ear ward and then as a graduate nurse in the Maximum Care Unit. She rotated to the new two-bed CCU in January 1963 when it opened. She began to work there full-time and became head nurse after Helen Haugh resigned. In 1966 she left the CCU and entered the Navy. Telephone interview by author, 13 November 2001; transcript in KC, CNHI.
43. Rose Pinneo, "Nursing Care of the Cardiac Patient," paper presented at the Third Clinical Nursing Conference, sponsored by the AHA Nursing Committee and the ANA Conference Group on Medical-Surgical Nursing, Miami Beach Florida, October, 1965; PC, CNHI.
44. Meltzer and Kitchell, "Grant," 8.
45. Lynn Warner, a 1963 diploma graduate of Presbyterian Hospital School of Nursing, worked in the first group of nurses who staffed the Presbyterian CCU. Her previous experience included a year of night shift work in the Maximum Care Unit at Presbyterian. Subsequently, she received a PhD in nursing. Telephone interview by author, 20 August 2001; transcript in KC, CNHI.
46. In addition to the primary study of the effectiveness of a CCU on MI mortality, Pinneo and Meltzer collected data on two smaller projects: the patients' reaction to CCU and nursing personnel. Pinneo, unpublished data, PC, CNHI.
47. Lufkin interview, 2001.
48. Rose Pinneo received her BA from Maryville College, Maryville, Tennessee, her diploma from Johns Hopkins Hospital, and her MS in Education from the University of Pennsylvania. She was Assistant Educational Director and Medical Nursing Instructor, West Jersey Hospital, Camden, New Jersey, and Medical-Surgical Instructor, University of Pennsylvania. Curriculum Vitae, Rose Pinneo, PC, CNHI; Pinneo interview, 2000.
49. Miki Iwata began working in the CCU at Presbyterian Hospital in Philadelphia in September 1963, after the unit had been open for about eight months. Iwata was one of the original six who worked in the unit. She was twenty-two and had one year of experience as a nurse after receiving her diploma from Presbyterian in 1962. She left in 1966 to enter the Navy. Later she attended the University of Pennsylvania, where she received a BSN in 1972. She was certified as a Family Nurse Practitioner at the University of San Diego in 1975, and as a Surface Warfare Medical Officer in 1993. She worked in the Navy Nurse Corps for 29 years and retired in 1995 as a captain. In the 1990s she was stationed on a ship in the Persian Gulf during Desert Storm.

Telephone interview by author, 30 October 2001; transcript KC, CNHI. Also Campbell interview, 2001; Warner interview, 2001; Lufkin interview, 2001.

50. Pinneo, unpublished data, 17. PC, CNHI.

51. Other nurses who worked in the CCU at Presbyterian included Mary E. Taglianerti, Diane Schmidt, Judith Litman, Sara Tuttle, Barbara P. Malkoff, Elaine L. Sellers, Teresa Vandiver Coffey, Helen L. Haugh Morita, Karen W. Campbell, Helen W. Jones, Janice M. Lufkin, Miki Iwata, Ann Tuckner, Donna Lauck, Sheila Hickey, and Lynn Warner. Pinneo, unpublished data, 17.

52. Pinneo interview, 2000.

53. Iwata interview, 2001.

54. Warner interview, 2001; Lufkin interview, 2001. According to an unpublished report, the data collected on the hourly status report included the following: (1) patient identification number; (2) day of the study, report number, and hour; (3) nurse on duty, type of nursing care administered; (4) emotional status of patient; (5) pulse rate and stability, blood pressure, temperature, respirations, clinical state, and state of consciousness; (6) procedures or intravenous fluid treatments administered; (7) food intake and elimination; gastrointestinal disturbances; (8) incidence of coronary and noncoronary pain; (9) presence of hospital staff and/or visitors; (10) type of drugs administered; distinction between routine and emergency drugs; (11) heart rhythm; presence of cardiac arrhythmias or conduction system disturbances and time of onset and course. M. Ferrigan, Rose Pinneo, Lawrence E. Meltzer, D. D. Yuu, and J. Roderick Kitchell, "Acute Myocardial Infarction: Methods of Data Accumulation," 6 December 1967, PC, CNHI.

55. Lufkin interview, 2001; Ferrigan et al., "Acute Myocardial Infarction."

56. Ferrigan et al., "Acute Myocardial Infarction," 1967. Basic laboratory studies included CBC, urinalysis, sedimentation rate, cholesterol, uric acid, enzyme studies, and prothrombin times. Meltzer and Kitchell, "Grant," 8.

57. Ferrigan et al., "Acute Myocardial Infarction."

58. Iwata interview, 2001.

59. Rose Pinneo, "Historical Perspectives of Coronary Care Units," speech given in Chicago, June 1981; PC, CNHI.

60. Rose Pinneo, "Mastering Monitoring". Nursing 72 (1972 reprint): 1–4. PC, CNHI.

61. Rose Pinneo, "Training of Personnel," undated manuscript of speech. PC, CNHI.

62. Lufkin interview, 2001.

63. Iwata interview, 2001.

64. Pinneo interview, 2000.

65. Pinneo interview, 2000.

66. Lufkin interview, 2001; Warner interview, 2000; Iwata interview, 2001.

67. Hughes Day, Training Manual on Basic EKG: Patterns for Nursing, Judith Stuart, RN, 1962, personal papers, Judith Stuart Collection, CNHI (hereafter cited as JS, CNHI).

68. Pinneo, "Mastering Monitoring," 4.

69. Campbell interview, 2001; Rose Pinneo, "Machines in Perspective: Nursing in a Coronary Care Unit," AJN 65, no. 2 (1965); Jean Hayter, "Acute Myocardial Infarction," AJN 59 (November 1959): 1602–4.

70. Lufkin interview, 2001.

71. Pinneo, "Mastering Monitoring."

72. Lawrence E. Meltzer, Rose Pinneo, and J. Roderick Kitchell, Intensive Coronary Care: A Manual for Nurses, rev. ed. (Philadelphia: Charles Press, 1972), 8.

73. Lawrence E. Meltzer and Arend J. Dunning, Textbook of Coronary Care, 2nd ed. (Philadelphia: Charles Press, 1972), 23.

74. Pinneo, "Machines in Perspective"; Lufkin interview, 2001; Warner interview, 2001.

75. Pinneo, "Nursing Care of the Cardiac Patient," 3.

76. Lufkin interview, 2001.
77. Warner interview, 2001; Lufkin interview, 2001.
78. Lufkin interview, 2001.
79. Warner interview, 2001.
80. Meltzer et al., *Intensive Coronary Care* (1970), 2.
81. Warner interview, 2001.
82. Rose Pinneo, "Cardiac Monitoring," *Nursing Clinics of North America* 7, no. 3 (1972): 457.
83. Lufkin interview 2001; Warner interview, 2001; Iwata interview, 2000.
84. Susan M. Reverby, *Ordered to Care: The Dilemma of American Nursing, 1850–1945* (New York: Cambridge University Press, 1987); Divina Allen, "The Nursing-Medical Boundary: A Negotiated Order?" *Sociology of Health and Illness* 19, no. 94 (1997): 498–520.

SECTION 4

Work and Knowledge

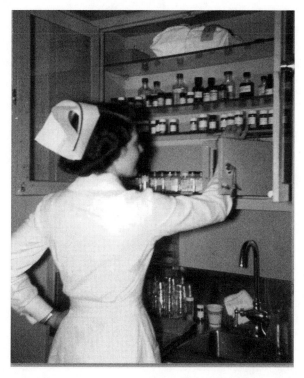

A nurse at St. Mary's Hospital in Rochester, New
York, circa 1950. Reprinted with the permission of the
Barbara Bates Center for the Study of the History of
Nursing.

Introduction

Joan E. Lynaugh

Four of the readings in this section span more than a century; each is a firsthand perspective on ideas influencing practice, changes in expectations placed on nurses, new demands for knowledge, nurses' changing self-image, and links between work, authority, and knowledge. The fifth reading offers a historical analysis of how specific elements of nurses' work are influenced by the context within which that work takes place.

We can see that at least three themes emerge from a review of nursing work and knowledge in the historical literature. First, there is the long series of experiments intended to protect patients from harm. Nurses tried to standardize the work of other nurses by setting rigid rules and detailed procedures. Then, with the same safety goal in mind, the emphasis changed toward developing nurses' critical thinking skills to individualize care and cope with novel clinical problems. The next theme is the search for acceptable ideals, values, and standards of conduct. Here the goal is to assure the public that nurses will conduct themselves in such a way that the public can have confidence in their work. The search for ideals, values, and standards began with nineteenth-century treatises on character and continued on to late twentieth-century nursing theories and definitions. And finally, we see in these chapters the continuing reality in which nursing work and knowledge may be slowed or stimulated but is inevitably directed by the context of the times. The readings are arranged more or less chronologically; that does not imply any kind of progressive change over time. It does suggest the permanence of these issues.

Let us start with Agnes Brennan, superintendent of the Training School at Bellevue Hospital, New York City. Speaking before the National Conference of Charities and Corrections in 1894, she sought to explain to her audience of government leaders and philanthropists that the goal of the Training School was to help pupils become thoroughly efficient nurses. Brennan struggled to convey her sense of the balance between theory and the work nurses did as she confronted the unspoken question of whether nurses needed special education at all. "An uneducated woman may become a good nurse, but never an intelligent one," "Theory in conjunction with practice is what we want," and, "Theory fortifies the practical: practice stimulates and retains the theoretical."[1]

Next, to sample the reconceptualization of the work of nurses during the middle years of the twentieth century, read Frances Reiter and Virginia Henderson. Frances Rieter, who coined the term *nurse-clinician,* worked to clarify and amplify the meaning of nursing. Her 1966 discussion was influenced by the then prevailing sense that nurses were not engaged in direct care and that technology separated nurses from patients; she tried to explain how nurses and physicians share responsibility for patients. Reiter's emphasis on coordination, continuity, and collaboration envisioned a highly responsible role for the educated and experienced nurse; a role that certainly transcended the expectations of the time.[2] Henderson, who was older than Reiter, reflected on her own career and how her philosophy of nursing developed. Her 1961 definition of nursing spelled out a distinct set of responsibilities for nurses in relation to their patients. She went on to detail what she called the unique function of the nurse and how that might relate to other caregivers in varying patient situations. This particular chapter is enhanced by its republication with a 1991 addendum reflecting Henderson's ideas 25 years after she originally published them.[3]

Margaret Sovie took aim at distractions nurses face in practice which she argued, undermined their ability to give quality care. In her 1989 article she targeted the then ubiquitous nursing care plans and "SOAP" notes as major time wasters. One of her main aims was to connect the caregivers and the patient using bedside documentation that was shared, useful, and significant. Implicit in her critique was the constant pressure to ensure high-quality nursing in a time of shortage. She found a solution through empowering nurses to use their knowledge free of impediments set up by administrative fiats and unexamined work rules. Sovie's comments highlight the continuing complex associations among nurse, patient, and institution and remind us that knowing how to nurse is not enough. Relationships, institutions, and leadership to fix problems are all necessary if knowledgeable care is to reach the patient.[4]

The first four chapters were all drawn from the literature of nursing. In contrast, the last paper in this group is a historical analysis of a clinical problem. Brush and Capezuti prove, using historical data, that an element of practice, i.e., using siderails on beds, is an outgrowth of legal and medical ideas rather than a nursing intervention. Their study of nursing literature and legal cases published in the nursing literature is an excellent example of how historical research can cast new insights on current problems in practice.[5] More historical work of this type is needed to help us better understand the why as well as the how of nurses' work.

It is often said that the creation of new knowledge and the interpretation of old knowledge defines scholarship. These chapters reveal how knowledge and nurses' work weave together, how new ideas change the work, and how it is the work that drives nurses to reexamine old ideas and discover new and better ways to care for others.

NOTES

1. Agnes Brennan, "Theory and Practice," Proceedings of the National Conference of Charities and Correction, Nashville, Tennessee, May 23–29, 1894. Ed. Isobel C. Barrows (Boston, Mass. 1894).
2. Frances Reiter, "The Nurse-Clinician," *International Nursing Review* 13, no. 4 (1966): 62–71 (also in AJN, February, 1966).
3. Virginia A. Henderson, "Development of a Personal Concept," *The Nature of Nursing: A Definition and Its Implications for Practice, Research, and Education: Reflections After 25 Years,* 9–33 (New York: National League for Nursing Press, 1991).
4. Margaret D. Sovie, "Clinical Nursing Practices and Patient Outcomes: Evaluation, Evolution, and Revolution," *Nursing Economics* 7, no. 2 (March/April 1989): 79–85.
5. Barbara L. Brush and Elizabeth Capezuti, "Historical Analysis of Siderail Use in American Hospitals," *Journal of Nursing Scholarship* 33, no. 4 (2001): 381–84.

CHAPTER 13

Theory and Practice

Agnes S. Brennan

Twenty-one years ago it was said in New York that "no refined, educated woman could go through the severe practical training required to fit her to enter the profession of a trained nurse," whereas today in some of our schools a faint echo of the cry for higher education of women is heard. We take it as a sign of the times, but hope that, when taking up the higher, the lower education of women will not be neglected. The young woman who enters a training school is supposed to do so for the purpose of becoming at the end of two or three years' training a thoroughly efficient nurse and an intelligent assistant to the attending physician or surgeon; and the aim of all good schools is in every way to help, assist, and train the pupils to become such.

Now, no woman of education and refinement would spend two years in a large city hospital (and only those who have done so can understand what that means) unless she had some compensation in the form of theoretical teaching and study.

An uneducated woman may become a good nurse, but never an intelligent one. She can obey orders conscientiously and understand thoroughly a sick person's needs; but, should an emergency arise, where is she? She works through her feelings, and therefore lacks judgment.

We have all heard of, and no doubt have met, the nurse who was "born, not made," as is the artist and musician. But it takes years of

Originally published in the Proceedings of the National Conference of Charities and Correction, 21st Annual Session, Nashville, Tennessee, May 23–29, 1894. Ed. by Isabel C. Barrows, Boston, 1894.

patient study in either profession before one can excel; and the cool hand
and light touch which are popularly supposed to belong to these heaven-
born nurses will count for little if they cannot mix solutions or give an
intelligent report of symptoms and results.

In this progressive age, training schools cannot afford to stand still
any more than other schools and colleges; and each year the graduates
should be more skilled, more cultured, and for this reason more practical.
A nurse can always take better care of a patient if she understands the
pathology of the disease her patient is suffering from. When typhoid,
under no consideration would she allow him to help himself, neither
would she in pneumonia turn him on his well side, etc.; and I hold that
all persons in charge of pupil nurses should strive to give a reason for and
explain why this is done or that is not done in each individual case.

The usual length of training is two years; and in that time much has
to be learned both practically and theoretically, but we must discriminate, and not sacrifice one for the other.

I have heard the study of the microscope advocated as necessary for
the thorough education of the pupil nurse. I acknowledge it to be a most
interesting and instructive study, but one that requires a great deal of time
and much patience. So, unless the hospital be a small one, and the
patients few, the pupil nurse will not have the necessary time to devote to
it, and would gain much more useful experience if she spent the half-hour
she had to spare for studying the character of the pulse, in the different
patients in the ward, or finding out just why some nurses can always see
at a glance that this patient requires her pillow turned or the next one her
position changed.

These are all simple things, necessary to the comfort and well-being
of the patient, wherein the microscope cannot help, no matter how proficient the nurse may be in its use. And, should the pupil practice her profession after graduating, she will find that even at a private case she has
no time to use it. Neither would the attending physician expect her to any
more than he would to diagnose the case or write prescriptions.

In the universities and colleges of the world the intention now is to
make the teaching far more practical than heretofore. This is particularly
so in medical colleges. We all know that the young physician (who most
likely has stood first, and taken all the honors of his class), when he enters
the hospital as *interne,* is utterly unfitted, in spite of his splendid theoretical knowledge, to put into practice what he can so fluently discuss.

Now, with the nurse it is different; and just here the word "trained"
comes in. From the very first day she enters the school, she begins with
the practical, and takes up the theoretical to enable her to give intelligent
care to her patients, and to expand her mind by contact with greater
minds, in lectures and books, not in any way to make her pedantic or

superficial, but to fit her for immediate usefulness when she is graduated. Theory in conjunction with practice is what we want; and, although it is undeniable that theory has done more to elevate nursing than any amount of clinical practice *alone* could have done, still we must remember that "too much reading tends to mental confusion."

Practice helps to impress and retain in the memory the knowledge obtained by theory, otherwise forgotten without the practical application. Any one who has been ill knows that the height of good nursing consists principally in what is done for the patient's comfort, outside of the regular orders. A theoretical nurse performs her duty in a perfunctory manner, and may carry out the doctor's orders to the letter; but the patient recognizes there is something lacking, and we know that it is the skilled touch, the deft handling, the keenness to detect changes and symptoms, the ready tact, the patience, the power of controlling her feelings and temper, self-reliance, the kindly sympathy for the sorrowing, and the peculiar power of soothing suffering which can be acquired only by much practice; and a nurse without these attributes, despite her wide theoretic knowledge and teaching, will never be a successful one.

Now, with our superior intelligence and advantages, we must not ignore the necessity of possessing a large amount of *good, plain common sense* to form a basis for the education of our nurses, which will hold the theoretical and practical training in a state of equilibrium. Theory fortifies the practical: practice strengthens and retains the theoretical.

CHAPTER 14

The Nurse-Clinician

Frances Reiter

Because this term is being discussed so widely today, the Journal asked the nurse who coined it to explore its meaning. Her beliefs about what a nurse-clinician could mean to the profession, based on the philosophy of nursing she has developed in her 35 years of experience, seem to us to hold one answer to that age-old question: "What is nursing?"

Some 23 years ago in a speech I was giving, I used the term "nurse-clinician" to describe a kind of nurse that I thought was needed by both patients and the profession. So far as I know, the term had not been used before. Today, however, as so many of us struggle to identify nursing's nature, its practice, and its directions, we hear the term "nurse-clinician" being used with increasing frequency.

Of course, not everyone means the same thing by it. I'm not even sure that I mean quite the same thing today by *nurse-clinician* as I did in 1943. For me, it is a concept that has been gradually evolving during my almost 40 years of nursing experience: a distillate of my ideas as they have been added to, enriched, tempered, and altered by those of others, I cannot present my concept of the nurse-clinician without also presenting some of the nursing philosophy that underlies it. I believe the time has come—may, indeed, be overdue—for us to reexamine our total

Originally published in *American Journal of Nursing* 66, no. 2 (February 1966): 274–80.

value system. So this discussion will necessarily include some of my own personal and philosophic nursing values. Paramount among these—and integrally associated with my concept of the nurse-clinician—is my unalterable conviction that *practice* is the absolute primary function of our profession. In recent years, however, I have found to my distress that it is necessary for me to identify what I mean by "practice." To me, it simply means the direct care of patients, but I find "practice" being more and more used to include administration, teaching, and supervision.

Now I admit that these three functions are essential underpinnings for good patient care and for total health services. But I consider them as secondary to patient care, and I deplore the tendency to use the word "practice" as encompassing these secondary functions. To me this is a devaluation of nursing's primary function: patient care. But, since this is the way the word is now used, I will alter my terminology accordingly and distinguish what I mean by referring to it as "clinical practice."

By clinical practice, I mean those personal services carried out at the patient's side—in contact with him and in behalf of him and his family. There are some indirect services in this category, too: those activities carried out in conjunction with other nurses or with other professions—away from the patient but still directly in his behalf.

In our present complex hospital situation, direct nursing care is—or, should be—the one area over which nursing has complete control. And it seems to me that, depending upon what we do in this area, we write our own destiny and that of the future of nursing. Hence, it is my conviction that the nurse-clinician, and the profession of nursing itself, must always remain closely identified with nursing practice.

CLINICAL COMPETENCE

Clinical competence, as I see it, has three dimensions—I call them ranges of function, depth of understanding, and breadth of services. Some of the personnel caring for patients will be prepared and proficient in one or more aspects of these several dimensions, but the nurse-clinician must be competent in all three.

Let's look at the ranges of function first. These I see as care, cure, and counseling. First, *care:* the fundamental things that we do to make a patient comfortable, the things that he is temporarily unable to do for himself. Early in my student days at Johns Hopkins, I became convinced that personal care of the patient is the heart of nursing practice. This care may be of a physical, palliative, protective, or rehabilitative nature, but it need never be less than personal. Nor need it be less than professional if we use and involve ourselves as we change the patient's position, give him mouth care, or support him as he coughs.

A little later in my career, when I studied at Teachers College, I realized more fully the importance of a second dimension to care—that of the use of basic sciences underlying this care—and I gained a deeper understanding of the rationale that governed what I was doing for my patients. I believe now that there is a body of knowledge underlying care and that we have hardly scratched the surface of it.

My basic nursing, as I had learned it, had of course included the specific treatments that nurses carried out: in those days, the irrigations, the compresses, the medications. But not until I became supervisor of ward teaching and staff education at the Massachusetts General Hospital (MGH) did my concept of this second range of clinical practice—curative nursing—become crystallized.

By curative nursing I mean much more than mere technical expertness in carrying out treatments and pouring medications. I refer, rather, to a much broader group of restorative and rehabilitative activities: to a sound knowledge of the principles on which they are based and of the goals to which they are directed. Curative nursing, as I see it, calls for a special approach—a perception of the medical and therapeutic goals so that nursing care can be tailored accordingly. If this curative range of nursing is to be practiced in close collaboration with the physician, it requires still more depth in the second dimension—understanding of clinical data and medical science.

Why did I become aware of this at MGH? Because I encountered there a kind of nurse, a kind of atmosphere, that I had not perceived before. I was not a peer of those MGH nurse supervisors, so far as cure was concerned. They had something I didn't; a clinical knowledge, competence, and approach that enabled them to function as professional colleagues of the medical staff.

THE NURSE-CLINICIAN

Take the neurologic supervisor, for instance. She not only knew neurologic nursing practice, she knew a great deal about neurology and neurologic medical practice. She worked closely with the chief of staff on patient management and care. She attended the departmental meetings. She was part of the group that planned each new therapy. Every door of knowledge was open to her.

Many of these doors she opened herself, as did the other clinical nursing supervisors there. They read the medical literature, they went on rounds; they sought out knowledge; they had to keep themselves informed about medical-surgical practice so that nursing practice could be integrated with it. Much of their study was self-impelled and self-disciplined. It derived from their own expectations of themselves, from the expectations of their medical colleagues, and from this atmosphere of interdisciplinary exchange, research, and practice.

This kind of knowledge, this kind of nursing, I felt, was exceedingly important so far as full-dimensioned clinical practice was concerned. I was secure in the "care" range of practice and I had thought I was secure in the "cure" range, but here I perceived a much greater span of curative influence. Combine depth of basic science with care and depth of clinical science with cure, I said to myself at the time, and you have a nurse-clinician.

However, as I turned this over in my mind during the next few years—years in which my own insight and understanding were being enriched by psychoanalysis—it became clear to me that there was still a third range to clinical practice. I call this range *counseling* and I know that it too must be based on a deep level of understanding—of perceptiveness and wisdom about the dynamics of human behavior.

By *counseling* I refer to the kind of emotional, intellectual, and psychological support that sometimes borders on the realm of social work but is still a part of professional nursing practice. Within this range, too, I see such nursing responsibilities as health promotion, preventive teaching, working with families, and the full therapeutic use of one's self in relationships with patients.

THE MOTHER ROLE

As the nurse cares for her patient throughout these three ranges—care, cure, and counseling—it seems to me that she is essentially acting as a mother substitute. She is trying to protect him from harm, teaching him to avoid it; she is doing for him only the things that he cannot do for himself; she is comforting him and making him comfortable when he is hurt or ailing; and she is encouraging him in doing the things that will help to grow. This may be oversimplified—but I believe that these mother-like ministrations represent the nucleus of nursing practice and are professional only when the second dimension, that of knowledge, plumbs the wisdom of human motivation.

Now, in the days when nursing was largely a matter of one nurse "specialling" one patient—often, even around the clock—competence in care, cure, and counseling, based on a relatively shallow dimension of nursing knowledge, may have been all the nurse needed in order to serve her patient well. Today, though, with so many separate disciplines involved in the patient's therapy, with so many kinds of personnel providing patient care, and with a complete turnover of these personnel every eight hours, I see a third dimension to clinical competence: the breadth of the services rendered.

Here, too, the services fall into a "three-C" division: coordination, continuity, and collaboration—all in relation to the kinds of programs and persons with whom nurses associate, and all in behalf of the patient.

Thus, it is my concept that nursing—perhaps in the form of the nurse-clinician—is responsible for *coordinating* all the various professional services relating directly to the patient's welfare. I see the nurse-clinician, too, as responsible for *continuity* of care: from one shift, one group of personnel, to another; continuity of care from the hospital to the home; and continuity of nursing care after patients have reached the point of maximum medical benefit—longterm nursing care and treatment.

Collaboration—the third of this group of C's—is, to my mind, the most significant of these services, so far as professional maturity and the development of the nurse-clinician are concerned. In fact, I would consider evidence of the ability to collaborate with medicine the most discriminating index of having attained the stature of nurse-clinician. By this I don't mean simply a capacity to "get along" well with the physician. I mean having the necessary knowledge, attitudes, and perceptions that will enable nursing to work in a collaborative relationship with medicine to achieve the therapeutic, restorative, and rehabilitative goals set for the patient.

Let me illustrate what I mean, and the illustration will cover all of the last three C's—coordination, continuity, and collaboration. There is, in practically all situations, one physician responsible for the medical management of the patient. He may be the patient's personal physician, the resident in charge of the service, or the chief of staff. Whoever he is, *he* is the one who determines the diagnosis and the tests that lead up to it, the therapies, the ultimate medical decisions. Essentially, he is responsible for all of the patient's professional services.

But, when we come to nursing, it is a *group* of nurses and ancillary personnel who are responsible for a patient's care around the clock and through the week. If a nursing decision must be made, there is no one nurse responsible for making it, as there is one doctor. Instead, it will in all likelihood be made by the nurse in charge on the shift when the need for the decision arises. It may not be the best decision, nor made by the best qualified nurse, nor necessarily followed through on successive shifts and days.

But suppose, on the other hand, that there was one nurse with authorized responsibility for nursing practice within a given area. Like the physician, she, too, might be on 24-hour call—for consultation and decision-making whenever nursing practice problems occur. (This idea has been tried at the University of Florida at Gainesville and found workable.) Obviously, she will have to be a very well-qualified nurse—a nurse-clinician.

I like to think of this nurse as a member of the school of nursing faculty. (Here, too, I think I reflect the philosophy of Dorothy Smith, dean of the College of Nursing and chief of nursing practice at the University of Florida College of Nursing; her title exemplifies what I am talking about.) To, me, it is highly appropriate that the faculty member combine these two responsibilities—for practice and for teaching, for I do not believe you can do one without the other.

Let's look a little further at the possible relationships that might exist between the physician and the nurse-clinician. These are based on another of my concepts: that the nature of nursing service is implementation of the total therapeutic regimen.

We have already noted that the doctor is generally considered responsible for all of the patient's varied professional services, even though studies of medical education point out that he isn't really prepared for this coordinating function. But the nurse-clinician, as I see her, is prepared to provide this needed coordination: She must be, if she is truly to implement the total therapeutic regimen. I would like to think of the nurse-clinician as having the abilities to serve as what might be called "clinical nurse associate" to a physician or group of physicians, being on call the same way the physician is and responsible for many decisions concerning the patient's welfare.

Actually, I believe that the nature of the relationship between the doctor and the nurse is different from that obtaining between the doctor and the member of any other professional discipline—social worker or diet therapist, for instance. The social worker has little or no responsibility for helping the diet therapist carry out her objectives, nor does the speech therapist have much to do with supporting the objectives of the social worker. Both doctor and nurse, on the other hand, share responsibility for the patient's total well-being, and this includes the need to coordinate and assess the specific contributions of these other specialties in the patient's best interest.

THE DOCTOR–NURSE RELATIONSHIP

I have already indicated that I think the essence of nursing is its mother-like ministrations. Now I would remind you that the doctor has always been thought of as the good "father" figure. Put these two concepts together and you will see that the relationship between doctor and nurse is—or might be—akin to a parental one: one wherein they share a mutual responsibility for the welfare of patients, just as actual parents do for their children.

This parental relationship between doctor and nurse, it seems to me, is something quite different from the relationship of either one with other members of the professional health family. It is a relationship which—if recognized, cultivated, and utilized—should provide the patient with care that is continuously evaluated and modified to meet his changing needs.

Not too many nurses are prepared to work in this type of interdisciplinary relationship, nor will all doctors welcome or make full use of the nurse-clinician who does have this capacity. But I maintain that only through such a collaborative working together can the patient be best served and nursing achieve its greatest potential.

Finally—and returning again to the breadth of the nurse-clinician's practice—it is not enough for her to be fully proficient in the care of the acutely ill patient, not even enough for her to enjoy the best kind of collaborative relationships in the acute setting. An additional criterion is that the nurse-clinician be competent in practice in all the stages of illness or wellness represented in the various settings in which we find patients today: not just the acute general hospital, but the home, the community, and the long-term facility, to mention the major ones.

It is on this latter setting—the care of the infirm, the aged, the disabled, the chronically ill—that I would place greatest emphasis. Here is the area with the greatest number of patients; here is the area with the smallest number of nurses, relatively and absolutely. Medicine may have done all it can do for these patients. Yet there is so much more to be done with them, so much that falls into the domain of independent nursing functions. I cannot conceive of a nurse-clinician as less than expert in assessing the needs of, and providing care for, patients within this category.

Now let me see if I can describe the nurse-clinician against this background of the dimensions of clinical practice. First, let me emphasize that *nurse-clinician* is a generic title, not a functional one. It describes a "state of being"—an accumulation of a depth of knowledge and experience that might be put to work in any number of positions—provided, of course, that the holder of these qualifications remains actively engaged in nursing practice.

The nurse-clinician, as I see her, is a master practitioner throughout all the dimensions of nursing practice. She is able to provide basic and technical care based on perceptive understanding of the patient's psychobiologic needs. Additionally, she brings to patient care a high degree of discriminative judgment in assessing nursing problems, in determining priorities of care, and in identifying the nursing measures necessary to achieve both immediate therapeutic objectives and long-term rehabilitative goals.

COMMITMENT TO EXCELLENCE

But even more fundamental than the intellectual qualifications of the nurse-clinician is her feeling of commitment to the provision of the highest quality of nursing care. In addition, I feel that she has a professional responsibility for extending her judgment and standards of care to larger and larger groups of patients. Obviously, there is never going to be a nurse-clinician available for total care of each patient. Therefore, it is all the more important that the nurse-clinician, in one way or another, ensure that truly professional nursing care—the full-dimensioned kind that she knows how to give—reaches every patient within her area of responsibility.

Let me explain what I mean. In our present system of patient services, nursing care is provided by what I call a "pyramid of personnel." The broad base of this pyramid is represented by the ever-growing numbers of ancillary personnel, the narrow apex by the relatively smaller number of professional nurse practitioners. It is the ancillary personnel who provide the bulk of direct care to patients. The contact of professional nurses with the patient today is, I submit, typically brief and intermittent: limited to such therapeutic tasks as giving medications or performing technical procedures, or to such administrative tasks as assigning, directing, and supervising the work of others.

This system, in my opinion, has resulted in a relative—and sometimes absolute—lack of professional nursing care for patients. It is almost literally impossible for patients to purchase professional nursing care at their bedside. The best they can get is the services of a "team" led by a professional nurse.

Depending on the team leader, the care the patient receives may or may not be of a professional quality. All too often, the team leader is at least one step removed from the patient; she is not involved in his direct care. Like the head nurse, she is a victim of our system that places emphasis on spreading available nursing service to all patients. She must be concerned with the *amount* of care. The nurse-clinician, by contrast, is concerned with the *kind* of care.

If I seem to be laboring this point, it is because I see it as a vital one. Nursing's gradual withdrawal or removal from direct nursing care has created a vacuum around the patient—one which is rapidly being filled by a variety of less well-prepared personnel. I can even visualize the day when we may be actually ruled out from giving direct nursing care.

"This is our job, not yours," I can hear the organized ancillary personnel saying to us, just as they said it to the nurses at Fairview, as reported in the January *Journal*.[1] It seems to me that if we continue our present patterns of nursing service, we may end up by giving away our very birthright.

Therefore, I see the nurse-clinician as a person with the abilities, the motivation, and the commitment to "hacking" her way down through the personnel pyramid so that her professional knowledge and judgment are exerted in behalf of every patient. Inevitably the question: just how is she going to do this? will be asked, and I will have more to say about this later on. For the moment, though, let me describe a pilot study we carried out at the New York Medical College, Flower–Fifth Avenue Hospital— one intended to explore ways to improve nursing care and to see how the competencies of the nurse-clinician could be utilized within the reality situation of a hospital unit.

Several nurse-clinicians—all members of our nursing school faculty— served as integral members of the nursing staff of a 61-bed medical-surgical unit for a 14-month period. They did not represent additional personnel; they served as clinical staff on the unit. We made sure that they were free of administrative and managerial responsibilities, functioning only in patient care and free to develop their own patterns.

Let me describe, for instance, how the nurse-clinician on the 3-to-11 shift functioned. First came the report from the nurse responsible for patient care during the previous shift. Under the leadership of the nurse-clinician, this report—rather than the usual flip through the Kardex to check doctors' orders, preps, and the like—evolved into a major device for teaching, supervising, and ensuring continuity of care. Questions asked by the nurse-clinician provided guidance to the other nursing personnel, improved their observations, enhanced their perceptions of patient needs, and helped them establish priorities.

Then the nurse-clinician made nursing rounds. This permitted her to evaluate the patients' status, determine their needs for medical attention, and make judgments as to needed nursing measures. As she made her rounds, the nurse-clinician provided nursing care and services as indicated: she might adjust the traction, instruct a patient in deep breathing, or get him a bedpan.

Now, these rounds served several purposes. First, the nurse-clinician was actually at each patient's side as a practitioner, using her informed judgment to determine his nursing needs. Some of these she met herself; otherwise, she worked closely with the person giving the care. Second, these rounds communicated to the patients a sense of caring and of safety; the nurse-clinician's services were always available to them and they knew it. In fact, they soon came to feel that nursing personnel cared not only *for* them but *about* them.

A final purpose—one that was served not only by the initial rounds but by the nurse-clinician's continuing involvement in patient care—was that, by observing the level of care being given, the nurse-clinician could evaluate the nursing staff's need for instruction and supervision. This she was able to provide on the spot—by demonstration and by serving as model. On the completion of this demonstration, we were able to say something like this: The nurse-clinician's, motivation, judgment, and visible and expert nursing care skills benefited both patients and staff, directly and indirectly. Patients benefited not only from the direct care the nurse-clinician gave, but from her informed perception of the care they needed as she passed this on to others. Her methods of giving care provided other nursing personnel with moral leadership and instruction by demonstration. And her own participation in giving care, coupled with the obviously high value she placed on this, gave real status to the provision of direct nursing care. Aides took more pride in their work, and other nurses no longer referred to bedside care as "aides' work."

This demonstration by a faculty of nursing represents only one possible pattern of utilization of nurse-clinicians. If we agree that this is a kind of nurse-practitioner we need, I am sure that many patterns of involvement will await her in the future.

I do not envision all future nurses as nurse-clinicians. To my mind, these will be the select members of our profession—the ones who will form the membership, perhaps, of our projected Academy of Nursing. We have not yet spelled out the criteria for admission to this body. When we do, I hope that among them will be the stipulation that members be those with responsibility for, and engagement in, practice—practice based on the extensive knowledge and clinical experience that should characterize the nurse-clinician.

QUALIFICATION

How should the nurse-clinician be prepared? Actually, I believe that at the present time in nursing education, there is no single avenue to becoming a nurse-clinician. Her background, though, should reflect a relatively long period of preparation in nursing, through a variety of formal and informal learning experiences: formal education, professional nursing education, familiarity with both medical and nursing principles and goals, and extensive clinical practice in a wide range of settings.

I do not believe that a degree alone, master's or doctoral, automatically makes a nurse-clinician. I have had on my own faculty, for instance, a person whom I considered fully qualified as a nurse-clinician in cardiac nursing—but she had no degree and had arrived at her point of clinical excellence through her own extensive study and practice.

Other things being equal, the nurse-clinician of the future will probably have at least a master's degree. But I don't want to run the risk, as we have in the past, of placing all our values on a degree without some substantive knowledge of what went into it. No matter how skilled a nurse may be in the teaching arts, for instance, I would not consider her a nurse-clinician unless she couples her teaching activities with continuing clinical practice. Nor can clinical specialization, in all of its various stages, be considered adequate preparation for the nurse-clinician unless it encompasses all the dimensions on which patient care is built.

I believe that it is possible to prepare a beginning nurse-clinician in a basic baccalaureate program, but there are three strings attached to this belief. The first is the emphasis on "beginning": breadth and depth of both knowledge and experience are essential for the nurse-clinician—more knowledge and more practice than she will have in her generic program. So, while the young graduate may be on her way toward becoming a nurse-clinician, she hasn't arrived there yet.

The second string concerns the nature of the generic program itself. This program, I believe, must be embedded in and radiate out from a medical teaching center—a center for multiprofessional education, practice, and research. Both faculty members and students must feel closely identified with the medical and nursing practice in that center, must feel part and take part in the interdisciplinary exchange that goes on there. Only when the student's home base for practice is such a center can she gain the professional maturity which is marked by the ability to establish collaborative relationships with other disciplines, to speak the same language, and to share the same perceptions, approaches, and values. To achieve this, she must learn, practice, and evaluate with others on the professional health team who are doing the same thing.

INVOLVEMENT

I do *not* believe she will be prepared, even as a beginning nurse-clinician, if her clinical practice experience as a student is offered in a variety of community settings with no real identification with any one of them. In this kind of setup the student does not have the opportunity to become a part of the total therapeutic team, to develop what might be called the *collaborative attitude*. Similarly, her instructor—functioning in the patient care setting only as a member of the university faculty—has no responsibility for, nor involvement in, the practice there, and therefore cannot pass this subtle value on to her students.

Patient management today—diagnosis, care, treatment, and rehabil-itation—is an interdisciplinary affair. The student must learn this from the very beginning; the faculty member must continue to be an active partner in it. Many nurses in baccalaureate programs today receive a fine type of higher education, but it is not professional education. The two are not the same thing, but I think nursing has often failed to recognize the distinction.

Finally, I believe that the student's spectrum of learning experiences must include all of the settings in which patient care is given: the home, the clinic, the ambulatory services, and the long-term care institutions. Without these experiences, especially the latter, the student's basic pro-fessional education is not complete. It is in the long-term area that the greatest numbers of patients needing care are concentrated. And it is also in this area, where so many ancillary personnel are employed, that the student can begin to learn how to extend her services and judgment down through the pyramid of personnel.

Some day in our hospitals I hope to see what might be called a "clin-ical nursing staff"—one with no responsibility for anything but patient care. Within such a staff I can visualize nurses with varying degrees of clinical knowledge and practice experience—some on their way to becoming nurse-clinicians, others satisfied to practice on the level they have already achieved.

Take, for instance, the nurse who is deeply interested in the care of sick children: she wants to know more about the medical and nursing practice in this field, to be expert in its care techniques, to learn all she can in this area. She is not a pediatric nurse-clinician, however, unless she is equally expert and knowledgeable throughout all the dimensions of pediatric nursing practice: the child with a chronic disease at home or in an institution, the one needing open heart surgery, the emotionally dis-turbed child, the adolescent.

Similarly, there may be nurses who are intrigued by the intricate medical-technical responsibilities that nurses carry today: operation of the artificial kidney, the cardiac monitoring devices, the various mechanical respiratory aids. This, to my mind, is curative nursing care carried to a high degree. Here we have another kind of nurse—what we might call the technical expert. This is fine, we need her, but she is not a nurse-clinician.

To recapitulate: I think there is more than one way to become a nurse-clinician. Some nurses, through self-impelled study and practice, may get there on their own. By and large, however, I believe that the most economic way to rapidly prepare a corps of beginning nurse-clinicians is through organized programs of graduate study in professional education. The student would enter such a program having had a liberal education culminating in a bachelor's degree. Her professional education could then concentrate on two things that would receive equal emphasis: (1) the necessary body of theory and clinical knowledge, and (2) the application of this in repeated, continuing practice which encompasses the full range of function and the full breadth of services.

All very fine, you may be saying. But how are we going to implement all these concepts? What about the changes in our patterns of nursing education, practice, and service that will be necessary to prepare this nurse-clinician, to enable her to practice in the way she is prepared to?

Unquestionably, changes will be necessary, especially within the organization of our present system of nursing services. But I think that we must first decide upon our ends before we worry about the means for achieving them. We need to take a look at where our present patterns have brought us—considerably removed from the practice of nursing—and decide whether this is where we want to remain.

THE ALTERNATIVES

The beginning of change and the beginning of wisdom must start with an idea, a value—in this instance, what is best for the welfare of those who are served by nursing. If others feel, as I do, that the nursing profession has to a shocking degree failed the public, has submitted to—or helped to create—a situation wherein professional nursing care and judgment are not available to those who need it, then we can set about in a concerted way to change things.

If we do not change, if we choose to maintain the status quo, then I think we are in danger of committing professional suicide: that nursing as a personal and professional service to patients may cease to exist.

NOTES

1. Lewis, E. P. The Fairview story. *American Journal of Nursing* 66: 64–70, Jan. 1966.

CHAPTER 15

The Development of
a Personal Concept

Virginia A. Henderson

My interpretation of the nurse's function is the synthesis of many influences—some positive, some negative. In chronological order I will identify those experiences I think most significant. First I would like to emphasize that I am not presenting my point of view as one with which I expect you to agree. Rather I would urge every nurse to develop her own concept, otherwise she is merely imitating others or acting under authority. In my own case I felt as though I were steering an uncharted course until I resolved certain doubts about my true function.

Most of my basic training was in a general hospital where, for the nurse, technical competence, speed of performance, and a "professional" (actually an impersonal) manner were stressed. We were introduced to nursing as a series of almost unrelated procedures, beginning with an unoccupied bed and progressing to aspiration of body cavities, for instance. Ability to catheterize a patient in this era seemed to qualify a

This text was originally published in 1966, in the first edition of Ms. Henderson's *The Nature of Nursing* (New York). The reprint given here, along with the addendum, is from a 1991 collection of articles. Notes and references have been renumbered for consistency. Originally published in *The Nature of Nursing: Reflections after 25 years*. New York: National League for Nursing Press (Pub. No. 15-2346): (1991) 9–33. Copyright National League for Nursing. Reprinted with permission.

student for so-called night duty, where, without any previous experience in the administration of a service, she might have the entire care of as many as 30 sick souls and bodies.

An authoritarian type of medicine was practiced in this hospital. Physicians who lectured to student nurses simply compressed and simplified the didactic instruction they gave medical students. They usually presented watertight diagnoses with textbook programs of therapy and cut-and-dried prognoses. In those days not even lip service was given "patient-centered care," "family health service," "comprehensive care," or "rehabilitation."

But there was, for me, an influence in those early student days that tended to negate this mechanistic approach. Annie W. Goodrich was dean of my school, the Army School of Nursing. Whenever she visited our unit, she lifted our sights above techniques and routines. With her broad experience in hospitals, in public health agencies, and educational institutions, she saw nursing as a "world-wide social activity," a creative and constructive force in society. Having a powerful intellect and boundless compassion for humanity, she never failed to infect us with "the ethical significance of nursing." This is the title she later chose for her collected papers, and it could not have been more apt for it was the essence of her teaching.[7]

Miss Goodrich often expressed full awareness of the physician's immeasurable contribution to social welfare and had a surprising knowledge of current therapies. Nevertheless, I attribute to her my early discontent with the regimentalized patient care in which I participated and the concept of nursing as merely ancillary to medicine. Although Miss Goodrich always presented us with the highest aim for nursing, she left us to translate it into concrete acts, and I needed someone to "show me"—as Liza Doolittle sang, when words had ceased to be enough for her. Dr. Osler's greatest contribution may well have been his insistence that medical students have the opportunity to see their teachers practice medicine. I seldom, if ever, saw graduate nurses practice nursing—never my teachers. Their teaching was in a classroom.

While it is true that as a student I was clinically self-taught for the most part, in the army hospital I had the privilege of nursing sick and wounded soldiers who were notably courageous and appreciative. I learned to serve in an atmosphere where the nurse, as a representative of society, felt indebted to the patient. The soldier patient demanded little, but the nurse felt that the most she could do was not enough, and therefore the nurse–patient relationship was a warm and generous one. The atmosphere in certain affiliated civil hospitals offered a distinct contrast, and so, in this respect, we thought our student nursing experience special, if not unique.

Professional and nonprofessional literature in recent decades abounds in criticism of hospitals. Their present burden is so great that it seems ungenerous to point to such publications. Some criticize the nursing care; others question many services hospitals offer. Elizabeth Barnes, in a small volume, *People in Hospital,* summarizes the findings of eighteen groups studying hospitals in Canada, Finland, France, Germany, Italy, Spain, Switzerland, the United Kingdom, and the United States.[8] Although this descriptive and judicial document shows up many weaknesses, it also notes that "hospitals contain and cope with the disorder and distress of illness which the community itself cannot tolerate."

Present-day hospitals as represented in this survey seem to offer a wide range of service by type and quality. For example, some permit families to move in with patients and help care for them, while others prohibit even parents visiting their children. One hospital is reported to have weekly interprofessional ward conferences attended by all members of the clinical team with, preferably, the head nurse presiding; but the statement follows that "meetings of this kind would be incompatible with the social structure of some hospitals." Certain hospitals represented have open days that encourage public interest and observation; others discourage public involvement.

Jan de Hartog has shown that in this decade conditions in a hospital of one of the wealthiest regions of the United States can rival in horror those found in the Dark Ages.[9] He does not, however, attribute the state of the hospital to the inhumanity of medical personnel primarily but rather to the apathy of the public and to the governing board that failed to provide conditions under which such personnel could operate effectively. He is as compassionate toward doctors and nurses as he is toward patients, for he sees all of them as victims of prejudice and a totally inadequate system.

No doubt many persons fear hospitalization, and others, unless they are desperately ill, feel apologetic about asking over-burdened doctors and nurses to care for them. Social scientists are vocal on this score. Esther Lucile Brown in a series of books with the overall title *Newer Dimensions of Patient Care* is an ardent and effective spokesman for the public.[10–12] These publications suggest changes in the general hospital that have been effected in certain psychiatric hospitals in which the goal is the establishment of a therapeutic environment.[13,14]

Medical and nursing faculties, realizing the limitations of institutional care, sporadically in the past and more generally at present, have offered their students (and some staff members) experience outside the hospital.[15–18] Programs that attempt to meet the total needs of patients as they move from inpatient to outpatient services demonstrate some of the gaps in hospital care as it exists today. The findings of Dr. George Reader, Doris Schwartz, and their associates at the New York–Cornell Medical Center seem to indicate that the ambulatory patients treated in the outpatient department are, to be quite specific, unable to use correctly at home the very drugs prescribed for them by the physician.[19,20] Other studies point to the relative inadequacy of written directions as a means of helping patients carry out prescribed therapy.

The president of a large university, speaking to me of medical education there, said that he and the medical and nursing faculties sometimes wondered whether medical personnel with a patient-centered approach could be produced within the hospital setting because so many of its practices are contrary to the best interests of patients. Esther Lucile Brown in *Newer Dimensions of Patient Care* suggests some radical changes that must be made in the hospital if it is to be patient-centered. Dr. Crew quotes Miss Nightingale as saying, "Hospitals are only an intermediate stage of civilization."[21] But this has been a digression on the limitations of our major institutions for medical care, and I should return to my student experiences.

Part of my preparation for nursing was in a psychiatric affiliation that might have supplied me with many of the human relation skills I needed—those, in fact, that all health workers need. There, hopefully, I might have seen an individualized program for patients that I failed to see in the general hospital. Actually, I learned names for supposed disease entities and treatments for them, most of which have been, or should have been, discarded. The chief value of this affiliation was that it gave me some appreciation of the extent and nature of mental illness. I acquired little or no understanding of the role a nurse might play in preventing or curing it. The following is an example of how completely I failed to grasp my function as a psychiatric nurse.

I was assigned the care of a large and very sick woman from a socially prominent family. We were alone in a short wing of the hospital. She was extremely negative and assaultive. She had attacked several nurses and had injured one by pinning her behind a door. I was frightened during this assignment until I found that by playing the part of a "handmaiden," speaking archaic English, and addressing my patient as "Your Majesty," I could get her to do anything. No one came to her aid—or mine—and so I left her even more deeply entrenched in the world of fantasy than she was when she fell into my ignorant hands. Only years later did I realize how untherapeutic my approach had been.

While my psychiatric nursing experience left me with a sense of failure, a pediatric affiliation with the Boston Floating Hospital had the opposite effect, for there I was introduced to patient-centered care, although this term was not used then. In that hospital we were regularly assigned patients, not tasks. Each of us cared for three sick infants or children. When the student with whom we were paired was "off duty," we would care for her three patients as well as our own. Under such circumstances we acquired considerable understanding of our charges and their needs, and we were greatly attached to them. The director of nurses and the able head nurses, who in this hospital were graduates, encouraged a warm relationship between patients and students.[1] Here we saw "tender loving care" before the label was invented. Unfortunately we did not see demonstrated the importance of bringing the mothers or fathers into the hospital with the sick child. While we glimpsed patient-centered care, it was not family-centered. We knew little or nothing of the parents or the home situation.[2]

A student experience I count as almost wholly positive was a summer spent with the Henry Street Visiting Nurse Agency in New York City. There I began to discard the formal approach to patients approved in the general hospital. In fact, I acquired a skepticism of medical care in hospitals that remains with me. Seeing the sick return to their homes following hospitalization, I began to realize that the seemingly successful institutional regimen often failed to change the patient's way of living that sent him to the hospital in the first place.

Because nursing in homes seemed so much more satisfying than hospital nursing, I became a visiting nurse after graduation. Several years later I left this field unwillingly to teach in a hospital school of nursing because I was made to feel that the need for instructors was so great. With no special preparation I was forced to learn as I taught in all areas of the curriculum. Over a five-year period I was the only nurse employed to teach in this institution. Fortunately for all concerned, I sensed my need for more knowledge and clarification of my ideas, and I went back to school.

Except for a brief period of clinical supervision and teaching in a basic university program, I remained at Teachers College, Columbia University, first as a student and then as a teacher, for twenty years. My concept of nursing during this period was not so much changed as clarified. It is impossible to identify all the persons and experiences that brought this about, but the following should be mentioned.

Caroline Stackpole based her teaching of physiology on Claude Bernard's dictum that health depends upon keeping the lymph constant around the cell. This emphasis on the unit structure taught me relationships in laws of health that, to me, had been unrelated up to that time. Miss Stackpole was a master teacher who was never satisfied until the student answered his own question. Jean Broadhurst, a microbiologist, had this same concept of teaching. From them, and through experimentation in the physiology course for medical students of the College of Physicians and Surgeons at Columbia University, I acquired an analytical approach to all aspects of care and treatment. This is more than justified by the articles and books by doctors who are now writing on pathology due to treatment (iatrogenic conditions).[22] As I read reports of malnutrition from therapeutic diets, emotional and physiological crises from endocrine therapy, drug-induced skin lesions, and the varied complications from cortisone administration, I think to myself, "The constancy of the intercellular fluids has been dangerously reduced." Ever since I grasped this danger, I have believed that a definition of nursing should imply an appreciation of the principle of physiological balance. It has made so vivid to me the importance of forcing fluids, of feeding the comatose in some way, or of relieving oxygen want. It became obvious that emotional balance was inseparable from physiological balance once I realized that an emotion was actually an interpretation of cellular response to fluctuations in the chemical composition of the intercellular fluids which produced muscle tension, changes in heart and respiratory rate, and other reactions. Mind and body have come to be inseparable in my thinking. Through this study of physiology, the way was paved for acceptance of psychosomatic medicine and all its implications for nursing. In order to understand physical and emotional balance, it has ever since seemed to me to be necessary to start with cell physiology. The man and the amoeba are points on a continuum.[3]

At Teachers College, Dr. Edward Thorndike's work in psychology provided some generalizations, or fixed points, in the psychosocial realm parallel to those I had acquired in the biological sciences. His investigations on the fundamental needs of man, including his research into how we spend our money and time, made me realize that illness was more than a state of disease and a threat to life. Too often it places a person in a setting where shelter from the elements is almost the only fundamental need that is fully met. In most hospitals the patient cannot eat as he wishes; his freedom of movement is curtailed; his privacy is invaded; he is put to bed in strange nightclothes that make him feel as unattractive as a punished child; he is separated from the objects of his affection; he is deprived of almost every diversion in his normal day, deprived of work, and reduced to dependence on persons who are often younger than he is, and sometimes less intelligent and courteous.

From the time I saw hospitalization in this light I have questioned every routine nursing procedure or restriction that is in conflict with the individual's fundamental need for shelter, food, communication with others, and the company of those he loves, for opportunity to win approval, to dominate and be dominated, to learn, to work, to play, and to worship. In other words, I have since conceived it to be the aim of nursing to keep the individual's day as normal as possible—to keep him in "the stream of life" to the extent that it is consistent with the physician's therapeutic plan.

If for too long we deprive a person of what he values most—love, approval, fruitful occupation—this condition of deprivation is often worse than the disease we are attempting to cure. If a person did not fear this complete dislocation of his life—this yawning abyss between himself and the healthy—sickness and even old age would lose many of their terrors.

Soon after this enlightenment I saw the work of Dr. George G. Deaver and the physical therapists associated with him at the Institute for the Crippled and Disabled and later at Bellevue Hospital, both in New York City. In these programs I found the implementation of many ideas I had been accumulating.[23,24] I noted that much of the effort of the expert in rehabilitation went into building the patient's independence—the independence of which hospital personnel had unwittingly deprived him, or had failed at least to encourage. Nothing has made my concept of nursing more concrete than the demonstrations and writings of these rehabilitation experts with their insistence on individualized programs and constant evaluation of the patient's needs and his progress toward the goal of independence. I believe the 1937 revision of the National League of Nursing Education's basic curriculum guide reflected these ideas and that ever since they have been part of the profession's lip service, if not its actual service, to the sick and disabled.[25]

Figure 15.1 makes the aim of rehabilitation concrete. It shows a list of the activities in daily living. Opposite are spaces in which members of the medical team record the patient's progress toward independence in the performance of these activities. After seeing this form in use, the goal behind it, for me, has been interwoven in the fabric of nursing.

My participation in preparing the 1937 curriculum guide, in the work of the NLNE's special committee on post-graduate clinical courses, and in the regional conferences associated with Miss Brown's study forced me to express in writing these evolving concepts of nursing.[26,27] It was not until the 1940s, however, that I could test my ideas in actual practice. It was then that we developed at Teachers College what was, at the time, a unique type of advanced study in medical-surgical nursing.

This course was unique because it was patient-centered and organized around major nursing problems rather than medical diagnoses and diseases of body systems. Related field experience gave the graduate nurse student an opportunity to increase her competence—for example, in helping a patient, and sometimes his family, to cope with a chronic condition; to help him prepare for, and recover from, surgical procedures; to help him to deal with a communicable disease that necessitates relative isolation, or with depression after the loss of a breast or a leg. It was one of the first advanced clinical courses that required students to actually nurse patients under a case assignment system and to conduct nursing clinics and interprofessional conferences around the care of the patients they nursed. The emphasis was on comprehensive care, and to the extent that hospital regulations permitted it, we were concerned with follow-up care.

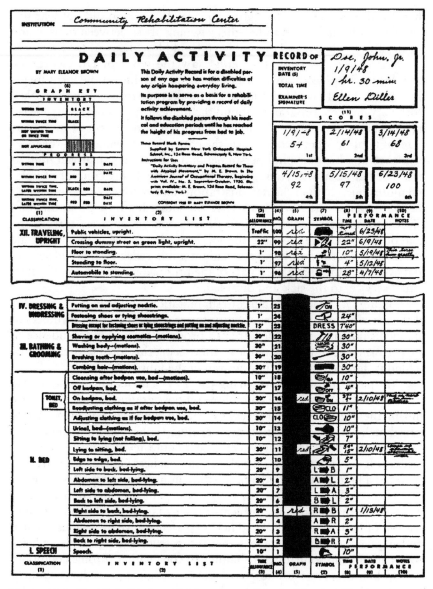

Figure 15.1   Record of daily activities prepared for handicapped persons during the period of rehabilitation. (Brown, Mary E.: "Daily Activity Inventory and Progress Record for Those with Atypical Movement," *Am. J. Occup. Therap.* 4: 195 [Sept.] 1950)

Associated with me in planning or teaching, or both, were Margaret Adams, Marion Cleveland, Ruth Gilbert, Marguerite Kakosh, Katherine Nelson, Frances Reiter (Kreuter), and Jean South. Exchanging views with these clinically able nurses and with students who were often experienced and expert, I gained immeasurably. When in the 1950s I revised the fourth edition of Bertha Harmer's and my text *The Principles and Practice of Nursing,* I could present what seemed to me a tested and specific definition of nursing.

Since that time the writings of psychiatric nurses, particularly those of Gwen Tudor (Will) and Ida Orlando (Pelletier), have made me realize how easily the nurse can act on misconceptions of the patient's needs if she does not check her interpretation of them with him.[28,29]

At the Yale University School of Nursing, where Miss Orlando was when she wrote *The Dynamic Nurse–Patient Relationship,* the faculty stated in 1959 this tentative definition of nursing: "The nurse's prime function is to enable the patients to utilize health measures which are available or prescribed."[30] The principal aim of teaching and research within this graduate program is "systematic study of the nature and effect of nursing practice." Most, if not all, members of this faculty believe that the analysis of the nurse's clinical experience, the identification of the effect on the patient of what she does, is the way to develop nursing theory, generalizations, or guidelines for action. Ida Orlando's book is a series of partial case histories around which she relates examples of patient behavior, as the nurse observes it, the nurse's related thoughts and feelings which she may share with the patient in her effort to get at the true meaning of the patient's facial expression, what he says or how he acts. Miss Orlando describes what the nurse does to meet the patient's need for help after he has confirmed her interpretation of his need, and how the nurse judges her effectiveness by whether the patient's need for help was met.

Ernestine Wiedenbach further clarifies this deliberative nursing process in her monograph *Clinical Nursing: A Helping Art.*[31] She also stresses the point that a worker's goal influences the way he or she works and that how the nurse functions depends upon her philosophy. Here I would like to make the point that these books and the numerous published reports of the Yale faculty and students reinforce Miss Orlando's conclusion that the most effective nursing involves continuous observation and interpretation of patient behavior, validation by the patient of the nurse's interpretation of his need for help, and action based on this validated inference.[32] Faculty discussions and study of their published and unpublished writings have contributed to my present concept of nursing. Faye Abdellah's study of the covert or concealed problems of the patient is related to the concepts just discussed, as is Helene Fitzgerald's work with Yale University students.[33,34] Unfortunately, it is impossible to mention all the nurses whose works have influenced my thinking.

In 1958 I was asked by the Nursing Service Committee of the International Council of Nurses to prepare a small pamphlet on basic nursing. I quote from this pamphlet, published by the Council in 1961, the following definition of nursing. It is an adaptation of the statement in my last revision of Bertha Harmer's text and represents the crystallization of my ideas:

> *The unique function of the nurse is to assist the individual, sick or well, in the performance of those activities contributing to health or its recovery (or to peaceful death) that he would perform unaided if he had the necessary strength, will, or knowledge. And to do this in such a way as to help him gain independence as rapidly as possible.* This aspect of her work, this part of her function, she initiates and controls; of this she is master. In addition she helps the patient to carry out the therapeutic plan as initiated by the physician. She also, as a member of a medical team, helps other members, as they in turn help her, to plan and carry out the total program, whether it be for the improvement of health, recovery from illness, or support in death. No one of the team should make such heavy demands on another member that any one of them is unable to perform his or her unique function. Nor should any member of the medical team be diverted by nonmedical activities such as cleaning, clerking, and filing, as long as his or her special task must be neglected. All members of the team should consider the person (patient) served as the central figure, and should realize that primarily they are all "assisting" him. If the patient does not understand, accept, and participate in the program planned with and for him, the effort of the medical team is largely wasted. The sooner the person can care for himself, find health information, or even carry out prescribed treatments, the better off he is.

This concept of the nurse as a substitute for what the patient lacks to make him "complete," "whole," or "independent," by the lack of physical strength, will, or knowledge, may seem limited to some. The more one thinks about it, however, the more complex the nurse's function as so defined proves to be. Think how rare is "completeness," or "wholeness," of mind and body. To what extent good health is a matter of heredity and to what extent it is acquired is controversial, but it is generally admitted that intelligence and education tend to parallel health status. If then each man finds "good health" a difficult goal, how much more difficult is it for the nurse to help him reach it: she must, in a sense, get "inside the skin" of each of her patients in order to know what he needs. She is temporarily the consciousness of the unconscious, the love of life for the suicidal, the leg of the amputee, the eyes of the newly blind, a means of locomotion for the infant, knowledge and confidence for the young mother, the "mouthpiece" for those too weak or withdrawn to speak, and so on.[35]

It is my contention that the nurse is, and should be legally, an independent practitioner and able to make independent judgments as long as he, or she, is not diagnosing, prescribing treatment for disease, or making a prognosis, for these are the physician's functions. But the nurse is the authority on basic nursing care. Perhaps I should explain that by *basic nursing care* I mean helping the patient with the following activities or providing conditions under which he can perform them unaided:

- Breathe normally
- Eat and drink adequately
- Eliminate body wastes
- Move and maintain desirable postures
- Sleep and rest
- Select suitable clothes—dress and undress
- Maintain body temperature within normal range by adjusting clothing and modifying the environment
- Keep the body clean and well groomed and protect the integument
- Avoid dangers in the environment and avoid injuring others
- Communicate with others in expressing emotions, needs, fears, or opinions
- Worship according to one's faith
- Work in such a way that there is a sense of accomplishment
- Play or participate in various forms of recreation
- Learn, discover, or satisfy the curiosity that leads to normal development and health and use the available health facilities.[4]

In helping the patient with these activities the nurse has infinite need for knowledge of the biological and social sciences and skills based on them. There are few more difficult arts than that of keeping a patient well nourished and his mouth healthy during a long comatose period, or that of helping the depressed, mute, psychotic individual reestablish normal human relations. No worker but the nurse can and will devote himself or herself consistently day and night to these ends. In fact, of all medical services nursing is the only one that might be called continuous.

This unique function of the nurse I see as a complex service. A Canadian physician, whose name escapes me, said there are two essentials: care (by the nurse) and cure (by the physician). He added, "I do not know which is nobler." Lord Horder, an English physician, speaks of nursing as a part of medicine. Dr. William R. Houston, late author of *The Art of Treatment,* points out that in some conditions nursing care is the only known therapy. He devoted a section of his text to patients who are to be "treated chiefly by nursing care."[5]

In emphasizing this basic, or unique, function of the nurse, I do not mean to disregard her therapeutic role. She is, in most situations, the patient's prime helper in carrying out the physician's prescriptions, and her very relationship with the patient can be itself therapeutic.

If we put total health and medical care in the form of a pie graph, we might assign wedges of different sizes to members of what we now refer to as "the team." It is, however, my contention that in some situations certain members of the team have no part of the pie, and the wedge must differ in size for each member according to the problem facing the patient, his ability to help himself, and whoever is available to help him. The patient and his family always have a slice, although that of the motherless newborn infant in a hospital nursery or the unconscious hospitalized adult are only slivers. In such cases the patient's very life depends on hospital personnel, but most particularly on the nurse. In contrast, when an otherwise healthy youth is suffering from a skin condition such as acne, he and his physician might compose the team, and they might divide the pie between them. When a patient is ambulatory with an orthopedic disability, the largest slice may go to the physical therapist or, in certain stages of adjustment to an amputation, to those who make and fit prostheses. When a sick child is cared for at home by the mother, or if we admit the mother to the hospital with the child, her share may be by far the largest. But of all members of the team, excepting the patient and the physician, the nurse has most often a piece of the pie, and next to theirs I believe hers is usually the largest share. Figures 15.2, 15.3, and 15.4 show conditions in which nurses play minor and major roles. Figure 15.5 shows how, with the same patient, the nurse plays a major role in one period and gradually assumes a diminishing role as other workers take over and as the patient acquires independence.

In talking about nursing we tend to stress promotion of health and prevention and cure of disease. We rarely speak of the inevitable end of life and what the nurse might do to help a person reduce its physical discomforts—to face death courageously, with dignity, and even bring to it an awesome beauty. Anthropologists and other critics of our European culture say we are prone to shrink from the thought and sight of old age and death. In fact, we exalt youth, hiding the signs of age in ourselves as long as possible. In this country, when the aged person loses his independence, we are likely to tuck him away in a nursing home. It is poorly named for it has few characteristics of a home and there is little nursing, as I describe it here. Such custodial care as the average nursing home offers is a national disgrace.

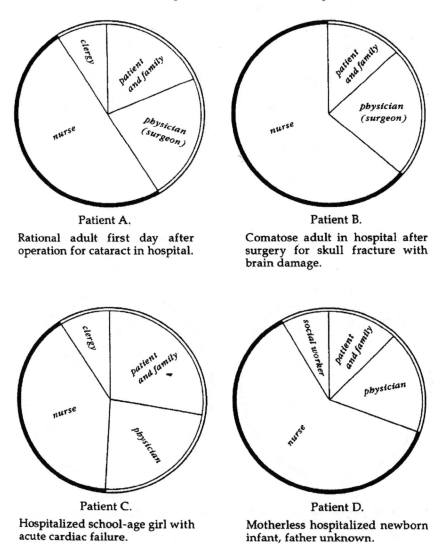

Patient A.

Rational adult first day after operation for cataract in hospital.

Patient B.

Comatose adult in hospital after surgery for skull fracture with brain damage.

Patient C.

Hospitalized school-age girl with acute cardiac failure.

Patient D.

Motherless hospitalized newborn infant, father unknown.

Figure 15.2   Conditions in which the nurse plays a major role.

For those who did not hear her speak when she was in the United States, I'd like to mention Cecily Saunders and her work in a London hospital.[38-40] Possibly because she is a nurse and a social worker, as well as a physician, she has developed a remarkable system of terminal care for cancer patients. Her institution provides an environment that appears to be cheerful and otherwise pleasing to the senses. More particularly she has

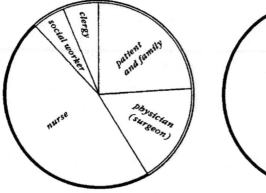

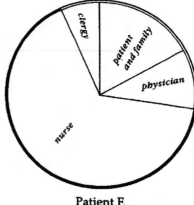

Patient E.

Mature rational hospitalized woman in body cast.

Patient F.

Elderly disoriented man in nursing
home.

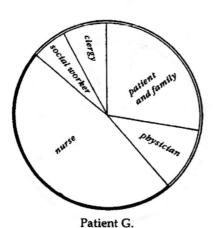

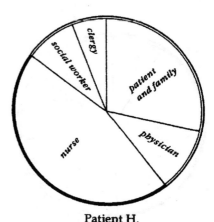

Patient G.

Depressed unwed mother living
alone. Referred to VNA by psychiatric clinic where patient fails to
keep appointments.

Patient H.

One-year-old baby with no diagnosed disease. Referred to VNA because he "fails to thrive."

Figure 15.3   Conditions in which the nurse plays a major role   (VNA = visiting
nurse association).

learned to give those who face death emotional support and to control
pain without producing coma, agitation, or the personality changes seen
with drug addiction. She shows one photograph after another of a person
eating a meal, sitting in a chair in the ward or on the terrace, knitting, or
occupied with a game, and she says, not without pride, that he or she died

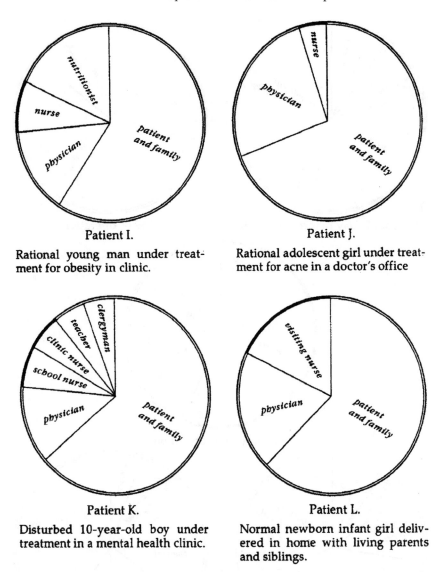

Patient I.

Rational young man under treatment for obesity in clinic.

Patient J.

Rational adolescent girl under treatment for acne in a doctor's office

Patient K.

Disturbed 10-year-old boy under
treatment in a mental health clinic.

Patient L.

Normal newborn infant girl delivered in home with living parents
and siblings.

Figure 15.4   Conditions in which the nurse plays a minor role (assuming that all
other persons contributing to patient care are available).

three days later, or, "He died peacefully the next day." After she spoke to
a large audience of medical students, physicians, and nurses in New
Haven, Dr. Saunders had a standing ovation.[6] It would be too bad if the
competences of the nurse and the physician must be literally embodied in

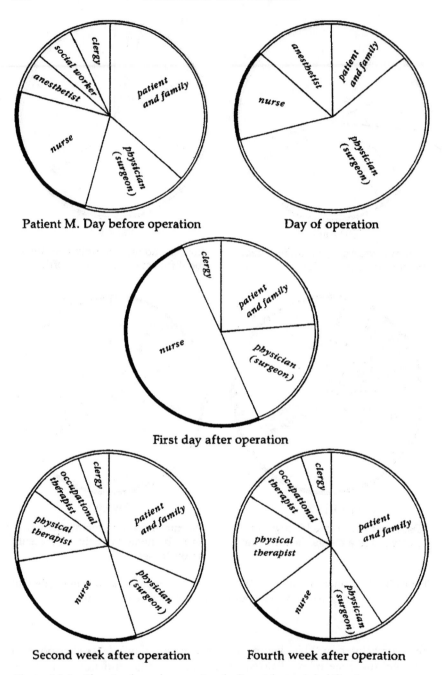

Patient M. Day before operation   Day of operation

First day after operation

Second week after operation   Fourth week after operation

Figure 15.5   Showing how the nurse's role dimmishes as rehabilitation progresses in the case of a young man having a leg amputated, for example.

one person to bring about their full engagement in the improvement of terminal care. But with or without prescriptions from the physician that reduce pain and coma to a minimum, the nurse can still do a great deal anywhere to keep the environment in which death occurs supportive and aesthetic; she can reduce the patient's discomfort with nursing measures and reduce his loneliness in death by facing it with him honestly and courageously. If the nurse has a religious belief akin to the patient's, she can reinforce his faith; but in any event she can see that he has the help he wants and needs from the minister of his choice.

In summary, I see nursing as primarily complementing the patient by supplying what he needs in knowledge, will, or strength to perform his daily activities and to carry out the treatment prescribed for him by the physician.

ADDENDUM

The nature of medical treatment has changed so greatly since 1966, and the technology employed by doctors and nurses has developed so rapidly, that my personal concept would undoubtedly reflect some aspects of those changes were I writing about health services today. Treatment has not only become more complex technically but, in this country, far more costly. This is especially true of hospital services, which has resulted in their being reduced in length with more and more emphasis put on home care.

The cost of nursing care—and all health care—has increased so much that it overrides other considerations. While I may not be informed enough to comment on this, I believe that the ownership of hospitals affects this practice. A hospital operated to make money operates differently from one that is not influenced by the financial return but rather by the therapeutic results for which it is known.

In the United States more than 12% of the gross national product is spent on health care. This expenditure is not the rule elsewhere in the world. Japan, for example, spends roughly half the U.S. amount and has better statistics for longevity, maternal and infant health, and deaths from heart disease than the United States can claim.

The United States is often cited as the only industrialized country, with the possible exception of South Africa, that has no universally available tax-supported health insurance. Medicare and Medicaid, which were created to provide for the needs of the elderly and the indigent, have both been so misused that they partially fail to meet their respective aims.

Military personnel, and governmental employees generally, have tax-supported health care. When speaking or writing about health care today,

I leave no doubt in the audience's mind that I think this should be universal. In 1966 I was not so aware of how peculiar the United States was in regard to providing all its citizens with the essential elements of health care. I now believe that without increasingly available tax-supported health care, nurses will find it impossible to provide the care implied in my personal concept. If writing today, I would put more emphasis on universally available care and on the preparation of citizens to assess their need for help and to help themselves effectively. I would stress that health care is a political subject.

Today I see the role of nurses as givers of "primary health care," as those who diagnose and treat when a doctor is unavailable, even as the midwife functions in the absence of an obstetrician. Nurses may be the general (medical) practitioners of tomorrow. Because of that, I also emphasize the extent to which not only doctors and nurses but all health care personnel share responsibility for providing care, particularly in underserved areas.

Writing today, I put more stress than I did in 1966 on the health record and the roles of health care consumers and providers in making and using it. I would advocate everyone having, as military personnel have, a personal copy of his or her health record. A lengthy medical record can now be put on a single microchip which can be kept with other essential records.

While I made no reference in 1966 to the role of the nurse in helping people have "a good death" when death is inevitable, I would now put more emphasis on the question of prolonging life beyond the period of its usefulness. The importance of working with families and the patient over issues of "the right to die" or dying with dignity are increasingly a part of nursing care. The development of hospices and the kind of terminal care they typify has affected the concept of the care of dying patients in all institutions and settings and certainly reflects a change since 1966.

NOTES

1. In this era, head nurses in many hospitals were, as I have noted, likely to be second- or third-year students.
2. It was interesting to find Dr. Veronica B. Tizza of this hospital reporting in 1956 that during the preceding ten years there had been a change of attitude which resulted in a visiting policy that encouraged daily visiting, and that there was an experimental living-in unit for parents.
3. Just so does Pierre Teilhard de Chardin, the Jesuit priest and scientist, in his *The Phenomenon of Man* (New York: Harper and Brothers, 1959, p. 318), in which he insists on the kinship of all matter, going beyond the cell back to the atom. He traces the first manifestations of life to the moment of "revolution" when on the surface of the earth the "biosphere"—or a layer of living cells—formed that new arrangement of mol-

ecules having, for the first time, the elusive principle we call "life." His theory, if I interpret it correctly, is a welcome antidote to cynicism. He sees in all matter a movement toward a higher, more complex, or perfect, arrangement of the elements of which it is composed. This universal quality establishes for him man's kinship not only with animals but with what we call inanimate things. His theory demanded of him a humility and universal sympathy that helps, I think, explain the piercing beauty of his countenance. It may be that future generations of scientists will find in the study of atoms a far greater enlightenment than past generations have experienced in the study of cells.

4. It is my belief that this list of activities can be used in evaluating nursing. In other words, the extent to which nurses help patients acquire independence in performing these functions is a measure of their success. Where independence is unattainable, evaluation may be based on the extent to which the nurse helps the patient accept his limitations or his death, when this is inevitable. No effort is made here to describe the way in which the nurse helps the patient with these daily activities. This is done briefly in the ICN pamphlet and more fully in *Textbook of the Principles and Practice of Nursing*, 5th ed.

5. Lydia E. Hall reports an experience at the Solomon and Betty Loeb Center at Montefiore Hospital, New York City, which illustrates this point. Patients are admitted to this unit because they need nursing care primarily. Physicians are called in by the nursing staff as the need for the services arises. Nursing is recognized as the main line of therapy. Hail, *Lydia E.: Project Report*. The Solomon and Betty Loeb Center at Montefiore Hospital. The Center, New York, 1960, p. 80.

6. Dr. Saunders always attributes to other members of the hospital staff, but particularly those of the religious nursing order there, much of the credit for patients seeming to feel safe, or at peace.

REFERENCES

7. Goodrich, Annie W.: *The Social and Ethical Significance of Nursing*. The Macmillan Company, New York, 1932, p. 401.

8. Barnes, Elizabeth: *People in Hospital*. Macmillan and Company, Ltd., London, 1961, p. 155. New York, St. Martin's Press.

9. de Hartog, Jan: *The Hospital*. Atheneum, New York, 1964, p. 337.

10. Brown, Esther Lucile: *Newer Dimensions of Patient Care. Part I. The Use of the Hospital for Therapeutic Purposes*. Russell Sage Foundation, New York, 1961, p. 159.

11. *Newer Dimensions of Patient Care. Part II. Improving Staff Motivation and Competence in the General Hospital*. Russell Sage Foundation, New York, 1962, p. 194.

12. *Newer Dimensions of Patient Care. Part III. Patients as People*. Russell Sage Foundation, New York, 1964, p. 163.

13. Jones, Maxwell: *A Therapeutic Community. A New Treatment Method in Psychiatry*. Basic Books, New York 1956, p. 186.

14. Greenblatt, Milton: *From Custodial to Therapeutic Patient Care*. Russell Sage Foundation, New York, 1955, p.497.

15. Weiskotten, H. G.: The Present and Future Status of the Hospital Phase of Medical Education. *J. Med. Ed.*, 38:737, (Sept.) 1963.

16. National League of Nursing Education and National Organization for Public Health Nursing, Joint Committee on Integration of the Social and Health Aspects of Nursing in the Basic Curriculum: *Bibliography on Social and Health Aspects of Nursing in the Basic Curriculum*. The Committee, New York, 1950, p. 14.

17. World Health Organization: *Training the Physician for Family Practice.* Technical Report Series No. 257, The Organization, Geneva, 1963, p. 39.

18. Snoke, P. S., and Weinerman, E. R.: *An Annotated Bibliography on Comprehensive Care Programs in University Medical Centers.* In preparation. Yale University School of Medicine, New Haven, Conn.

19. Schwartz, Doris, *et al.*: The Nurse, Social Worker and Medical Student in a Comprehensive Care Program. *Amer. J. Nurs.,* 58:39, (Jan.) 1958. 30.

20. *Interim Report on a Study of Nursing Needs of Chronically Ill Ambulatory Patients, over the Age of 60, in a General Medical Clinic.* The Cornell-New York Hospital Medical Center, New York. Research Memorandum No. 10, Series B, (May) 1960, p. 10.

21. Crew, F. A. E.: Nursing as a National Service. The Second Revolution. *Nurs. Times,* 51:483, (6 May) 1955.

22. Spain, David M.: *The Complications of Modern Medical Practices: A Treatise on Iatrogenic Diseases.* Grune & Stratton, New York, 1963, p. 342.

23. Severdlik, Samuel S., *et al.*: Fifty Years of Progress in Physical Medicine and Rehabilitation in New York State. *New York J. Med.,* 51:90, (Jan.) 1951.

24. Buchwald, Edith (in collaboration with Howard A. Rusk, George G. Deaver, and Donald A. Covelt): *Physical Medicine for Daily Living.* McGraw-Hill Book Co., New York, 1952, p. 183.

25. Williams, Edna: The Patient Profile. *Nurs Res.,* 9:122, (Summer) 1960.

26. National League of Nursing Education. Special Committee on Postgraduate Clinical Courses (Elizabeth K. Porter, Chairman): *Courses in Clinical Nursing for Graduate Nurses. Basic Assumptions and Guiding Principles. Basic Courses. Advanced Courses.* The League, NewYork, 1945, p. 12.

27. National League of Nursing Education: *A Curriculum Guide* for *Schools of Nursing.* The League, New York, 1937, p. 689.

28. Tudor, Gwen E.: A Sociopsychiatric Nursing Approach to Intervention in a Problem of Mutual Withdrawal on a Mental Hospital Ward. *Psychiatry,* 15:193, (May) 1952.

29. Orlando, Ida Jean: *The Dynamic Nurse-Patient Relationship: Function, Process and Principles.* G. P. Putnam's Sons, New York, 1961, p. 91.

30. Yale University School of Nursing: *Self-Evaluating Report of Yale University School of Nursing.* The School, New Haven, 1964, various paging.

31. Wiedenbach, Ernestine: *Clinical Nursing: A Helping Art.* Springer Publishing Co., New York, 1964, p. 118.

32. Dumas, Rhetaugh, *et al.*: Validating a Theory of Nursing Practice. *Amer. J. Nurs.,* 63:52, (Aug.) 1963.

33. Abdellah, Faye: Methods of Identifying Covert Aspects of Nursing. *Nurs. Res.,* 60:4, (June) 1957.

34. Hathaway, John S., and Fitzgerald, Helene: A New Dimension to the Nurse's Role. *Nurs. Outlook,* 10:535, (Aug.) 1962.

35. Henderson, Virginia: Basic Principles of Nursing Care. International Council of Nurses London, 1961, p. 42.

36. Nursing. *Nurs. Times,* 49:1049, (17 Oct.) 1953.

37. Houston, William R.: *The Art of Treatment.* The Macmillan Co., New York, 1936, p. 744.

38. Saunders, Cecily: Should the Patient Know? *Nurs. Times,* 55:954, (16 Oct.) 1959.

39. Control of Pain in Terminal Cancer. *Nurs. Times,* 5:1031, (23 Oct.) 1959.

40. Mental Distress in the Dying. *Nurs. Times,* 55:1067, (30 Oct.) 1959.

CHAPTER 16

Clinical Nursing Practices and Patient Outcomes: Evaluation, Evolution, and Revolution

Margaret D. Sovie

Today's environment demands revolutionary as well as evolutionary changes in practice patterns. All clinical practices must be critically examined in terms of their contributions to quality patient outcomes, and their effects on nurses' time and morale.

The current nursing shortage may be the best thing yet to confront the profession of nursing and the institutions that are dependent on nurses to manage as well as provide the required health care to patients and families. Some describe it as a crisis; and as Dr. John Romano (1964) reminded us, "crisis" when written in Chinese is done so in two characters: one meaning danger; and the other, opportunity. Nurses have to seize this opportunity and revolutionize selected structures and processes in nursing and the health-care delivery systems as well as assist consumers of

---

This chapter is based on a presentation made during the Fifth Annual Nursing Economics Conference, Washington, DC, October 22, 1988. Reprinted with permission.
Originally published in *Nursing Economic$*, 1989, Volume 7, Number 3, pp. 79–85.
Copyright Nursing Economic$. Reprinted with permission of the publisher, Jannetti Publications, Inc.

nursing services to modify some of their traditional expectations of nursing services. "Revolutionize" means to bring about a radical change or to alter extensively or drastically, as contrasted with "evolutionary," which means gradually changing or progressing.

Today's problems are too severe and the demands too extreme to depend on evolution or gradual change. The continuous turbulence on the health-care scene, particularly in hospitals, has produced a prolonged tension with pressures that demand revolutionary change. These same tensions and pressures provide a readiness and receptiveness to change, new approaches, and revisions in structures and processes that will maximize the time nurses have to provide care for patients and families. The focus is certain—high quality patient/family care. To achieve and maintain it requires change.

Everyone in nursing must be empowered to help create new and better ways of providing nursing care to patients and families. We must critically examine what needs to be done, what difference it makes in patient outcomes, and the best way to do it to produce the desired results. There should be nothing that escapes scrutiny, examination, and, evaluation. There should be no sacred cows. We should discard what does not work or what does not produce the desired results and design and implement new approaches that do. Nurse administrators and managers need to legitimize the slaughtering of sacred cows and facilitate the radical changes as well as support the continuous evolutionary changes that are required to maximize nurses' time for quality care. The doors to change need to be opened wide. Practicing nurses can lead the way in a partnership for change—a partnership with patients, physicians, other health-care providers, and the administrators, regulators, and payers of the health-care organizations in which all work side by side to accomplish the mission of high quality, individualized care.

REEVALUATING NURSING CARE PLANS

If practicing nurses are to lead the way, we should begin by looking at what we as nurses do and what difference it makes in patient outcomes. I suggest that the first targets are the sacred cows called the nursing care plan and the nursing problem-oriented SOAP notes. The revolution needs to start here. More time is devoted to trying to get nurses to complete care plans and nursing problem lists as currently structured than to any other aspects of nursing. And when nurses are so little motivated to comply with JCAHO regulations as well as nursing's own standards of practice, it should tell us something is wrong. Valuable time is devoted to nursing a system's structural component and policing that component—time that could better be devoted to nursing the patient and family. Furthermore, we have little, if any, evidence that patient outcomes are affected positively or negatively when a completed nursing care plan is in the patient record and "supposedly" guiding the nursing care interventions of all nurses.

Ferguson, Hildman, and Nichols (1987) examined the effects of three types of nursing care planning systems on selected patient outcomes: length of stay; number of readmissions within 30 days; patient satisfaction; number of nosocomial infections; incident reports related to patient safety; medication or treatment errors by nurses; number of analgesics/narcotics administered to patients; and acuity level upon discharge. The three types of nursing care planning systems studied were: (a) a printed Kardex with physicians' orders and menu of nursing tasks; (b) standardized nursing care plans with provision for individualizing same on the chart; and (c) a Kardex that was a permanent part of the chart with inclusion of nursing diagnoses and nursing orders as well as physician dependent functions. Data were collected over a 7-month period. Essentially, no significant differences were found on any of the outcome variables. In other words, the type of nursing care plan had no effect on patient outcomes. These investigators concluded that written care plans with identified nursing diagnoses and nursing outcomes are not essential to deliver individualized quality care. They urged more research and if these results are validated, a revision in JCAHO requirements.

Written care plans may be an extremely valuable way to teach undergraduate nursing students. However, they may not be an essential activity in guiding professional nursing practice or ensuring quality patient outcomes. In fact, it could be that they are consuming valuable time as well as space in both the record and the computer and that they are not contributing to patient outcomes. This sacred cow needs to be targeted, if not for slaughter—for revolutionary transformation.

I believe that practicing nurses have been demonstrating with their overwhelming lack of enthusiasm for compliance to the nursing care plan standard that written care plans (as now construed) are not essential to quality patient care. I once thought that generic or standardized care plans were the answer. At least with the latter, the nurse only had to review and individualize to the patient. Even this approach has not found acceptance. The nurses may pull the generic care plan and place it in the record, but it is not uniformly individualized and, more troubling, probably not even read. This should provide us with insights. Nurses are continuing to give individualized care, and patients are responding and getting better. De La Cuesta (1983) identified the conflict between nursing education and practice as it relates to the care plan:

> It is necessary for educational purposes to break down in detail the elements of the problem-solving method and to expect from nursing students written and formalized reports on what they are doing at, each

stage as a training exercise to heighten their consciousness of what is required in detail. However, once the nurse is qualified, has been educated in the approach, has mastered the skills . . ., it may not be necessary to continue the extensive obligation to record. (p. 370)

Benner (1982), in her outstanding work *From Novice to Expert,* has described how different levels of nurses function and perceive clinical situations. The five levels of proficiency in acquiring and developing skills call for different approaches to guiding and directing care.

McHugh (1986) also examined the nursing process in terms of its relevance for the novice or the expert. Using Benner's five levels of skill proficiency, McHugh concluded that the written nursing process or care plan serves the novice or advanced beginner. However, more advanced practitioners and experts may be frustrated at best by a system more suitable for beginners.

Virginia Henderson (1982) has challenged us to distinguish between nursing and the nursing process. She states that the latter is an analytical process that should be used by all health-care providers who are problem-solving. Henderson suggests that the nursing process evolved from the movements to "individualize nursing care, identify and help people with their psychosocial as well as their physical problems, emphasize the science of nursing as opposed to the art of nursing, and establish the right of the nurse to an independent, professional and unique role" (p. 104). Henderson states that the best health care is patient/family focused; and that since 1937, she has been stressing planning with rather than for the patient and family. She states:

I question the nurse's identifying a patient's problem and making a plan to solve it, although he or she can help the patient and the family do both, just as he or she can help them implement and evaluate the programme.

She concludes her critique of the nursing process with these words:

While the nursing process recognizes the purpose of the problem-solving aspects of the nurses' work, a habit of inquiry and the use of investigative techniques in developing the scientific basis for nursing, it ignores the subjective or intuitive aspect of nursing and the role of experience, logic and expert opinion as bases for nursing practice. In stressing a dominant and independent function for the nurse, it fails to stress the value of collaboration of health professionals and particularly the importance of developing the self-reliance of clients. (p. 109)

All of these studies should help us in leading this one revolutionary change—removing the mandate that each patient have a nursing care plan as now required by our own ANA and JCAHO standards. Let's experiment, promote, and test different approaches!

Zander's (1988) nursing case management is a collaborative model of strategic management by nurses and physicians of episodes of illness. Her results are exciting. In ischemic stroke patients, this case management approach resulted in a 29% reduction in length of stay and a 46% reduction in ICU days. Zander describes the "critical path" as an abbreviated, one-page version of a case management plan and states that these critical paths, once individualized by the primary nurse and physician, are used to plan and monitor patient care. Interestingly, Zander's model combines the plan and the documentation, thus eliminating redundancy and promoting efficiency in recording. Zander states:

> Nurses have always been managers of care, but have labored with outdated management tools (such as nursing care plans) and shift-centered management systems. (p. 7)

The case, in my opinion, has been made. The sacred cow of nursing care plans must be slaughtered and a new and better something put in its place.

NURSING PROBLEM-ORIENTED RECORDING AND SOAP NOTES

The next sacred cow on my target list is the problem-oriented recording system with a nursing problem list, SOAP notes, and SOAPIER notes. The time that nurses spend recording on patient and hospital records must be reduced. Again, this time must be freed to focus on patient care activities that will be related to desired patient outcomes. At least five basic guidelines (if fully implemented) could considerably reduce time spent in documentation:

1. **Document at the source of data collection, at the patient's side.** Flow sheets to capture routine care and completed treatments, vital sign records, intake and output sheets, and medication administration records could all be kept in the patient's room or in the immediate area. Everything on these records can be used in the process of making the patient and family informed partners in the care process.
2. **Avoid redundancy in recording.** If the data are recorded once on a permanent record, they should not be recorded again.

3. **In the progress notes, record only significant observations and changes in the patient's condition or response**—those that are critical for evaluating the patient's progress and clinical decision making. I do not believe that it is necessary to identify the specific problem and then give the subjective and objective symptoms, followed by the assessment, and then the plan for each entry, or to compound it further with the description of the intervention, and the evaluation of the response. Treatment records and/or flow sheets can be designed to capture many of these critical data elements.

4. **Forcing the generation of a separate nursing problem list should be eliminated.** Without even going near a patient, I can predict that in 9 out of 10 patients, I will find a knowledge deficit on the problem list. I wonder how valuable this problem or diagnosis is as it relates to guiding nursing interventions and the results in patient outcomes. I suggest that the competent nurse, as well as proficient and expert level nurses, will all teach the patient as an integral aspect of their nursing care. The very essential aspects of patient teaching (including the assessment of learning needs, teaching, and response) can be documented on patient education flow sheets.

5. **Where separate nurses' notes remain, discontinue their use and move rapidly to having the nurses record significant observations on the progress record integrated along with the physician and other professional care givers.**

These five guidelines will help conserve time. To capture more time-saving approaches and maximize the creative talents of the staff, create a Documentation Revision Team and charge them with the responsibility to find new and better ways to capture essential patient care data while conserving nursing time. Then establish pilot units and test the revised approaches.

New documentation methods are being tested around the country, and those that have merit will survive and deserve replication. The PIE method (Problem Identification, Intervention and Evaluation) incorporates the plan of care into the nursing progress notes, eliminating the need for a traditional care plan according to Buckley-Womack and Gidney (1987). The system includes a comprehensive flow sheet where routine interventions and assessments are documented. Siegrist, Dettor and Stocks (1985) have illustrated what they believe to be the major advantages of the PIE system with a case study. I found their Daily Patient Assessment Sheet very interesting and one that could be helpful to nurses interested in flow sheet innovations.

Matthewman (1987) and a committee of staff nurses created a combined care plan and Kardex in their efforts to streamline documentation. Murphy, Beglinger, and Johnson (1988) eliminated problem-oriented records in their 600-bed private hospital and created a system of charting by exception that includes a nursing/physician order flow sheet, a patient teaching record along with a graphic record, and the nurses' notes. In their pilot unit, registered nurses (RNs), using the traditional charting method, averaged 44 minutes per shift in documentation activities. In the new system of charting by exception, the average dropped to 25 minutes, a decrease of 44%. There were different time savings for licensed practical nurses (LPNs) and unit secretaries. In all, the time savings in this institution with charting by exception equaled *100 hours per day,* the equivalent of *12.5 additional 8-hour shifts* each day.

These examples illustrate that a revolution has begun, and we need to help spread the change. Our patients and their families will be the central beneficiaries in addition to the nurses who will experience increased satisfaction and less stress due to standards that do not serve them or their patients. Kramer and Schmalenberg (1987) in their revisit of 16 magnet hospitals reported the stress that some forms of nursing documentation have created:

> . . . written nursing care plans. "I hate them. I hate them. I hate them. They really take time away from my patients . . . drudgery, repetition, and time-consuming writing out of a care plan. No other professional group has to write out in such detail what they plan to do. Why do nurses have to do so?" (p. 34)

Legitimizing revolutionary changes in planning and documenting care will help maximize nurses' time for quality patient care. Virginia Henderson (1987) summarizes with these words:

> Nothing would more radically improve health care than simplifying the form and language of the health record, identifying its, essential content, and making a copy of it available to the patient. To best serve the public interest, health-care providers must work with recipients and their families. They must also collaborate with each other in helping citizens prevent diseases, recover from illnesses, cope with handicaps, and die peacefully when death is inevitable. (pp. 17–18)

Let's create a patient care plan and eliminate the current nursing care plan. In this newly designed patient care plan, the patient/family and the physician as well as the nurse and other care providers will focus together on the problems to be addressed in this episode of care and the care that will follow.

PATIENT CARE PROGRAMS

The patient and family need to become central partners on the health-care team and, wherever possible, become more actively involved in the care and treatment program. Hospital systems and procedures will have to change, and nurses and other providers will have to learn new behaviors. Self-administration of medications, including patient controlled analgesics, should become a norm rather than the exception. Perhaps every bedside stand should have a medication drawer where all individual medications are maintained and dispensed.

Patient/family education programs need creative work and creative materials that will assist nurses in the teaching of critical information and skills. Media specialists and writers could be employed for a designated period, along with a librarian, to get materials prepared, catalogued, and ready for use. Volunteers could help deliver software and brochures. Closed circuit television could be used to greater advantage. Some nursing staff vacancy money may need to be used to produce technological tools to assist and complement the nurse with essential aspects of patient care.

Standard and routine care procedures must be examined. Are they necessary in the frequency and format in which they are currently administered? If not, what is essential to the desired outcome, and how do we change it to create the desired outcome? A classic example is incentive spirometry. More nursing and patient time have been wasted on a treatment with little or no value for a large number of patients. Equipment as well as time have been squandered. Making certain that treatments are appropriate to the patient's specific needs is a good beginning.

The routine taking of temperature and vital signs when there is no indication of need also needs to be questioned. Daily monitoring data may be appropriate for all patients in an acute care hospital, but more frequent measurements, without specific indicators of need, are useless rituals.

In this important area of patient care programs and procedures, the nurses who are primarily involved in delivering the care must be empowered to critically examine their routines and challenge those activities of questionable merit. Of course, where patients are directly involved, caution must be exercised as changes are evaluated. Carefully controlled demonstrations or pilot programs are warranted, and patient outcomes must be continually monitored as the changes are introduced.

Hobson and Blaney (1987) have identified three additional areas where change can cut costs and not care: inefficient use of patient care supplies; ineffective motivation and teaching of patients; and poor patient scheduling. The point I want to underscore is that it cannot be business as usual. Nurses have too much to do, and patients are in great need of effective and efficient services.

EXQUISITE TEAMWORK NEEDED MORE THAN EVER BEFORE

To meet the increased demands with existing staff requires exquisite team work, and that means everyone needs to work closely together.

- **Physician/nurse joint practice or collaborative practice is essential.** There is no time for parallel play. Joint planning, management, and evaluation of the patient's care and progress are essential.
- **Support services must deliver their services in a timely and responsible manner.** Medications must be there when needed as well as patient care supplies and equipment. Nurses' time cannot be squandered on the telephone chasing after required services. Nurses cannot be expected to make up for inadequate support services. If this belief exists, it too must be slaughtered.
- **Unit support services, such as housekeeping functions, may need to be restructured.** Housekeepers need to be responsive to the needs of the patient units, and head nurses must be able to establish priorities for housekeeping in order to meet patient care needs. This desired outcome may call for revolutionary structural changes with all staff who work on a unit being made responsive to the head nurse as well as to their respective department heads.
- **The time may have finally come when 24-hour, 7-day a week secretarial services** are absolutely essential requirements to support the nurse's ability to care for patients. Again, the shortage and vacant position dollars may be considered for adding the required support staff to manage the system and free the nurse to care for patients.
- **New unit services should be explored and tested.** A hospital concierge may provide many useful services that once fell within the domain of nurses. The concierge could get the newspapers, arrange for telephone or television service, order special meals for family members, arrange sleeping accommodations for the families of critically ill patients, and the list goes on. All of these vital patient care services need to continue, but they can be done by someone other than the professional nurse.

STAFF MIX

The nursing shortage has demanded an adjustment to the nursing staff mix. Some may say that it has created a demand for revolutionary change. I disagree. This is one area where I believe evolution is indicated. Here are the facts on the shortage as summarized by the Delaware Valley

Hospital Council in an August 1988 statement before a Pennsylvania Subcommittee on Health:

- The major cause of the current shortage is increased demand as opposed to a contraction of supply.
- The output of nurses increased by 55% between 1977 and 1984, compared to an 8% growth in population.
- Nurses are not leaving their profession. Almost 80% of RNs are actively employed.
- Ratios of nurses to patients in hospitals increased from 50:100 in 1972 to 91:100 in 1986.
- The proportion of RNs in the hospital nursing staff changed. In 1968, RNs were 33% of the nursing staff mix; in 1986, RNs were 58% of the nursing staff mix.
- RN employment in Medicaid and Medicare certified nursing homes increased 22% from 1981 to 1986.
- RN Medicare home health visits increased 60% between 1980 and 1987.
- The supply is at risk. Undergraduate enrollments in baccalaureate and associate degree programs have experienced a 30% decline since 1983.

What do these facts portend for staff mix? Certainly the movement to an all-RN staff has been halted. And maybe this too will serve nursing's desired future. The supply conditions have forced hospitals and other users to examine staffing and support services and identify new approaches to maximizing nurses' time for patient care. The roles of nursing assistants and LPNs are being explored with renewed interest. How can these auxiliary personnel complement the registered professional nurse so that quality care at controlled costs is achieved? The more than 400 tasks that have been identified as being performed by nurses are being reviewed and parceled out to ancillary staff including unit secretaries and other support service staff.

Having LPNs and nursing assistants become part of a unit's staffing complement does not have to interfere with primary nursing. Yet some say primary nursing may not survive. My belief is that every patient deserves a primary nurse just as every patient has an attending physician. Primary nursing has demonstrated its worth. Marie Manthey (1988), an originator of the primary nursing model, makes the following statement in the article Myths that Threaten:

The essential ingredient of the [primary nursing] delivery system is the establishment of a responsibility relationship between a nurse and a patient. . . . The primary nurse's decisions are carried out by those who care for the patient in her absence. . . . The shortage of RNs does not have to mean a loss of professional progress. (p. 55)

We will have to focus more attention on team building and ancillary staff supervision. With careful mix changes, we can identify the best assistance roles that will support primary nursing and quality patient care.

RETENTION OF STAFF

The essential element in accomplishing clinical practice analyses and evaluation is the retention of professional nurses who feel empowered to examine the relationships of clinical practices to patient outcomes and who will help us identify the critical components for potential change. Shared governance and participative management are features of a professional practice model that must be woven into the hospital fabric. Nurses need to be in control of their own practice and active participants in the management of patient care services and activities.

Hinshaw, Smeltzer, and Atwood's (1987) study of organizational and individual factors predicted to influence job satisfaction and turnover of nursing staff found that job stress buffered by satisfaction led to reduced turnover. The major stressors to be buffered were lack of team respect and feelings of incompetence while the primary satisfiers were professional status and general enjoyment in one's position, which correlated significantly with the ability to deliver quality nursing care (p. 14). These investigators identified the following strategies that can provide the satisfiers:

- Orientation and cross-training must be provided to help nurses feel competent in the care they are expected to deliver.
- Group cohesiveness must be fostered.
- Professional growth opportunities must be provided, including continuing education, research development and projects, tuition reimbursement, professional recognition for achievements, committee responsibility, and career mobility.
- Control over professional nursing practice within the institution must be achieved.
- Autonomy in the nurse's own professional practice must be felt. (pp. 14–16)

Institutions and their executives will do well to concentrate on retention of existing staff. Competent, proficient, and expert level nurses will help achieve the needed revolutionary and evolutionary changes. Their value needs to be recognized with financial differentiation for experience as well as special longevity benefits and perquisites. Furthermore, they deserve the added prestige of having their value recognized by membership and leadership in the participative management and shared governance structures that are in place or are being developed. Finally, the nurses must have strong administrative leadership and backup support, including head nurses and directors who are supportive, available, flexible, and who have excellent business skills they are willing to share. There is no doubt that nurses will continue to be excellent care givers and knowledgeable business partners as the evolutionary and revolutionary changes unfold. Yes, the shortage is real. The crisis is now. But the opportunities are many. The future is bright!

REFERENCES

Benner, P. (1982). From novice to expert. *American Journal of Nursing, 82,* 402–407.

Buckley-Womack, C., & Gidney, B. (1987). A new dimension in documentation: The PIE method. *Journal of Neuroscience Nursing, 19,* 256–260.

De La Cuesta, C. (1983). The nursing process: From development to implementation. *Journal of Advanced Nursing, 8,* 365–371.

Ferguson, G. H., Hildman, T., & Nichols, B. (1987). The effect of nursing care planning systems on patient outcomes. *Journal of Nursing Administration, 17,* 30–36.

Henderson, V. (1982). The nursing process. *Journal of Advanced Nursing, 7,* 103–109.

Henderson, V. (1987). Nursing process—a critique. *Holistic Nursing Practice, 1,* 7–18.

Hinshaw, A. S., Smeltzer, C. H., & Atwood, J. R. (1987). Innovative retention strategies for nursing staff. *Journal of Nursing Administration, 17,* 8–16.

Hobson, C. J., & Blaney, D. R. (1987). Techniques that cut costs not care. *American Journal of Nursing, 87,* 185–187.

Kramer, M., & Schmalenberg, C. (1987). Magnet hospitals talk about the impact of DRGs on nursing care_Part II. *Nursing Management, 18,* 33–39.

Manthey, M. (1988). Myths that threaten. *Nursing Management, 19,* 54–55.

Matthewman, J. (1987). Combining care plan and Kardex. *American Journal of Nursing, 87,* 852–854.

McHugh, M. (1986). Nursing process: Musings on the method. *Holistic Nursing Practice, 1,* 21–28.

Murphy, J., Beglinger, J. E., & Johnson. (1988). Charting by exception: Meeting the challenge of cost-containment. *Nursing Management, 19,* 56–72.

Romano, J. (1964). And leave for the unknown. *Journal of the American Medical Association, 190,* 282–284.

Siegrist, L. M., Dettor, R. E., & Stocks, B. (1985). The PIE system: Complete planning and documentation of nursing care. *Quality Review Bulletin, 11,* 186–189.

Zander, K. (1988). Nursing case management: Strategies management of cost and quality outcomes. *Journal of Nursing Administration, 18,* 23–30.

ADDITIONAL READINGS

Aiken, L. (1988). Put nurses on hospital boards. *Health Management Quarterly, 10,* 6–8.

Fields, W. L., & Loveridge, C. (1988): Critical thinking and fatigue: How do nurses on 8- and 12-hour shifts compare? *Nursing Economic$, 6,* 189–191.

Friedman, L. H., Oberg, B. J., Dansby, M. M., Sanders, J., Leonard, S., & Davis, B. (1988). Cost-effectiveness of a self-care program. *Nursing Economic$, 6,* 173–204.

Greiner, L. E. (1972): Evolution and revolution as organizations grow. *Harvard Business Review,* 37–46.

Helt, E. H., & Jelinek, R. C. (1988). In the wake of cost cutting, nursing productivity and quality improvement. *Nursing Management, 19,* 36–48.

"Johnson Pew Foundations Commit Millions to Nursing Initiative." Program brochure. *AHA Convention Daily,* 1988.

Manthey, M. (1988). Can primary nursing survive? *American Journal of Nursing, 88,* 644–647.

Silver, M. B., & Tubbesing, B. (1988). Nursing director: Creator of culture. *Nursing Management, 19,* 64.

York, C., & Fecteau, D. L. (1987). Innovative models for professional nursing practice. *Nursing Economic$, 5,* 162–166.

CHAPTER 17

Historical Analysis of Siderail Use in American Hospitals

Barbara L. Brush and Elizabeth Capezuti

Throughout most of the twentieth century, the use of siderails as safeguards against patients' falls from hospital beds has spurred debate. Although researchers and practitioners have argued the merits and pitfalls of siderail use, few have explored how use of siderails evolved and gradually became embedded in nursing practice. Raising bed siderails remains the most frequently used intervention to prevent bed-related falls and injuries among hospitalized patients and institutionalized older adults (Capezuti, 2000; Capezuti and Braun, 2001).

Examining the social, economic, and legal influences on siderail use in American hospitals, we explored the centrality of the hospital bed to the mission and purpose of nursing and the shifting focus of bedside care from patient comfort to patient safety. We argue that use of siderails has been based more on a gradual consensus between law and medicine than on empirical evidence for nursing practice. Nonetheless, nurses, as hospital employees, adopted siderail use as part of their standard of bedside care (Barbee 1957).

Social-historical research methods were used to collect and interpret data. Thus, the pattern of siderail use, the value attached to siderails as an example of benevolent care, and attitudes about raising siderails were examined as they evolved and shifted over time. Primary sources included medical trade catalogs, hospital procedure manuals, newsletters, photographs, and other archival materials from the New York Academy of Medicine, the College of Physicians in Philadelphia, and the Center for the Study of the History of Nursing at the University of Pennsylvania. Journal articles, government documents, published histories of hospital bed design, and nursing and medical texts provided additional sources of data.

THE HOSPITAL BED AS CENTRAL TO NURSING'S MISSION

In 1893, Isabel Adams Hampton made clear, in a chapter devoted entirely to hospital beds, that nurses were the overseers of beds and their occupants. As she put it, "A nurse who works over [beds] daily ought to be a fair judge of what is required in the way of a bed for the sick" (Hampton, 1893, p. 751). Hampton charged nurses to coordinate bed type to patient condition, maintain a neat and uniform bed appearance at all times, and ensure patient comfort during the period of recuperation.

In Hampton's day, the ideal bed was 6 feet 6 inches long, 37 inches wide, and 24 to 26 inches from the floor (Hampton, 1893). Although similar in length and width to standard twin beds in homes, hospital beds were approximately 6 to 8 inches higher to facilitate patient care and prevent unnecessary strain on nurses. Because beds were a fixed "nursing" height, stools were often used to accommodate patients as they transferred from bed.

Bed height, more than any other bed dimension, has consistently influenced bedside nursing care in American hospitals and long-term care facilities. Bed height and the outcomes of bed-related falls in hospitals have been the basic issues underlying numerous legislative and practice initiatives in the twentieth century. Despite changes meant to remedy injurious outcomes from bed-related falls, however, patients falling from high beds are deemed at risk for increased morbidity and mortality (O'Keeffe, Jack, and Lye, 1996). Bed siderails, initially used as a temporary means to prevent confused, sedated, or elderly patients from falling from bed, are now permanent fixtures on most institutional beds (Braun and Capezuti, 2000; Capezuti and Braun, 2001). Their increased use in the latter half of the twentieth century reflects a shifting emphasis from patient comfort to patient safety as hospitals, evolving from charitable institutions to modern medical centers, became increasingly subject to litigation (Stevens 1989).

"RENDERING THE OBSTINATE DOCILE"

Bed siderails were rarely available on adult hospital beds until the 1930s. More common were cribs or children's beds equipped with full or partial crib sides, which, similar to siderails, were meant to protect infants and young children from falling from or leaving beds unattended. The primary intervention for agitated, confused, or other adults considered at risk of falling from bed was nurses' provision of "careful and continuous watchfulness" (Merck Manual, 1934, p. 36).

Haigh and Hayman's (1936) study of 116 "out of bed" incidents at the University Hospital of Cleveland, however, provided early evidence of siderail use to control adult patient behavior and prevent deleterious outcomes. The authors reported that in 31% of bed-related falls at the study institution, patients climbed over siderails, and an additional 7% removed a physical restraint and then proceeded over the rails before falling. Although siderails, as well as rails in combination with restraints, were ineffective in preventing falls or deterring patients from leaving beds unassisted, the nurse and physician authors concluded that siderails were a reasonable precautionary measure against falls from bed as well as necessary adjuncts in "rendering the obstinate docile" (Haigh and Hayman, 1936, p. 45).

When first used, siderails, also known as sideboards or side restraints, were not permanently fastened to hospital beds. Instead, they were accessories that nurses physically attached to beds when they deemed necessary or when prescribed by a physician (Tracy, 1942). Securing these devices was a time-consuming and cumbersome procedure that often required at least two people (Manley, 1944).

In the 1940s, siderail use on adult hospital beds gradually became the subject of legal action against personal injury and death. In 1941, for example, the parents of 21-year-old Edgar Pennington sued Morningside Hospital after their son fell from bed and sustained a fatal head injury (*Morningside Hospital v. Pennington et al.*, 1941). When Mr. Pennington was initially hospitalized, his bed siderails were raised because of his irrational behavior. A few days later and presumably calmer, his side rails were removed and his left leg was chained to the bed instead. The plaintiffs argued that the nurses' failure to maintain side rails on their son's bed caused him to sustain his fatal fall. Whether his leg was still chained to the bed when he was found "with his bloody head on the concrete floor" was unsubstantiated. Ultimately, the case was dismissed.

A year earlier, the surviving husband of Jennie Brown Potter sued the Dr. W.H. Groves Latter-Day Saints Hospital for his wife's fall-related death, claiming that the hospital's failure to attach side boards to her bed constituted negligence. As in *Morningside Hospital v. Pennington et al.*,

(1941), the court ruled for the defendant, citing lack of evidence that standard of due care required the hospital to place sideboards on patients' beds (*Potter et al. v. Dr. W.H. Groves, 1940*).

THE NURSE'S ROLE IN HOSPITAL SAFETY

By the 1950s, siderail use became more visibly linked to institutional liability. Numerous factors contributed to this transition. First, many states adopted laws overturning charitable hospitals' immunity from the negligence of their employees, necessitating hospitals' purchase of expensive insurance policies (Hayt, Hayt, and Groeschel, 1952). Second, a severe postwar nursing shortage limited nurses' ability to provide previous levels of watchfulness over patients in their charge (Lynaugh and Brush, 1996). Finally, bed manufacturers expanded their focus in advertising to include patient safety along with patient comfort and rest. Consequently, institutional beds equipped with permanent full-length siderails became more readily available (Hospitals, 1954). Nurses raised siderails on patients' beds to reassure the public and hospital administrators that even if nurses were in short supply, at least patients were secure in their beds (Aberg, 1957; Barbee, 1957).

Ludham (1957) reinforced this notion in one of the first reported studies of hospital insurance claims involving bed incidents. In his study of 7,815 "out-of-bed" incidents in California hospitals, Ludham found that although 63% (4,893) of reported incidents occurred when siderails were raised, claims paid by insurance companies increased tenfold when falls occurred in the absence of raised siderails. The imbalance in jury awards was largely attributed to the perception that raising siderails was a demonstrable effort, however unproved, to protect patients from falls and serious injury. With no supporting evidence, Ludham nonetheless echoed previous claims (Aston, 1955; Price, 1956) that out of-bed incidents with raised siderails caused less severe injury because patients had something to grasp when falling. He recommended that hospitals establish standing orders or policies requiring siderail use with certain types of patients (e.g., sedated, confused, "older") as a national standard of hospital practice. Locally, the Council on Insurance of the California Hospital Association urged its hospitals to permanently attach siderails to every bed "as rapidly as possible" (Ludham, 1957, p. 47).

Professional journal articles and nursing texts also regularly encouraged nurses to use siderails as part of their therapeutic actions (Aberg, 1957; Harmer and Henderson, 1952; Price, 1954), especially because of the claim that "bedfalls, together with hot-water bottle burns account for more lawsuits involving nurses than all other risks combined" (Hayt, Hayt, Groeschel, and McMullan, 1958, p. 206). Although the standard hospital bed height was "not always comfortable to the patient [but] convenient for the nurse and the doctor" (Harmer and Henderson, 1952, p. 126), siderails, defined as restraints or restrictive devices, were advocated in the prevention of falls and injury from these high beds (Hayt et al., 1952; McCullough and Moffit, 1949; Price, 1954).

Meanwhile, bed manufacturers continued to sell to "safety-minded hospital administrators" (Hospitals, 1954, p. 197). The Hard Manufacturing Company's "Slida-Side" offered permanent siderails on every hospital bed, and the Inland Bed Company guaranteed portable siderails to "provide safety for your patients, protection for your hospital" (*Hospitals,* 1954, p.197). Both the Hall Invalid Bed and the Simmons Vari-Hite bed could be manually lowered from the standard height of 27 inches to the "normal home bed height" of 18 inches (*Hospitals,* 1950). They were considered safer for two reasons: They eliminated the need for "slipping, tilting footstools" and they allowed patients to get up from a familiar bed height without calling for the nurse (Advertisements, 1950, 87, 102). Thus, and most important, the Simmons Company reported, the Vari-Rite bed reduced "the likelihood of falling and serious injury" (Hospitals, 1950, p. 87).

The Hill-Rom Company also advertised its Hilow Beds as the pinnacle of modernization and fall prevention because the crank-operated bed could be lowered to 18 inches, making patients less likely to misjudge the distance to the floor, lose their balance, and fall (Hospitals, 1955). To make their point that lower beds eliminated the need for full siderails to prevent bed-related falls and injuries, advertisements depicted the Vari-Rite and Hall Invalid beds without siderails and the Hilow Bed with a half rail meant to assist patients to transfer independently.

Despite the availability of lower and variable height beds that eliminated the need for siderails, that were comfortable for patients, and increased nursing efficiency, fixed "nursing height" beds with permanent full-length siderails were used more regularly than were these new inventions (Smalley, 1956). The "commonsense" notion that siderails were safety devices led to hospital-wide policies that standardized their use. Because nurses and hospital administrators failed to question siderail efficacy in preventing bedside falls, they also failed to use alternatives. Gradually, hospital-based nurses in the 1950s raised siderails to substitute for their physical presence at the bedside and to protect hospitals' legal interests.

THE STANDARD OF GOOD NURSING PRACTICE

An escalating nurse shortage in the 1960s and 1970s, coupled with changes in hospital architecture from multi-patient wards to semiprivate and private patient rooms, prompted the continued use of siderails, as well as other physical restraints, as substitutes for nursing observation. By the 1980s, falls, especially from beds, were identified as a major hospital liability issue (Rubenstein, Miller, Postel, and Evans, 1983). In 1980 the National Association of Insurance Commissioners reported that falls represented 10% of all paid claims between 1975 and 1978; absence of siderails was identified as a principal justification. As a result, "routine use of bedrails" became "the standard of good nursing practice" (Rubenstein et al., 1983, p. 273).

As siderail use became common nursing practice, particularly to prevent falls among older patients, its scientific rationale was brought into question. Rubenstein and colleagues (1983) at Harvard Medical School labeled the continued use of siderails, in the absence of supporting data, an example of "defensive medicine" (p. 273). In other words, raising siderails was practice based on consensus rather than on scientific evidence. Based largely on legal action against hospitals and their personnel, siderail use became a means to promote patients' "right" to safety during hospitalization and nurses' "responsibility" to keep patients safe (Anonymous, 1984; Horty, 1973).

Shifting decisions about patient safety to nurses shifted liability from physicians to institutions. As a result, institutions took greater precautions to ensure that patients, especially the elderly, did not fall. Raising siderails for individuals deemed vulnerable to injury or death, in addition to using physical restraints for immobilization, reinforced the opinion that siderails and restraints were benevolent interventions (Cohen and Kruschwitz, 1997; Strumpf and Tomes, 1993). Although nurse attorney Jane Greenlaw found medication to be a major cause of negligence related to siderail use, she also noted the importance of a patient's mental state in determining liability. She noted, "Where it can be shown that a patient was senile, irrational, confused, or otherwise impaired, this can affect the hospital's duty to safeguard the patient" (Greenlaw, 1982, p. 125), and, "Nursing responsibility to evaluate each person's safety and to act accordingly, regardless of whether the attending physician has done so" (Greenlaw, 1982, p. ,127).

The nurse's duty to render independent judgment about siderail use was evident in the 1977 fall and injury case of John Wooten. Eighty-three-year-old Wooten suffered a severe head injury after falling at the Memphis, Tennessee Veterans Administration Hospital. During the evening, Wooten had risen from his bed unattended and walked a short distance before falling. Before the fall, Wooten's physician deemed him "stable" and gave an order for "bedrest with bedside commode and up in chair three times per day" (Anonymous, 1984, p. 4). Despite the physician's medical opinion, the U.S. District Court of Tennessee ruled that hospital personnel were negligent in caring for Wooten because his condition "mandated the use of siderails" (Anonymous, 1984, p. 4). The court held that raised siderails were a reminder for patients to call nurses when they needed assistance to transfer from bed. Moreover, because Wooten was "older," he was at greater risk for confusion and disorientation. The court awarded $80,000 in damages.

In 1981, 80-year-old Esther Polonsky was injured during her stay at Union Hospital in Lynn, Massachusetts, upon attempting to use the bathroom during the night. Several hours before the incident, the nurse had administered 15 milligrams of Dalmane to Polonsky to aid sleep. The Appeals Court of Massachusetts found that because the nurse failed to raise her bed siderails, a confused and disoriented Polonsky fell and fractured her right hip. She recovered $20,000 in damages (Regan, 1981).

While Polonsky's fall was directly linked to her medication, the case of Catherine Kadyszeski, like that of Wooten, illustrates the ageism often associated with siderail use (Tammelleo, 1995). Kadyszeski was 67 years old in 1985 when she fractured her left hip in a bathroom-related fall at New York's Ellis Hospital. Although heavily sedated with Demerol, Vistaril, and Phenobarbital, Kadyszeski did not win her claim on the basis of oversedation. Rather, the hospital was found negligent for failing to comply with its own rule that siderails be raised for all patients over age 65.

The continued use of siderails and restraints in the 1980s and 1990s sharply contrasted with new ideas about the importance of mobility during recuperation from acute illness or surgery (Allen, Glasziou, and Del Mar, 1999.). The trend toward decreasing bedrest and increasing ambulation in hospitalized patients did not translate to the care of frail elders (Creditor, 1993; Sager et al., 1996). While younger patients' beds were equipped with half- instead of full-length siderails to facilitate transfers, older patients continued to be immobilized in bed, in large part because nurses equated full siderail use with greater patient protection (Rubenstein et al. 1983). Even as negative consequences of immobilizing hospitalized elders, such as deconditioning, pressure ulcers, and pneumonia, were reported in the literature (Creditor, 1993; Hoenig and Rubenstein, 1991; Inouye et al., 1993; Sager et al., 1996), the use of siderails in this population did not abate.

IMPLICATIONS FOR CURRENT PRACTICE

Reports of siderail-related entrapment injuries and deaths over the past decade (Food and Drug Administration, 1995; Parker and Miles, 1997; Todd, Ruhl, and Gross, 1997) continue to challenge perceptions of siderails as safety devices. Many legal claims are now being won against hospitals for siderail misuse (Braun and Capezuti, 2000; Capezuti and Braun, 2001).

The Health Care Finance Administration (HCFA) has issued surveyor guidelines redefining siderails as restraints when they impede the patient's desired movement or activity, such as getting out of bed (U.S. Department of Health and Human Services, 2000). The fundamental goal of these guidelines is to deter health care providers from routinely using siderails. Instead, they encourage a thorough assessment of patients' individualized needs and consideration of alternative interventions to siderail use (Capezuti et al., 1999; Capezuti, Talerico, Strumpf, and Evans, 1998). More broadly, the HCFA guidelines will likely influence siderail use by hospitals accredited through the Joint Commission on Accreditation of Healthcare Organizations (JCAHO, 1996). Because JCAHO must, at a minimum, meet applicable federal law and regulations, new standards consistent with HCFA regulations likely will be promulgated in the near future (Capezuti and Braun, 2001).

The acceptance and use of alternatives to siderails, however, will depend on a new consensus among health care providers, hospital administrators, bed manufacturers, insurers, attorneys, regulators, and patients and their families. To reach consensus, all parties need to understand how and why siderails became common practice in the first place and why, despite evidence to the contrary, they remain firmly entrenched as acceptable bedside care. Rethinking siderail use, especially with the elderly, will require new incentives for their discontinuation. The new guidelines by HCFA (U.S. Department of Health & Human Services, 2000) are a beginning step in this direction.

Bed manufacturers have also reintroduced adjustable low-height beds, similar to the models first proposed in the 1950s. These "new" beds, as well as siderails with narrower rail gaps, will be on the market over the next few years. Financing the purchase of this equipment and retrofitting outdated bed systems will likely raise new concerns about siderail-related liability (Braun and Capezuti, 2000; Capezuti and Braun, 2001). Nurse researchers are in key positions to evaluate how legislative and manufacturing trends affect clinical outcomes.

Given the gradual evolution of siderail use in American hospitals, nurses can anticipate that attitudes and practices about use of siderails will not change quickly or easily. Changing views and practices of siderail use will require reinterpretation of nursing care standards and benevolent care. Given the evidence of these shifting ideas and practices now (Braun and Capezuti, 2000; Capezuti and Braun, 2001; Capezuti, 2000; Donius and Rader, 1994), new perceptions and habits will develop. Those changes should be based on empirical outcomes rather than on untested consensus.

ACKNOWLEDGMENTS

This study was supported by a grant from the *Xi* Chapter of Sigma Theta Tau International. The authors thank Deborah J. Swedlow, MSS, MLSP, JD, for assistance with obtaining and interpreting legal sources.

REFERENCES

Aberg, H. L. (1957). The nurse's role in hospital safety. *Nursing Outlook, 5,* 160–162.

Allen, C., Glasziou, P., & Del Mar, C. (1999). Bed rest: A potentially harmful treatment needing more careful evaluation. *Lancet, 354,* 1229–1233.

Anonymous. (1984). Hospital policy re: "siderails" nurses' responsibility. *Regan Report on Nursing Law, 24,* 4.

Aston, C. S., Jr. (1955). Grasping bars means added safety. *Hospitals, 29,* 102–104.

Barbee, G. C. (1957). More about bedrails and the nurse. *American Journal of Nursing, 57,* 1441–1442.

Braun, J. A., & Capezuti, E. (2000). The legal and medical aspects of physical restraints and bed siderails and their relationship to falls and fall-related injuries in nursing homes. *DePaul Journal of Healthcare Law, 3,* 1–72.

Capezuti, E. (2000). Preventing falls and injuries while reducing siderail use. *Annals of Long-Term Care, 8,* 57–63.

Capezuti, E., Bourbonniere, M., Strumpf, N., & Maislin, G. (2000). Siderail use in a large urban medical center (abstract). *Gerontologist, 40,* 117.

Capezuti, E., & Braun, J. A. (2001). Medicolegal aspects of hospital siderail use. *Ethics, Law, and Aging Review, 7,* 25–57.

Capezuti, E., Talerico, K. A., Cochran, I., Becker, H., Strumpf, N., & Evans, L. (1999). Individualized interventions to prevent bed-related falls and reduce siderail use. *Journal of Gerontological Nursing, 25,* 26–34.

Capezuti, E., Talerico, K. A., Strumpf, N., & Evans, L. (1998). Individualized assessment and intervention in bilateral siderail use. *Geriatric Nursing, 19,* 322–330.

Cohen, E.S., & Kruschwitz, A. L. (1997). Restraint reduction: Lessons from the asylum. *Journal of Ethics, Law, and Aging, 3,* 25–43.

Creditor, M. C. (1993). Hazards of hospitalization of the elderly. *Annals of Internal Medicine, 118,* 219–223.

Donius, M., & Rader, J. (1994). Use of siderails: Rethinking a standard of practice. *Journal of Gerontological Nursing, 20,* 23–27.

Food and Drug Administration. (1995). FDA *Safety Alert: Entrapment hazards with hospital bed side rails.* Rockville, MD: U.S. Dept. of Health and Human Services, Public Health Service, Center for Devices and Radiological Health.

Greenlaw, J. (1982). Failure to use siderails: When is it negligence? *Law, Medicine and Health Care, 10,* 125–128.

Haigh, C., & Hayman, J. M., Jr. (1936). Why they fell out of bed. *Modern Hospital, 47,* 45–46.

Hampton, I. A. (1893). *Nursing: Its principles and practice.* Philadelphia: W. B. Saunders.

Harmer, M., & Henderson, V. (1952). *Textbook of the principles and practice of nursing.* New York: Macmillan.

Hayt, E., Hayt, L. R., & Groeschel, A. H. (1952). *Law of hospital and nurse.* New York: Hospital Textbook Co.

Hayt, E., Hayt, L. R., Groeschel, A. H., & McMullan, D. (1958). *Law of hospital and nurse.* New York: Hospital Textbook Co.

Hoenig, H. M., & Rubenstein, L. Z. (1991). Hospital-associated deconditioning and dysfunction. *Journal of the American Geriatrics Society, 39,* 220–222.

Hospitals. (1950). Hall Invalid Bed; Simmons Vari-Rite [Advertisements]. *Hospitals, 24,* 86–87, 102.

Hospitals. (1954). Inland Bed Company; Hard Slida-Side [Advertisements]. *Hospitals, 28,* 19, 197.

Hospitals. (1955). Hill-Rom Hilow Beds [Advertisement]. Hospitals, *29,* 161.

Horty, J. F. (1973). Hospital has duty to maintain premises, but employees have duty to be cautious. *Modern Hospital, 120,* 50.

Inouye, S. K., Wagner, D. R., Acampora, D., Horwitz, R. I., Cooney, L. M., Hurst, L. D., et al. (1993). A predictive index for functional decline in hospitalized elderly medical patients. *Journal of General Internal Medicine, 8,* 645–652.

Joint Commission on Healthcare Organizations (JCAHO). (1996). *Comprehensive accreditation manual for hospitals (restraint and seclusion standards plus scoring: Standards TX7.1–TX7.1.3.3,191–193j).* Oakbrook Terrace, Ill.

Ludham, J. E. (1957). Bedrails: Up or down? *Hospitals, 31,* 46–47.

Lynaugh, J. E., & Brush, B. L. (1996). *American nursing: From hospitals to health systems.* Cambridge, Mass.: Blackwell.

Manley, M. E., & The Committee on Nursing Standards, Division of Nursing, Department of Hospitals. (1944). Chapter VI: Preparation and care of beds. In *Standard Nursing Procedures of The Department of Hospitals City of New York,* (pp. 109–125). New York: Macmillan.

Merck and Company. (1934). *The Merck manual of therapeutics and materia medica,* 6th ed. Rahway, NJ.

McCullough, W., & Moffit, M. (1949). *Illustrated handbook of simple nursing.* New York: McGraw-Hill.

Morningside Hospital & Training School for Nurses v. Pennington et al., 189 Okla. 170, 114P.2d 943 (1941).

National Association of Insurance Commissioners. (1980). *Medical claims: Medical malpractice closed claims, July 1, 1975, through June 30, 1978,* Vol. 2. Brookfield, Wis.

O'Keeffe, S., Jack, C. I., & Lye, M. (1996). Use of restraints and bedrails in a British hospital. *Journal of the American Geriatrics Society, 44,* 1086–1088.

Parker, K., & Miles, S. H. (1997). Deaths caused by bedrails. *Journal of the American Geriatrics Society, 45,* 797–802.

Potter et al. v. Dr. W .H. Groves Latter-Day Saints Hospital, 99 Utah 71, 103 P.2d 280 (1940).

Price, A. L. (1954). *The art, science and spirit of nursing.* Philadelphia: W. B. Saunders.

Price, A. L. (1956). Short side guards are safer. *Hospital Management, 82,* 86–89.

Regan, W. A. (1981). Legal case briefs for nurses. *Regan Report on Nursing Law, 21,* 3.

Rubenstein, H. S., Miller, E. H., Postel, S., & Evans, H. B. (1983). Standards of medical care based on consensus rather than evidence: The case of routine bedrail use for the elderly. *Law, Medicine and Health Care, 11,* 271–276.

Sager, M. A., Franke, T., Inouye, S. K., Landefeld, C. S., Morgan, T. M., Rudberg, M. A., et al. (1996). Functional outcomes of acute medical illness and hospitalization in older persons. *Archives of Internal Medicine, 156,* 645–652.

Smalley, H. E. (1956). Variable height bed: A study in patient comfort and efficiency in care. *Hospital Management, 82,* 42–43.

Stevens, R. (1989). *In sickness and in wealth: American hospitals in the twentieth century.* New York: Basic Books.

Strumpf, N. E., & Tomes, N. (1993). Restraining the troublesome patient: A historical perspective on a contemporary debate. *Nursing History Review, 1,* 3–24.

Tammelleo, A. D. (1995). Siderails left down-patient falls from bed: "Ordinary negligence" or "malpractice"? *Regan Report on Nursing Law, 36,* 3.

Todd, J. E, Ruhl, C. E., & Gross, T. P. (1997). Injury and death associated with hospital bed side-rails: Reports to the U.S. Food and Drug Administration from 1985–1995. *American Journal of Public Health, 87,* 1675–1677.

Tracy, M. A. (1942). *Nursing: An art and a science.* St. Louis: C. V. Mosby.

U.S. Department of Health and Human Services. (2000). Health Care Financing Administration, guidance to surveyors. Hospital conditions of participation for patients' rights (Rev. 17). Retrieved from http:// www.hcfa.gov/quality/4b.htm

Index